DOING PLAY THERAPY

Creative Arts and Play Therapy

Cathy A. Malchiodi and David A. Crenshaw
Series Editors

This series highlights action-oriented therapeutic approaches that utilize art, play, music, dance/movement, drama, and related modalities. Emphasizing current best practices and research, experienced practitioners show how creative arts and play therapies can be integrated into overall treatment for individuals of all ages. Books in the series provide richly illustrated guidelines and techniques for addressing trauma, attachment problems, and other psychological difficulties, as well as for supporting resilience and self-regulation.

Creative Arts and Play Therapy for Attachment Problems
Cathy A. Malchiodi and David A. Crenshaw, Editors

Play Therapy: A Comprehensive Guide to Theory
and Practice
David A. Crenshaw and Anne L. Stewart, Editors

Creative Interventions with Traumatized Children,
Second Edition
Cathy A. Malchiodi, Editor

Music Therapy Handbook
Barbara L. Wheeler, Editor

Play Therapy Interventions to Enhance Resilience
David A. Crenshaw, Robert Brooks, and Sam Goldstein, Editors

What to Do When Children Clam Up in Psychotherapy:
Interventions to Facilitate Communication
Cathy A. Malchiodi and David A. Crenshaw, Editors

Doing Play Therapy: From Building the Relationship
to Facilitating Change
Terry Kottman and Kristin K. Meany-Walen

DOING
PLAY
THERAPY

From Building the Relationship
to Facilitating Change

Terry Kottman
Kristin K. Meany-Walen

Series Editors' Note by
Cathy A. Malchiodi and David A. Crenshaw

THE GUILFORD PRESS
New York   London

Library of Congress Cataloging-in-Publication Data

Names: Kottman, Terry, author. | Meany-Walen, Kristin K., author.
Title: Doing play therapy : from building the relationship to facilitating
    change / Terry Kottman, Kristin K. Meany-Walen ; series editors, note by
    Cathy A. Malchiodi and David A. Crenshaw.
Description: New York : The Guilford Press, 2018. | Series: Creative arts and
    play therapy | Includes bibliographical references and index.
Identifiers: LCCN 2018022678| ISBN 9781462536115 (hardback) | ISBN
    9781462536054 (paperback)
Subjects: LCSH: Play therapy. | Psychotherapy. | Therapist and patient. |
    BISAC: PSYCHOLOGY / Psychotherapy / Child & Adolescent. | MEDICAL /
    Psychiatry / Child & Adolescent. | SOCIAL SCIENCE / Social Work.
Classification: LCC RJ505.P6 K642 2018 | DDC 618.92/891653--dc23
LC record available at *https://lccn.loc.gov/2018022678*

As usual, I dedicate this book to Jacob (who is the world's best kid, even though he technically isn't a kid anymore) and to Rick (who is supportive, patient, and loving, and reads everything I write before I send it to the publisher— which might make him a bit crazy, in addition to being my definition of the world's best husband).

—TERRY

I dedicate this book to my husband, Terry, and my children, Skyler, Parker, Zoey-Anne, Bennett, Lake, and Ryder! You make my life meaningful, fun, and a wonderful sort of crazy.

—KRISTIN

About the Authors

Terry Kottman, PhD, NCC, RPT-S, LMHC, founded The Encouragement Zone, in Cedar Falls, Iowa, where she provides play therapy training and supervision, life coaching, counseling, and "playshops" for women. Dr. Kottman developed Adlerian play therapy, an approach to working with children, families, and adults that combines the ideas and techniques of Individual Psychology and play therapy. She writes about play therapy and regularly presents workshops nationally and internationally. Dr. Kottman is a recipient of Lifetime Achievement Awards from the Association for Play Therapy and the Iowa Association for Play Therapy.

Kristin K. Meany-Walen, PhD, LMHC, RPT-S, is Assistant Professor of Counseling at the University of North Texas. She was previously in private practice, where she worked with a variety of clients who reinforced her belief in the significance of play and creative expression. Dr. Meany-Walen regularly publishes and presents on play therapy with children and adolescents. She conducted the first Adlerian play therapy study, which was instrumental in Adlerian play therapy becoming recognized as an evidence-based treatment for reducing behavioral problems in children.

Series Editors' Note

The central role of play is now recognized by mental health professionals as an important developmental experience. Through play, not only are children encouraged to create and imagine, they also have opportunities to master stressful or overwhelming situations and practice healthy interactions with others. For people who have experienced trauma, crises, or loss, play is a way to rehearse new behaviors and use symbol and metaphor to communicate perceptions about events, feelings, and relationships.

Play therapy is the systematic and formalized application of play to help prevent or resolve psychosocial challenges and achieve optimal growth and development. It is predicated on many different theoretical models and approaches, but in all cases its goal is to support therapeutic communication through the use of toys, games, props, and other media. Above all, play therapists provide clients with a safe and attuned relationship through which they can master troubling emotions, practice new skills and responses, and experience positive attachment.

Up until now, there has been no book that clearly defines just how to go about applying play therapy and, more importantly, how to cultivate an effective and successful relationship through play therapy principles. Fortunately, *Doing Play Therapy: From Building the Relationship to Facilitating Change* fills this gap in current play therapy literature—a practical and timely text that articulately explains methods and best practices. While many play therapy books focus on a single theory or application, this volume not only masterfully integrates multiple approaches, but also addresses key questions that most practitioners have about successfully using play therapy methodology to accomplish two critical tasks: how to establish and support a therapeutic relationship through play and ways to strategically apply play therapy principles to effect positive change.

The appeal of this volume begins with the authors. Terry Kottman is a recipient of the most coveted recognition given by the Association for Play Therapy: a Lifetime Achievement Award. Dr. Kottman is an acclaimed presenter at play therapy conferences statewide, nationally, and internationally. Terry founded The Encouragement Zone in Cedar Falls, Iowa, where she has treated countless children and families and trained numerous play therapists. As a teacher and presenter, she is known for her unfailing sense of humor. If you go to a play therapy conference and you hear gales of laughter coming from one of the rooms, Terry is the likely presenter. Both authors' humor is laced throughout this volume, making it even more enjoyable to read.

Kristin K. Meany-Walen is a highly respected scholar and researcher, currently teaching at the largest play therapy training program in the world, at the University of North Texas. She is a prolific writer and scholar and provided the scientific data that led the Substance Abuse and Mental Health Services Administration in 2017 to recognize Adlerian play therapy as an evidence-based modality. As if this were not enough to keep Kristin busy, she also manages to be the mother of six children.

Our book series, *Creative Arts and Play Therapy*, highlights action-oriented therapeutic approaches that utilize art, play, music, dance/movement, drama, and related modalities. Emphasizing current best practices and research, experienced practitioners show how creative arts and play therapies can be integrated into overall treatment for individuals of all ages. As coeditors of the series, we feel fortunate to include this seminal book on play therapy by Drs. Kottman and Meany-Walen. This highly readable volume will greatly enhance the therapeutic skills of graduate students and will serve as a foundational text for play therapy, counseling, and psychotherapy courses. Although crafted as a comprehensive text, seasoned practitioners will find a wealth of clinical knowledge throughout, including play therapy strategies that can be immediately applied to address a variety of situations and challenges.

CATHY A. MALCHIODI, PhD
DAVID A. CRENSHAW, PhD

Preface

Between the two of us, we have taught introductory play therapy classes an innumerable number of times. (Okay, it's not really *innumerable*, but it's *a lot*.) And both of us have longed (yes, *longed*—not just wanted or wished to have—but *longed*) for a different kind of introductory play therapy book designed for folks who wanted either to learn play therapy or to deepen their play therapy expertise. We longed for a book that helped readers to examine their own beliefs about people and how they change—as a vehicle for helping them choose a theoretical orientation that would serve as a foundation for their play therapy practice. We longed for a book that featured practical information about the various skills, strategies, and techniques that make up play therapy. We longed for a book that addressed using play therapy with children, adolescents, adults, families, parents, and teachers. We longed for a book that described tools for building a relationship with clients; exploring their issues and underlying dynamics; helping them gain insight into their issues and underlying dynamics; and working with them to make changes in cognitive, emotional, behavioral, interpersonal, attitudinal, and bodily patterns. We longed for a book that inspired play therapists to be intentional and systematic in their work with clients. We longed for a book that gave readers permission to give themselves permission to adapt techniques for specific clients and to "make stuff up" for the playroom. We knew that was a lot, and we believe all of those elements are essential for exemplary practice of play therapy. We never found such a book, so we decided to write it. This is the book you have in your hands (or on your tablet if you are e-reading).

We framed this book around the story of Zan, a student (or maybe an experienced mental health or school professional) you'll meet in the prelude who wanted to learn play therapy. She (or maybe he—we want to acknowledge that not all play therapists are female, and alternating pronouns is confusing, so we are just using the feminine pronoun for simplicity) represents our students and the readers of this book. She is meant to embody our desired audience—learners who, like Zan, love to tell stories, have adventures, dance, hear stories, make up songs, build worlds in the sand, do art, and generally love to play—folks who want to learn to use all those loves to help clients through the process of play therapy.

In working to help you learn how to do play therapy (or how to deepen your practice of play therapy), we first wanted to explicate the basics of play therapy (the what, who, where, and how)—that's in Chapter 1. We also wanted to cover counseling theories applied to play therapy— we think having a theoretical orientation or a systematic way of conceptualizing clients and developing treatment plans is important to becoming an effective play therapist. In order to help you explore this approach, we have included a chapter on theory applied to play therapy and on how to decide on a theory that will work for you (Chapter 2). Chapter 3 contains an overview of the broad strategies that play therapists can use throughout the play therapy process—we have techniques from each of those broad strategies in the five chapters that are about some things you can do in the playroom (Chapters 4, 5, 6, 7, and 8). In Chapter 4, we describe the basic play therapy skills and techniques for building the relationship in play therapy, which is foundational for everything else you do, regardless of your approach to play therapy. Chapter 5 is about exploring clients' interpersonal and intrapersonal issues—deciding whether and how to go about investigating "what's up" with your clients. For those play therapists who believe it is important for clients to gain insight into their patterns of thinking, behaving, and feeling, Chapter 6 is designed to give you ideas for helping clients begin to understand themselves (and maybe even others) better. Chapter 7 is about helping clients make changes; it is filled with skills and techniques designed to give you a plethora of directive (and some not-so-directive) methods for assisting clients to move forward with shifts in behavior, thinking, feeling, attitudes, and so forth. There is also a chapter (Chapter 8) with practical suggestions and activities for including parents and families (and teachers, when appropriate) in the play therapy process. Chapter 9 covers what to do when challenging situations come up in the playroom. Interspersed between the chapters, we have also included small bites of knowledge (or maybe even wisdom—we aren't sure which) on a number of topics designed to inspire you to be present, intentional, creative, and innovative; we called these small bites "Interludes."

As far as the techniques/activities go, certain things were important to both of us: (1) providing activities that could be used across several theoretical approaches to play therapy; (2) keeping the "mechanical communication" (S. Riviere, personal communication, September, 2015) aspect of each technique as the primary focus of the intervention—paying attention to what the client is *doing*; (3) encouraging readers to be intentional in their play therapy process—to think about what they want to accomplish with each activity they use with their clients; (4) supporting play therapists in balancing goal-directedness and flexibility both within and across sessions; (5) providing enough concrete detail in our descriptions that you can actually use these interventions in your practice; (6) creating an atmosphere of permission so you feel comfortable adapting the activities to your population and your practice; (7) challenging you to keep in mind the interests, talents, preferences, passions, likes, and dislikes of your clients as you choose activities tailored to appeal to and work with individual clients; (8) encouraging/inspiring you to invent your own activities; and (9) modeling how, with some clients and some interventions, asking questions can facilitate optimal growth, and with other clients and other interventions, not asking questions can facilitate optimal growth.

There are many, many skills and techniques/activities scattered throughout the book. We want to remind you (probably over and over and over again) not to consider the skills and techniques as recipes. There is no "right way" to do an activity. How each technique should be delivered "depends." It depends on you (and your ideas about how people grow and change) and on the client (and what is going on with him or her right then in the session and in general). Even though we have provided you with skills and intervention techniques, it is up to you to custom-design the application for the specific clients with whom you are working. We believe a big part of the play therapist's job is to tailor interventions to meet the needs and interests of individual clients. It is our conviction that paying attention to what is important to specific clients, paying attention to their preferred ways of expressing themselves, and paying attention to the best way to engage them in directive activities are all key elements to being successful and congruent in play therapy.

Acknowledgments

Our thanks to Rebecca Dickinson, Jill Thomas, Melissa Wehr, and John Young for answering our call to friends and students to contribute techniques to the book. A note of gratitude to all of our clients, our play therapy teachers, our colleagues, and our students for helping us figure out how to do play therapy so we could teach it to you. We also want to thank the baristas at Cup of Joe and Cottonwood Canyon in Cedar Falls, Iowa, and Island Joe in North Padre Island, Texas, for creating safe spaces for us to write.

Contents

Contents

Prelude

Once Upon a Time

*O*nce upon a time . . . well, maybe it might have been kind of recently, actually . . . in a kingdom kind of like ours (though not exactly like ours), there was a child named Zan. Zan was a delightful child—filled with joy and love and laughter. (And sometimes tears and anger and frustration and disappointment and hurt . . . Zan was like a lot of other kids—filled with lots of different feelings.) Zan liked to tell stories and have adventures and dance and hear stories and make up songs and build worlds in the sand and do art—Zan loved to *play*!

Now, as Zan grew up, some hard and scary things happened to Zan. Maybe Zan's parents got a divorce, and Zan thought she had to decide which one she loved most . . . Or maybe Zan's mom (or dad) got drunk and hit her . . . Or maybe the other kids in Zan's school made fun of her for being different than they were . . . Or maybe Zan's parents told her they didn't love her and didn't want her . . . Or maybe school was hard for Zan, and she felt like she was stupid and couldn't learn like the other kids . . . Or maybe sometimes Zan was so scared and sad, even though she didn't know why, she didn't want to get out of bed . . . Or maybe . . . Or maybe . . . Or maybe . . . (You get the idea . . . some hard and scary things happened to Zan—you know, like in real life hard and scary things happen to kids (and sometimes even teenagers and grownups.)

Nobody really seemed to notice that Zan had stopped telling stories and having adventures and dancing and hearing stories and making up songs and building worlds in the sand and doing art and playing. Zan felt that nobody really cared that she was struggling with the things that happened to her, and she often felt sad and lonely. She wished she had someone in her life who would help her understand what was going on with her and maybe even help her feel a little better . . . about herself and about her life.

One day (finally), Zan's school counselor did notice that she was struggling and arranged for her to work with a play therapist—someone who used play and stories and adventures and dance and music and art to create a safe space for Zan to tell her story. The play therapist had special training to be able to hear and see her (her whole self), to be her companion on her journey to reclaim the parts of herself she had lost, to create a safe space where she could tell stories and have adventures and hear stories and dance and make up songs and build worlds in the sand and do art to help her begin to heal herself. Play therapy helped Zan figure out some things about what had happened to her; it helped her to learn new ways to express her feelings and thoughts; it helped her to learn to understand herself and her feelings better. By giving her permission to use play to express herself, play therapy reminded her how much she loved playing.

Zan got older (as people do), going through puberty and adolescence (never an easy journey for anyone). As a teenager, she struggled . . . feeling lonely and isolated . . . feeling like no one else had ever experienced the hard times, the difficult situations she had suffered. Recognizing that she needed help getting through the tough times, she went back to play therapy. The play therapist used all of the amazing play therapy tools to create a safe space for Zan to tell her story—it might have been a retelling of the story she had to tell when she was younger, and it might have been a new story she had to tell. Again, play therapy helped Zan figure out some things about what had happened to her, helped her to learn new ways to express her feelings and thoughts, helped her to learn to understand herself and her feelings better. By giving her permission to use play to express herself, play therapy reminded her how much she loved playing.

As Zan got older, moving into adulthood, she recognized that she wanted to find a way to help other kids (and maybe even teenagers and grownups) who were struggling like she had struggled. She wanted to help children (and teens and grownups) who felt sad and lonely and needed someone to help them understand what was going on with them and maybe even help them feel a little better about themselves and their lives. She remembered how much she liked going to play therapy and telling stories, having adventures, dancing, hearing stories, making up songs, building worlds in the sand, and doing art—how much she loved to *play* with the play therapist when she was younger. She also realized she still loved doing all those things and thought, "Maybe I can learn to use all of those things I love to help other people."

Zan became very curious about how people get the way they are . . . why they think the things they think . . . why they feel the things they feel . . . why they do the things they do. . . . The more curious Zan got about what caused people to struggle, what helped them learn to express their thoughts and feelings, how to create safe spaces for them to tell their stories, the more Zan explored and studied. As Zan matured, going to college, going out into the world after she graduated, she set out to find a way she could use all her loves (for hearing stories, having adventures, dancing, telling stories, making up songs, building worlds in the sand, doing art, and playing) to connect with kids (and maybe even teenagers and grownups) and maybe even help them understand what is going on with them and maybe even help them feel a little better about themselves and their lives. And she decided the best pathway to help others, doing the things she loved, was to study play therapy. . . . She set out to learn about play therapy. She knew if he could learn to be a companion/ mentor/witness/healer/teacher/play therapist, she could help other kids (and teens and grownups) to rediscover their joy and delight again. (Not that anyone could make what happened to them and their lives go away, but having a companion/mentor/witness/healer/ teacher/play therapist could start them on the journey back to gladness and playfulness.)

So . . . she started her search for knowledge and wisdom, looking for a teacher (or two)—someone who could answer some of her questions about play therapy. (And she had a *lot* of questions.)

Luckily, she found us . . . and we happen to be teachers . . . who happen to know something about play therapy . . . and love using play therapy as the foundation of our relationships with kids (and teens and grownups) on their journey. The following few hundred pages are our attempts to answer Zan's questions as she studies how to use play therapy as a tool for connecting, facilitating understanding, and supporting growth. We hope you love taking this adventure with her as much as we have loved writing this book to teach her (and you, of course) many of the things you need to know about how to use play therapy as a healing modality.

CHAPTER 1

An Introduction
to Play Therapy

If you are someone who loves to hear stories and have adventures and dance and tell stories and make up songs and mess around in the sand and do art, and if you might be interested in exploring ways to use play to work therapeutically with children, welcome to the world of play therapy! This is the introductory chapter, wherein we lay out the basics of play therapy. In this chapter, we have outlined multiple definitions of play therapy, danced through a brief explanation of the various approaches to play therapy, described possible clients who would be appropriate for play therapy, delineated the personal and professional qualifications of people who want to be play therapists, described various settings for play therapy, explained some ideas about how play therapy works, and defined some of the logistics involved in play therapy.

WHAT, EXACTLY, IS PLAY THERAPY?

As the title suggests, this is a book designed to teach you how to do play therapy. Before we get into the nitty-gritty details, though, we thought it would be good to explain what play therapy is. Keep in mind, though, that it is a little tricky to answer the question posited in the heading of this section of the chapter ("What, exactly, is play therapy?") because there are a lot of different ways to define play therapy.

The *Merriam Webster Dictionary* (n.d.) defines play therapy as "psychotherapy in which a child is encouraged to reveal feelings and conflicts in play rather than by verbalization." According to the British Association for Play Therapy (2014a), "Play Therapy is the dynamic process between child and Play Therapist in which the child explores at his or her own pace and with his or her own agenda those issues, past and current, conscious and unconscious, that are affecting the child's life in the present. The child's inner resources are enabled by the therapeutic alliance to bring about growth and change. Play Therapy is child-centered, in which play is the primary medium and speech is the secondary medium" (para. 13). Wilson and Ryan's (2005) definition focused on children and adolescents: "Play therapy can be defined as a means of creating intense relationship experiences between therapists and children or young people, in which play is the principal medium of communication" (p. 3). Landreth (2012), in *Play Therapy: The Art of the Relationship,* suggested that play therapy can be useful for people of any age when he defined play therapy as "a dynamic interpersonal relationship between a child (or a person of any age) and a therapist trained in play therapy procedures who provides selected play materials and facilitates the development of a safe relationship for the child (or person of any age) to fully express and explore self (feelings, thoughts, experiences and behaviors) through play, the child's natural medium of communications, for optimal growth and development" (p. 11). According to the Association for Play Therapy (2017), play therapy is "the systematic use of a theoretical model to establish an interpersonal process wherein trained play therapists use the therapeutic powers of play to help clients prevent or resolve psychosocial difficulties and achieve optimal growth and development" (para. 1). (Sounds like a definition made by a committee, doesn't it ?) If we synthesize and summarize all of these definitions, play therapy can be best described as a modality of therapy in which trained professionals use a theoretically based, consistent way of understanding and communicating with their clients through *doing* rather than just *talking.*

In our very broad definition of play therapy, we would describe play therapy as a therapeutic modality that uses a wide variety of methodologies to communicate with clients, including adventure therapy, storytelling and therapeutic metaphors, movement/dance/music experiences, sand tray activities, art techniques, and structured play experiences in addition to free, unstructured play. To us, interactions in play therapy should always allow for and even encourage self-expression, creative representation, and imagination. Simply put, play therapy is a relationship in which a trained therapist creates a safe space for clients to explore and express themselves through telling stories, having adventures, dancing, hearing stories, making up songs, messing around in the sand, doing art, and playing.

APPROACHES TO PLAY THERAPY

There are many different approaches to play therapy. Some of these approaches are based on major models of counseling and psychotherapy (e.g., Adlerian, person-centered, object relations, existential, cognitive-behavioral, Gestalt, Jungian, narrative, psychodynamic, prescriptive/integrative). Other approaches were developed specifically for play therapy (i.e., dynamic play therapy, experiential play therapy, synergetic play therapy, schema-based play therapy, Autplay, Somaplay, release play therapy, ecosystemic play therapy, and Theraplay). Recently, there has been a major upsurge in the development of additional approaches to play therapy. Each of these approaches has underlying philosophical assumptions about people, how they develop their personalities, how dysfunction develops, how people grow and change, how clinical interventions can be helpful. Adequately describing all of these approaches to play therapy is beyond the scope of this book (and beyond the capacity of our brains), so we have chosen certain widely used approaches to explicate. (See Chapter 2.) We did want you to know that there are many, many different ways to approach play therapy—if you are interested, please explore . . .

WHO ARE PLAY THERAPY CLIENTS?

We believe play therapy is for everyone . . . for people of all ages and in any configuration that works best for clients and their families: individual, family, and group. It's for children, teens, and adults who've experienced loss, divorce, sadness, anxiety, guilt, anger, fear, or hurt. It's for people who are uncertain. It's for people who have been abused or neglected. It's for individuals, groups, or families. Play therapy is for people who are having a hard time at school or work, struggling with their families, or spending a lot of time in hospitals. It's for scared people, brave people, lonely people, loved people, artsy people, shy people, and anyone else who has goals of living a more fully alive and functioning existence.

While play therapy is often done with children under the age of about 12, there is a growing body of literature that supports the use of play therapy and play strategies with clients who are older (sometimes significantly older) than 12 (e.g., Ashby, Kottman, & DeGraaf, 2008; Frey, 2015; Gallo-Lopez & Schaefer, 2005; Gardner, 2015; Green, Drewes, & Kominski, 2013; Ojiambo & Bratton, 2014; Schaefer, 2003). Because we believe play therapy is appropriate for all ages, we made the conscious decision to broaden the scope of this book to include skills, strategies, and techniques you can use with children, adolescents, adults, and families.

WHO DOES PLAY THERAPY?

There are some specific personal qualities that are important in being a play therapist, and there are professional training and experiences that are essential in preparing people to become play therapists. The British Association for Play Therapy (2014b) has provided a list of personal characteristics desirable for play therapists. They believe play therapists must be empathic, sincere, honest, respectful, ethical, knowledgeable, self-aware, self-responsible, congruent (authentic and genuine), compassionate, critically reflective, and committed to personal and professional development. According to Kottman (2011), effective play therapists should like children and treat them with respect and kindness, have a sense of humor and be willing to laugh at themselves and with others, be fun-loving and playful, be sufficiently self-confident not to depend on positive regard from other people to bolster their self-worth, be open and honest, be flexible and able to deal with ambiguity and uncertainty, be accepting of others' perceptions without feeling vulnerable or judgmental, and be willing to think of play and metaphor as vehicles for communication with others. They should also be relaxed and comfortable being with children and have experience building relationships with them, be capable of firmly and kindly setting limits and maintaining personal boundaries, be self-aware and able to take interpersonal risks, and be open to considering their own personal issues and the impact of those issues on what transpires in play therapy sessions and relationships with clients and their families (Kottman, 2011).

In general, we think it's important for those who practice play therapy or want to become play therapists to be creative, cognitively flexible (physically flexible is nice and not a requirement, especially since only one of us is physically flexible—that would be Kristin, not Terry), fun, passionate, caring, trustworthy, and responsible. This isn't a whole lot different from counselors or therapists who do other types of therapy. We think an important consideration for professionals who do play therapy is a willingness to enter into the creative world of the client and to think symbolically. These qualities are important because your primary "tool" in play therapy is you—the person who loves to play—the person who loves to listen to stories and have adventures and dance and tell stories and make up songs and mess around in the sand and do art.

If you have already been trained as a traditional counselor, social worker, psychologist, or other mental health professional and you want to be a play therapist, it is also essential that you are open to thinking about the play (or what the client does), rather than words (what the client says), as the healing channel—the path for communication and facilitation of movement and growth. You must be willing to jump the chasm of the paradigm shift from focusing on talk as the vehicle for building relationships, exploring dynamics, helping folks gain insight, and facilitating them in making changes to the understanding that play can be an effective medium for those same therapeutic processes—in play therapy, the play *is* the therapy.

The Association for Play Therapy (APT) also has some important (okay, okay—necessary) standards as well. (The APT is the national professional society founded in 1982 to foster contact among mental health professionals interested in exploring and, when developmentally appropriate, applying the therapeutic power of play to communicate with and treat clients.) APT has defined a set of standards and requirements for a professional helper to become a registered play therapist (RPT). They have recently added the option for school counselors and school psychologists to become registered as well. (See Appendix C for the rules for becoming a registered play therapist, a school-based registered play therapist [SB-RPT], and a registered play therapist-supervisor [RPT-S].)

APT provides detailed information about each of these points and the biannual continuing education requirements of RPTs. Because the credentialing process is subject to change, we don't want to provide you with specific nitty-gritty details that might be outdated as you read this book. A major area to note is that the RPTs and SB-RPTs are licensed professionals before they are RPTs. That is, they must be licensed in their state before they can hold the RPT designation. We recommend that you clarify the expectations required of you to become an RPT and continuously review them as you start your journey so that you will not get blindsided with changes.

Recently, the Center for Play Therapy at the University of North Texas also established standards for becoming certified in child-centered play therapy (CCPT) and in child–parent relationship therapy (CPRT). The certification in CCPT involves two levels. Both levels have specific requirements that include licensure as a mental health professional, specific hours of education related to CCPT, an examination over CCPT, supervised experience conducting child-centered play therapy sessions, and self-evaluation papers. There are three levels to the certification for CPRT, and they have similar requirements. The details of these requirements can be found on the website for the Center (*http://cpt.unt.edu*). We are in the process of developing a certification program in Adlerian play therapy, and we suspect that other approaches to play therapy may have similar evolutions in their futures.

WHERE IS PLAY THERAPY DONE?

The short answer to this question is that you can do play therapy anywhere. While this is true, it helps to have a space that is private and (in a perfect world) sound-proof because play therapy can get loud! Often it is not loud in ways that are problematic, but consider toys hitting the floor (accidentally or on purpose), lions roaring, clients (or therapists) singing karaoke, or laughing. Aside from the ethical obligation of confidentiality, any of these might be considered concerning, or disruptive, for people in adjacent rooms. Rooms that are a bit bigger than a standard bedroom are ideal. This gives you enough space for the toys and materials and you and the client. However, we have worked in a room that used to be the janitor's closet (it's a good thing we're not very tall). For several years, I (Terry) worked in a cubby outside the elevator in an elementary school and a playroom that was huge in counseling office standards (30 feet by 30 feet); now I have a corner of a (very generous) school counselor's office. What we're trying to say is that you can make any location work—remember, your clients have very seldom read a textbook describing what kind of space is needed as a playroom. As my (Kristin's) children say, "You get what you get, and you don't throw a fit."

There are no "rules" about where you can do play therapy, and if you agree with the way we define play therapy, you might find play therapy taking place in locations that seem a bit unorthodox for counseling. Typically speaking, play therapists work in private practice settings, community agencies, schools (we both volunteer at schools), hospitals, camps, or clients' homes. You can also do play therapy outdoors—on nature trails, lakes or rivers, or rope courses. (We've even done sand tray play therapy on a beach!) As long as the space allows for confidentiality and/or the client (or guardian) understands the risks to confidentiality (i.e., in a park or nature trail you can't guarantee privacy), play therapy can take place anywhere. There might be some limitations or restrictions on what you can do in different settings (for instance, it's hard to play with toys or do directed art activities while you're kayaking). And we want to invite you to think creatively about location and about the "stuff" you use for the therapeutic process. (Because, remember, you, yourself, and your love of hearing stories, having adventures, dancing, telling stories, making up songs, messing around in the sand, and doing art are the only "tools" you need.)

HOW DOES PLAY THERAPY WORK?

It's important to remember that the foundation of play therapy rests on the therapeutic powers of play—the inherent powers that exist when people are in a relationship in which they are free to be creative, accepted, and safe. As a creative and artistic modality of counseling, play therapy allows for the expression of thoughts, emotions, and experiences in a variety of ways. Schaefer and Drewes (2014) delineated twenty therapeutic powers of play, which they labeled as self-expression, access to the unconscious, direct teaching, indirect teaching, catharsis, abreaction, positive emotions, counterconditioning fears, stress inoculation, stress management, therapeutic relationship, attachment, social competence, empathy, creative problem solving, resiliency, moral development, accelerated psychological development, self-regulation, and self-esteem. (If you are interested in being inspired by reading about all of these superpowers, read *The Therapeutic Powers of Play: 20 Core Agents of Change* [Schaefer & Drewes, 2014].)

Play, in and of itself, is a primal human activity. Brown and Vaughn (2009) described the power of play: "Most obviously, it is intensely pleasurable. It energizes us and enlivens us. It eases our burdens. It renews our natural sense of optimism and opens us up to new possibilities" (p. 4). Young children often lack the capacity to use language adequately to describe their emotions, experiences, and thoughts required for talk therapy and are typically more comfortable expressing themselves through play and metaphor (Kottman, 2011; Nash & Schaefer, 2011). Specifically, for young clients, play has been described as children's language (Kottman & Meany-Walen, 2016; Landreth, 2012; Moustakas, 1997; Ray, 2011). For children, play therapy facilitates communication, fosters emotional wellness, enhances social relationships, and increases personal strengths (Schaefer & Drewes, 2014). For adolescents and adults, play facilitates relationships, ignites creativity, reduces resistance, deepens insight, and helps bridge abstract ideas to day-to-day situations for clients (Gallo-Lopez & Schaefer, 2005; Gardner, 2015; Green et al., 2013).

Emerging research and publications have offered us more information about the "Why play therapy?" and "How does play therapy work?" questions. Important in today's climate of evidence-based practices, play therapy has a rich body of literature to substantiate the "why?" of play therapy. There is empirical research that supports the efficacy of play therapy in reducing clients' behavioral problems related to aggression, anxiety, conduct disorders, depression, and symptoms related to attention-deficit/hyperactivity disorder (ADHD), such as disruptiveness and inattentiveness. Play therapy has also been found to be useful for improving clients' symptoms related to adoption, abandonment, autism, divorce, homelessness, learning disabilities, trauma, and academic or social problems (e.g., Blanco & Ray, 2011; Bratton, Ray, Rhine, & Jones, 2005; Carnes Holt & Bratton, 2015; Dillman Taylor & Meany-Walen, 2015; LeBlanc & Ritchie, 2001; Lin & Bratton, 2015; Meany-Walen, Bratton, & Kottman, 2014; Meany-Walen, Kottman, Bullis, & Dillman Taylor, 2015; Ojiambo & Bratton, 2014; Ray, Armstrong, Balkin, & Jayne, 2015; Schottelkorb & Ray, 2009; Swan & Ray, 2014). This is an abbreviated list to give you just a taste of the ways play therapy has shown effectiveness.

Recently, Adlerian play therapy, Theraplay, filial family therapy, CPRT, and CCPT were added to the National Registry of Evidence-Based

Programs and Practices (NREPP) managed by the Substance Abuse and Mental Health Services Administration (SAMHSA). Adlerian play therapy was found to be effective in reducing disruptive disorders and behaviors and promising for building positive self-esteem. Theraplay was designated effective in internalizing problems, and promising for helping clients with autism spectrum disorder and symptoms. Filial family therapy was found to be effective in enhancing family–child relationships and promising for reducing unspecified mental health disorders and symptoms, enhancing personal resilience/self-concept, improving parenting behaviors, and upgrading social functioning/competence. CPRT was declared to be effective in improving family cohesion and in helping clients with disruptive disorders and behaviors, and promising for internalizing problems. CCPT was established as promising in the enhancement of general functioning and well-being, and in the treatment of anxiety disorders and symptoms and disruptive disorders and behaviors.

Here's what we've learned so far about how play therapy works. (*Disclaimer:* We are not experts on interpersonal neurobiology. We don't even play experts on TV. This is merely a summary of how we understand it with our limited knowledge. Please seek additional information for more thorough explanations of this important topic if you are interested in how play therapy works from a brain development perspective.)

During the early ages of life, the brain builds upon itself in a relatively hierarchical fashion (Gaskill, 2010). The brain stem and diencephalon are the first areas of the brain to begin to develop and are responsible for functions such as metabolism, hyperarousal, sensory perceptual problems, and emotional arousal. The cortex, which is the rational executive part of the brain, develops later. Trauma impacts the part of the brain that is currently under construction, which means that when children experience trauma, the organization of the brain stem and diencephalon is disrupted, which can have negative effects on the areas controlled by those brain regions. Furthermore, the growing brain is developing upon a disorganized foundation, which can negatively impact a person's ability to think rationally and conduct him- or herself in a way that is socially expected and accepted throughout life.

Play therapy intersects the level of the brain affected by the insult, particularly if the trauma happened early in life (such as with kids or adults who experienced trauma as children). Because play therapy can be nonverbal or less reliant on insight and reasoning than talk therapy, it can help clients with affected brain regions to process their experiences and communicate about their thoughts and feelings (Gaskill, 2010). Play therapy responds to the developmental level of the person and the area of the brain impacted by the distressing event or events. Play therapy is different from "just playing" because the presence of an empathic and attuned witness helps clients process their experiences, feelings, and thoughts.

LOGISTICS OF PLAY THERAPY

There are many things to consider when you examine the logistics of play therapy: stages of play therapy; skills, strategies, and techniques; toys and play therapy materials; explanation of play therapy for parents and clients; the first session; what to do in sessions; how to end a session; course of treatment, and termination. (This section could be a whole book by itself. As you explore, one of the things you will discover is that logistics can unfold in a multitude of ways—depending on your theoretical approach to play therapy, your setting, and your personal preferences. We don't believe there is just one way to do anything connected to play therapy, so give yourself permission to evolve all of these elements in ways that will work for you.)

Stages

Each of the various approaches to play therapy uses different words or phrases to label the different stages of play therapy—some of them focused on the behavior of the client, some on the actions of the therapist, and some on the relationship. Since this book is designed to teach you how to do play therapy, it seemed expedient to have a way to organize our presentation of the unfolding of the play therapy process with a focus on what the play therapist does. We wanted a cross-theoretical method of discussing the skills and techniques you need to learn to be able to use play therapy as your therapeutic modality. We decided to present the play therapy process as unfolding in four overlapping phases. Since every approach to play therapy has unique labels for the phases of therapy, we have tried to just give them a name that labels what the therapist does in the phase: (1) building the relationship (this one keeps on going throughout the process because even after you have established a connection with the client, you will need to do some maintenance to keep things rolling); (2) exploring the interpersonal and intrapersonal dynamics of the client; (3) helping the client gain insight into his or her patterns of thinking, feeling, and behaving; and (4) facilitating the client's ability to make desired changes in thoughts, emotions, and behavior. The different approaches to play therapy put varying emphases on these phases (some of them skip one or more of these phases altogether, but we will get to that later). Because this is meant to be a cross-theoretical book, we have included all four of these phases, along with play therapy skills and techniques for each one.

Skills, Strategies, and Techniques

We make a distinction between play therapy skills, play therapy strategies, and play therapy techniques. Play therapy skills are the basic building blocks used in play therapy by practically every approach to play therapy. Some of the basic *play therapy skills* include tracking, restating content, reflecting feelings, returning the responsibility to the client, questioning, observing, and setting limits, which are used to build the relationship with the client (described in Chapter 4), and it is important to remember that they are used throughout the process as a way to maintain the relationship. We use play therapy skills of questioning and observing during the phase of therapy in which we explore the interpersonal and intrapersonal dynamics of the client (described in Chapter 5). To help the client gain insight into his or her patterns of thinking, feeling, and behaving, some play therapy approaches use more directed play therapy skills, and some theoretical approaches to play therapy do not use these skills because there isn't an emphasis on gaining insight in those approaches. For those approaches that emphasize gaining insight, interpreting, using the client's metaphors, confronting discrepancies, and designing custom therapeutic metaphors are skills used in this phase (described in Chapter 6). In addition to the skills we've used throughout the other phases of therapy, the skills used in the last phase of play therapy, helping the child gain insight, are paying attention to timing, looking at secondary gain, being realistic and helping others to be realistic, and teaching (described in Chapter 7). For play therapists who work with parents and teachers, many of the skills used in working with play therapy clients are useful, plus there are even skills used specifically in the consultation process with parents and teachers: reframing, conveying understanding and compassion [yes—important with all clients—we just wanted to make a special case for it with parents, especially because we have both needed it in interactions with counselors and teachers about our own children], avoiding judgment (okay, we know this is important with clients, too, but sometimes it is more difficult with parents and teachers, so we just wanted to emphasize it as a skill with them), helping define "stake in the ground." All of these skills, along with family play therapy, are described in Chapter 8.

Play therapy strategies are broad areas of expertise that can be applied in every part of the play therapy process. We have labeled the various broad categories of play therapy strategies as adventure therapy; storytelling and therapeutic metaphors; movement, dance, and music experiences; sand tray activities; art techniques; and structured play experiences. You'll find thorough explanations, descriptions, and examples of these play therapy strategies in Chapter 3. We also want to acknowledge that several of these strategies are actually separate professional disciplines as well as methods you can use in play therapy. (Quietly dancing through the tulips here—we don't want to step on anyone's toes.)

Within each of these broad strategies are a plethora of individual *play therapy techniques*—activities that the play therapist can use as tools and interventions throughout the process. You'll find the play therapy techniques nestled within each of the strategies throughout Chapters 4, 5, 6, and 7. Our intention was that this book be informative and practical, so that you could come back to these chapters as a reference or launching pad for intervention ideas. We wanted to be sure we included techniques that use play as the primary vehicle for communication, allowing clients to communicate in what Scott Riviere (personal communication, October 2016) described as "mechanical communication" (using their bodies and their actions without having to use their words). We think it is important to keep the focus on the play as communication because otherwise, you wind up doing talk therapy in a playroom. (There's nothing wrong with doing talk therapy in the playroom; it just isn't what we want to teach you to do.)

Toys and Play Therapy Materials

Toys and materials are the "things" that you can use to do play therapy. How many and the kinds of toys and materials you have are going to depend on you, your "style" of play therapy, and your setting—in several approaches to play therapy (ecosystemic play therapy and Theraplay—we will get to those in the next chapter), play therapy happens in an empty room with the therapist choosing specific toys or materials for what he or she wants to accomplish in a particular session.

Kottman (2011) described five broad categories of materials that many play therapists choose to have in their playrooms: family/nurturing, scary, aggressive, expressive, and pretend/fantasy. Family/nurturing toys provide opportunities for clients to develop a relationship with the therapist, explore family dynamics, and express relational experiences, wants, or needs. Toys in this category might be a dollhouse; doll families (with different colored skin tones); baby doll and accessories such as bottles, blankets, cradles; stuffed toys; sandbox; doctor kit; tool kit; and kitchen with pans, dishes, utensils, empty food containers such as cereal box, peanut butter jar (plastic), and sour cream containers.

Scary toys provide opportunities for clients to deal with and overcome fears. These toys might include snakes, insects, sharks, dragons, and other animals commonly considered scary or frightening. Animals should come in a variety of sizes and textures, (e.g., a plush snake, a puppet alligator, a plastic insect family with several very large members and several smaller members). For clients who have experienced trauma or medical emergencies, ambulances, firetrucks, police cars, and the like might be scary.

Aggressive toys allow clients to express and process anger, aggression, protection, or control issues. Using aggressive toys, children can symbolically explore these feelings, which is typically discouraged in other environments such as school or home. These toys can include dart or ray guns, handcuffs, rope, bop bag, swords or knives, soldiers, or shields.

You might include small pillows that can be used for pillow fights or for practicing ways of appropriately expressing anger (punching or yelling into a pillow).

Expressive toys provide opportunities for clients to express themselves in ways that other materials don't. They can enhance feelings of mastery and provide opportunities to practice problem solving and be creative. Examples of these materials are arts-and-craft materials such as watercolors, crayons, markers, clay, tape, scissors, glue, glitter, paper punch, stapler, stickers, paper, construction paper, feathers, pompoms, straws, pipe cleaners, egg cartons, and newspapers and magazines. (These are substantially harder to find now than they used to be. Doesn't anyone read anything in print anymore?)

Pretend/fantasy toys invite clients to express themselves and their desires. They can practice a variety of roles, experiment with different behaviors or attitudes, and act out situations within the safety of the playroom. Materials can include dress up clothes (ties and sports jacket, capes, high heels, a lab coat, and/or dresses), hats (army, fire fighter, police officer, cowboy/cowgirl, or wizard), masks, magic wands, and crowns. You can also have family sets of animals (farm, zoo, safari, ocean, etc.), puppets, cars, trucks, planes, telephones (at least two), blocks and building materials, and so on.

In addition to the toys and materials listed in the categories, there are a few other items to consider. We like having an easel. A free-standing (as opposed to a table-top) easel is ideal, with at least four different colors of tempera paints. It is helpful to use paper or foam cups inside of the plastic paint cups, filled with only a bit of paint because if there is a catastrophe, it will be kind of a small mess. (We learned this from not-so-pleasant experiences.) Add a few drops of dish soap to the paint. This helps to wash out paint from clothes or walls . . . or hair. It also makes the paint smoother and more slippery, a kinesthetic benefit for clients. We have found that having a puppet theater or something that can serve as a puppet theater is fun. Clients can hide, perform plays, or use it as a way to separate themselves from the therapist if needed. (Sometimes a puppet theater is more than a puppet theater.) A table or desk that doesn't take up your entire space can also be nice. Clients can use this to work with expressive materials, and it can be more comfortable than working on the floor. We recommend having a chair that rolls or something that can support your back if you choose to sit on the floor. Wheels allow you to easily maneuver around the room, if needed. If you sit on the floor, you might consider a gaming chair or a "back jack" that helps you not sit hunched all day. (We both have bad backs, so just thinking of sitting unsupported for any amount of time makes us hurt.)

Also know that not all practitioners agree with what you should or should not include in your play therapy tool kit. The use of technology in the playroom is a hot topic right now (Snow, Winburn, Crumrine, Jackson, & Killian, 2012)—even between the two of us. Some play therapists (including Terry) think it's perfectly fine to have a tablet or laptop in their play space and believe that using technology with clients who are "gamers" can actually facilitate connection and encourage them to practice skills like anxiety management or anger control using their preferred mode of playing. Others (including Kristin) think that anything that has a battery has no place in the playroom, believing that it limits creativity and free expression.

To include a bop bag or to not include a bop bag is another conversation among play therapists. Some argue that the inclusion and use of bop bags encourage aggression (Charles Schaefer, personal communication, 2015), while others believe that using a bop bag to express anger is necessary and does not increase aggression or anger in children (Ray, 2011). As you are thinking about whether to invest in a bop bag, consider that they are not limited to being punched. We've had clients ride them like horses, hug them, and practice frustration tolerance and mastery as they find ways to keep the bop bag from returning to the upright position. (Again, we come down on different sides of this issue—Kristin has a bop bag in her playroom and Terry doesn't—which illustrates that there is no right answer here—or if there is, we don't know what it is.)

We should also talk about having toy guns and other weapons in a playroom. Play therapists tend to feel very strongly one way or another about having toy weapons in playrooms. You need to consider your own comfort level with and beliefs about toy guns and kids using them in various ways. It is also important to consider the locale in which you want to do play therapy—schools or other settings might also have rules about having guns (even toy ones) on the property. One of my (Kristin's) favorite play therapy stories is of a young girl who picked up the dart gun, pointed it at her head and started blow drying her hair. To her, the gun wasn't a gun; it was a hair-styling tool! It was a great lesson for me about creativity and imagination. Overall, we believe it's not so important "what" you have in the playroom as long as you have a rationale for its being in the playroom and as long as your rationale is based on training, experience, human development, and theory. (We'll get to that in the next chapter.)

There's no doubt about it: furnishing a playroom can be costly. We've learned along the way that most clients do not care if toys are new or used. In fact, many kids prefer the used toys as it invites playfulness without setting an expectation of keeping things neat and kept. Go to thrift shops, garage sales, and maybe your children's toy box to look for unused, old toys. Make things with clients or with your own family members, kids in the neighborhood, or your friends. You can make sock puppets instead of buying, for example. My (Kristin's) husband and oldest son made my puppet theater and doll house. It was a fraction of the cost of purchasing new. Another cost saver is to use items across categories. For example, the small pillows that we described for pillow fights could also be used in the nurturing category with baby dolls. Egg cartons listed in the expressive toys category can be used for nurture/family play in the kitchen area, aggressive play for tearing up, pretend play for clients who are acting like a chef (or hen?), or maybe even scary play for a client with egg allergies. (I guess what we're saying is, "Save all your egg cartons. You'll use them!")

Explaining Play Therapy to Parents and Clients

Think about this: How did you learn about play therapy? What were your initial thoughts about what it is and how it's done? What helped you to better understand and find value in play therapy? Many of the clients with whom you'll work will already have some beliefs about play therapy. Some of those ideas may be accurate, and others may be inaccurate. Some people will feel positively about play therapy, and others might think it's frivolous. When you start working with new clients, you'll want to be sure that you don't assume that others know what play therapy is or what you'll be doing in therapy. It is most helpful to describe play therapy to clients in a way that they understand and don't mistake play therapy with "just play-ing." We have given you three different ways of explaining play therapy (to parents and teachers of child clients, children, and adults/adolescents) because the way we go about explaining play therapy to each of these populations varies.

Explaining Play Therapy to Parents of Child Clients (and Teachers When Appropriate)

When we first meet with parents and teachers, we believe it is important to have meetings with them without the child present. We want a chance to meet and get to know them and for them to get to know us a bit. Another advantage of not having kids present during our first session with these important adults is that we want parents to be free to share whatever information they want without having to filter in front of their child (either on their own accord or on our request for them to not talk poorly about a child in front of the child). During this time, we explain what play therapy is, what they can expect, and how we anticipate the process going.

We give brief and concise information about child development and how play connects to children's mode of communication. The classic description of "toys are their words and play is their language" might be used to help explain the process and rationale. Sometimes we talk about the idea that children communicate with their bodies and what they do more than their words. We might show them a playroom or hold our "explaining session" in the playroom so they can see the area in which the child will be doing therapy. Here's an example of what we would tell a parent or teacher who is just learning about play therapy

> "For lots of young children, they don't know how to tell us about their problems with words in the same way that adolescents or grown-ups do. Instead, they tend to show us what is going on in their lives by playing or interacting. My job as a play therapist is to listen with my ears, my eyes, and my heart. I watch children, interact with children, and try to figure out how they are feeling, what they are thinking, and what's going on in their lives.
>
> "I also work with parents (and sometimes teachers and other family members) to help me understand the child better and for them to make adjustments in the way they think about the child and shift their interactions with the child to support his or her progress. I'll give you information about what I notice about the child's patterns of thinking, feeling, and behaving in our sessions and share ideas about what you can do to help the child. I believe that, when a child has a problem, everyone in the family has a share of that problem, so I expect that everyone in the family will have a share in working toward making things better for the child and for themselves. Or for teachers (I believe that, when a child has a problem, the teacher and everyone in the classroom can help work toward making things better for the child and themselves)."

With parents, we discuss expectations about how the child should dress, scheduling of sessions, length of sessions, number of sessions, inclusion of other important adults, and confidentiality. We encourage parents to bring their child to play therapy in play clothes that can get ruined. (Not that we are going to try to ruin a kid's clothing, and better safe than sorry—sometimes parents dress kids up in their "going to the doctor" fancy clothes and that is just a disaster waiting to happen.) We explain that in play therapy we use paint, sand, water, and other materials that might be messy, and we don't want a child to feel restricted or to get in trouble for getting clothes messy during play therapy. As play therapists, we don't wear our nicest clothes either. You'll often find us in t-shirts and leggings or jeans. This is not typical "professional" attire, so we tell parents that we wear these types of clothes so we can be comfortable playing and moving, and we don't want our energy consumed by a worry about our clothes being damaged.

The scheduling of sessions, as well as their length and number, are an important part of your discussion in the first meeting with parents and teachers. Unless you work in a school setting, it is likely that many of your parents will want to schedule sessions after school hours, and often kids have extracurricular activities such as sports, scouts, church/faith groups, and music lessons. These might be obstacles you and the parents will need to consider. Sometimes the child's inclusion in these activities can contribute to the presenting issue, particularly when children are over-scheduled or parents have expectations beyond their child's interests or capabilities. Sometimes these activities are an asset and should be encouraged, which means you will have to schedule around them.

The length of your sessions will depend on your schedule, the child's needs, the needs of the organization (such as in schools or hospitals), and other variables. For example, in school-based counseling, we usually see kids for 30-minute sessions so that they are not removed from the class for long periods of time. Sometimes we see them twice a week. In our private practices, our sessions are usually about 45–60 minutes. A portion of the longer sessions includes time to consult with parents. Younger children or children with particular needs might benefit from briefer sessions. Older children can usually benefit from lengthier sessions. Whatever you determine is best and appropriate for your situation, you'll want to communicate that to the parents.

Many parents (and teachers) want a guesstimate of the number of sessions or length of time we anticipate will be necessary for the child. We are clear with them that we cannot guarantee any particular number of sessions. We also share with these adults that play therapy and working with children is rarely a brief process. It typically takes several sessions to build a therapeutic relationship with children, understand their unique dynamics, and help them to make changes. We also communicate that we are not here to "fix" the child (in fact, we don't believe they are "broken"), and then we describe our philosophy about what children need and our beliefs about how change happens. (Chapter 2 is designed to help you explore your own philosophy about what people need for change to occur and to invite you to develop your style of play therapy.) We've worked with some children for just a few sessions with successful results, but we see most of our clients for 4–6 months. In a few cases, we might even work with a client for a year or more.

We work with parents frequently and let them know up front that we will meet with them regularly to discuss play therapy themes, progress, strategies to use at home, or other topics as they become relevant. We do family play with many of our clients as well, and so we discuss the why and how of doing family play therapy with various family members throughout the process. If you work with other adults in the child's life, such as teachers, it will be important to describe to the parents your reasons for wanting to include teachers and gather any consent forms needed for your setting.

Confidentiality is an important concept to explain and to ensure it's understood by parents. We explain that play therapy is like talk therapy for adults, and we want to create and honor a relationship of trust and privacy. We explain that, while we do not tell anyone every detail of what is played or discussed in play therapy, we do share with parents (and, in some cases, teachers) the key themes that emerge and strategies that we believe could be helpful for them to use with their child. For example, let's say that I (Kristin) am working with 6-year-old Tay and notice that she consistently plays out relationship themes and seeks nurturing either through play metaphors or from me. I would share this observation with her parents, process this a bit with them to try to get a better understanding of family dynamics, and work with them to find more ways to nurture their child or respond to her needs.

We are also very clear that we follow the ethical codes and legal requirements of our profession, which include breaking confidentiality in the case of suspected abuse or neglect, harm to self or others, or legal matters in which records are subpoenaed by the courts. If you are under supervision, you should add a statement about consulting with other professionals as a routine and safe practice, and should report that you don't use client names when you consult about particular cases. Here's an example of what you could say to parents regarding confidentiality.

> "It's important that Cooper feel safe and trust that he can share with me without fearing that I will report everything to anyone. So, I won't be repeating everything that Cooper does or says in our sessions, and I will talk to you about the patterns I notice in the playroom. I'll also share my observations and understanding of Cooper so that we can create ways for you to support him. If I come across something that I believe is really important for you to know, I'll be sure to tell you. Also as part of my job, I am ethically and legally responsible to break confidentiality and inform the proper authorities if I suspect abuse or neglect or if I fear he is at risk for harming himself or others. Sometimes I consult with a supervisor, as a routine practice, to make sure that I'm not missing something about a client or to brainstorm ideas. What questions do you have about any of this?"

Because many parents are uncertain or haven't yet thought about how they'll explain to their child that he or she is coming to play therapy, we initiate this conversation and give the parents some prompts or a script to use with their child. Mostly, we instruct parents to say something like the following:

> "You're going to see Terry and play with her in her playroom. Lots of kids go see her when they are [sad, mad, angry, confused, lonely, having a hard time making friends, etc.]."

You might add a sentence about it being okay to play and to talk or ask questions of the play therapist. Typically, the younger the client, the shorter the explanation. Not too many kids listen much after "you get to play with . . ." because they are already on board by the time parents say that. You can coach parents on what to say to their kid so that it doesn't sound like a punishment or feel scary. I (Terry) lend *A Child's First Book about Play Therapy* (Nemiroff & Annunziata, 1990) to parents (or teachers if the play therapy is taking place at a school) and ask them to read it with their child before the child's first session. This book gives a clear and concrete description of play therapy and clarifies certain aspects of play therapy.

There is a lot of information to give in the initial meeting. At some point in your career, you'll have this stuff memorized and rattle it off without thinking much about it. It'll be important for you to remember that, even though you have become very confident in starting play therapy sessions, most parents (and many teachers) aren't familiar with play therapy. More importantly, by the time you're meeting with these adults they are usually pretty freaked out—they are often stressed, concerned, worried, at their wit's end, full of self-doubt about their ability to be a good parent or a good teacher. Their ability to hear, digest, and remember all of the information you provide is probably a bit impaired. (Have you ever tried to study for a test while you were stressed and overwhelmed with a number of other responsibilities? How well did you remember all of the details for that test?) Because you're a caring and compassionate therapist, you could create a handout to give to parents (or teachers) with key things to remember such as appointment time and length, phone number to the office, a reminder about wearing play clothes, key statements to use with the child about coming to play therapy, and limits to confidentiality.

Each of you will want to develop your own personal style of talking to parents and teachers about what play therapy is and how the process will unfold. You will need to formulate what you talk about in that first session with parents and teachers based on how you are going to proceed in your interaction with them. As you will see in Chapter 2, the various approaches to play therapy handle working with these important adults differently. There is also a lot of information about working with parents, families, and teachers in Chapter 8.

Explaining Play Therapy to Clients

When we talk to children about play therapy, we use pretty much the same language that we suggest parents use with them. We say something like, "In here, you can play in many of the ways you want to play. You can dance, sing, tell stories, ask questions, get answers to questions, mess around in the sand—there are lots of things to do." We provide information about play therapy, what it is, and what we do in session, using developmentally appropriate language. Talking with kids about what play therapy is can feel a bit awkward at first. I (Kristin) remember not wanting children to feel as if they were in trouble, had done anything wrong, or had something wrong with them. I remember learning (or at least interpreting) that many children had limited understanding of certain concepts and might not understand what therapy entails. I would trip over my words trying to be as concrete and simple as possible, undoubtedly complicating the whole thing. After several tries, I decided to just tell the young clients something like:

> "Hi, I'm Miss Kristin, and we are going to play together. (Surely, they quit listening at this point, but I persist.) Your mom (or dad, or teacher, or grandparent, etc.) told me that your family just moved and you're missing your friends and feeling sad (or whatever the presenting problem is). She (or he) thought you'd feel better by coming to play therapy."

This is usually enough—kids accept this explanation and move forward with the process. At some point within the first few minutes of being in the room, we say something about confidentiality.

> "This is a really special place where kids come to play. I don't have to tell anyone everything that we do in here or talk about unless you want me to. Sometimes I might tell your parents (or teacher) ideas I have for them to help you at home. You can tell them anything you want about what we do in here."

We're careful to add the last part so as to not imply that we are keeping secrets. Speaking of "secrets," we avoid the word "secrets" used in this context because children who have been abused usually have been told to keep "secrets." We also tell kids, "One of my jobs is to make sure you are safe, so if you share with me that someone has hurt you, I'd have to tell people who can help." Depending on the child's response, we might ask a child to tell us in his or her own words what we've said, we might ask if he or she knows what confidentiality means, or we might ask if he or she has any questions. We want to be sure that the child understands confidentiality and its limitations.

More and more adults and adolescents are engaging in play therapy, so it behooves you (if you want to work with them) to have a way of talking about play therapy and what it is to this population too. In thinking about play therapy with adult and adolescent clients, it is important for you to remember that play therapy is not just playing with toys—though sometimes that is the perfect intervention for teens and grownups. It can include telling stories and having adventures and dancing and hearing stories and making up songs and messing around in the sand and doing art. Most of the time, in explaining play therapy to adolescents and adults, that is exactly what we tell them! We also give an elevator speech about why creative activities and play interventions are advantageous. Here's an example of an elevator explanation of why we use creative activities and play interventions with adolescent and adult clients. (Cue the elevator music . . .)

> "Play or creative expressions can tap into our unconscious and bring up memories, feelings, or ideas that we don't always access through talking through things. People are often surprised by the symbolism expressed through creative therapies and find them to be a helpful launching pad for seeing things differently and/or making changes in their lives. Because most of us learn better through doing than we can through just talking about something, play interventions can provide an active way for people to experience and explore new ways of thinking, feeling, and behaving."

We also use our own experiences to help inform our older clients of play therapy strategies that could be interesting and helpful. Here's an example of something we could say to an adult or adolescent client who might be interested in play therapy:

> "I've used play therapy activities such as creative arts or music with clients your age, and they really seemed to enjoy it. Since you described enjoying Broadway plays and listening to the soundtracks, I wonder if you'd like to try some play therapy activities. I thought it would be interesting and fun for you to come up with the title track of a Broadway musical based on your life. [You can expand this idea to include drawing pictures of the album cover, making the playbill, writing scripts, acting out scenes, etc.]"

Some adults and adolescents are ready to rock and roll—jumping right into the process. Others are a bit more reluctant to let down their hair and play. We have noticed that when we are able to suggest a broad strategy and intervention that matches their interests, we have better results. As compared to children, adults tend to worry more about doing the activity "right." So, we say (and sometimes repeat, and repeat, and repeat once again) that the goal is not to create a perfect song (or picture, clay figure, or poem), and there is no right or wrong way to complete the task. In some cases, we'll ask clients to draw or paint with their nondominant hand or to do a drawing in a minute or less to help reduce any performance anxiety, and emphasize the importance of the process rather than product.

We gave you lots and lots of information about introducing play therapy to clients. As with many things in this book, the ideas we shared are not the "only" way to introduce and explain play therapy, and our way might not even be the "best" way to do it. We suggest you practice giving explanations before you have to do it with real clients. Role-play with your family, your pet, or your friends; rehearse in your car or in front of a mirror. Having practiced verbalizing some of these things will help you to be more comfortable in session.

The First Session

When you meet a child client for the first time, you'll kneel or squat down to get on eye level, and introduce yourself.

> "Hi, Courtney. I'm Kristin, and I'm so happy to meet you. I see you wore a shirt with a kitty on it; it's got pink fluffy hair! Today, we're going to play together in the playroom. Let's go check it out together."

A couple of things we've learned along the way:

1. Do not ask questions you do not want answers to. Do not ask the child if he wants to come back to your playroom. Do not ask if she's excited or ready to go play. If you do ask those kinds of questions and the child says, "no," you'll really be in a pickle. Instead, announce that you are going to the play space together. In the event that there is resistance, you can handle that as it comes up. For example, for a child who doesn't want to leave Mom, you could invite Mom to come back for 5 minutes, or some limit of time that seems reasonable. You could also ask Mom to leave her keys with the child so the child feels connected or trusts that Mom won't leave. Sometimes we've used string to connect the parent and child. The child holds one end, the parent holds the other, while in the waiting room. (Clearly, this only works in particular settings where a string can lay on the floor between the waiting room and your office without tripping anyone or getting in the way of someone/something else.) The child or parent can tug on the string occasionally to check-in with the other person or remind the other person that he or she is still there.

2. Notice something about the child to initiate a quick connection. A quick mention of a character on the child's shirt or how his or her hair is styled (i.e., spikey Mohawk, curly pigtails, purple highlight) will do. This communicates that you notice the child and are interested in him or her. Kids who are uncertain of coming to play therapy can start to feel more confident in your ability to play and be cool.

3. Be semi-enthusiastic or theatrical in your tone of voice. We're not suggesting that you talk in baby-talk (that would be a bad idea, actually). From the perspective of children, the tone of your voice sends a message about your willingness to connect with children and separates you from other "stuffy" adults they might know.

4. You do not have to confine yourself to simply walking to the play-room. For kids who are hesitant to go with you, you can find more fun ways to get to your office (assuming it's allowed in your setting and is safe). Perhaps you skip, walk backwards, have duck tails (hands behind your back near your bum), or are soldiers. Maybe you say the alphabet backwards, sing a song, or run in slow motion (*Bay Watch* style—without the bikinis) as you go down the hall. These are also helpful tricks when you're trying to leave a playroom with children who are not keen on leaving the session. (We will get to that later in this chapter.)

Assuming you've gotten the child into your play space, you'll intro-duce the first session with a brief description of what you'll be doing. Many play therapists (including most child-centered play therapists) initi-ate the first few sessions with something like, "This is our playroom. In here, you can play with all the toys in many of the ways you'd like." Notice the intentionality of the language. Children can play with *all* of the toys in *many* of the ways they would like. They cannot play with toys any way they wish (i.e. breaking them, painting on them, taking them home, or other creative ways children might imagine playing with some of the toys that would be against the rules). Adlerian play therapists could say something like, "This is our playroom. Sometimes you'll get to decide what we play, and other times I'll get to decide what we play. Today, you can play with any of the toys in many of the ways you'd like." A play therapist who works from a cognitive-behavioral perspective might start a session by saying, "This is our playroom. In here, we'll do activities together to help you to _____." Play therapists from other theoretical orientations might not even have a playroom full of toys, and they will use a completely different introduction to the play therapy room.

We are often curious about what a child knows about play therapy and his or her reasons for coming to play therapy. So, lo and behold . . . we ask the child, "What have you been told about coming to play therapy?" Sometimes children have no idea why they are coming to play therapy. In this case, we tell them something similar to what we would tell parents to tell the child.

"Sometimes kids who feel really nervous about going to school (or whatever the client's reason is) come to play with me. We can play and talk, and we will find some ways for you to not feel so nervous. What do you think about that?"

For kids who do have an idea of why they are coming to play therapy, we usually explore how they feel or what they think of that explanation. What we really want to know is if they agree or disagree with what they've been told about coming to play therapy and if they have different ideas about it and if they have a negative belief about the reason they have been sent to work with us. If they do, we try to reframe the presenting problem and reassure them that we do not think they are a problem.

Imagine for a moment that you are a child and you enter a room filled with toys and an adult who just gave you permission to play with them. What might you think? (This is the equivalent of giving Terry free rein in a library and saying, "It's yours! It's all yours! Do as you wish!" She would probably lose her mind with excitement.)

For children in this position, there could be a flood of emotions ranging from feeling tricked, excited, uncertain, elated, nervous, cautious, happy, eager, curious, tentative, and on and on and on. (This scenario involves a playroom in which all or most of the toys are made available to the children. There are some play therapists who do not have a room filled with toys, and that will be described later.) For play therapists who have a filled playroom, we usually allow the first session to be relatively nondirective (even for those theories that would allow for directed activities) in order for children to familiarize themselves with the space and start to build a relationship with the therapist. Some children need no prompting to explore the toys and materials. Other children stand in the room like statues and feel overwhelmed with where to start. You can track the child's actions (i.e., "You're looking at all the toys in here"), reflect the child's feelings (i.e., "You're unsure of what to play with first"), or make guesses about his or her choosing to stand still and not play (i.e., "I'm guessing you're not sure what to do and you're wondering if I'm going to tell you what to do"). If you choose to be more direct, you can invite a child to play something with you, or you might give several suggestions about what the child could play. "There are so many toys, and it can be hard to decide where to start. You could play with the blocks, we could draw a picture together, or maybe you have something else in mind." Nondirective play therapists would not give the child ideas about what to do and instead would simply acknowledge what is going on with the child at that moment: "There are so many toys, and it can be hard to decide where to start."

Throughout the remainder of the first session, you'll use your play therapy skills. (See Chapter 4 for skills and ideas for how to build a relationship with clients.) As you end the first session, you can reinforce your enjoyment of working with the client and state that you're looking forward to next time. You might mention some of the things that you did during the first session and remind the client about the date of your next session, assuming the child is old enough to understand concepts of dates. Here's an example:

"Di'Metre, our time is up, and it's time to meet your dad in the waiting area. I'm happy I got to meet you today and look forward to our next time together. I noticed you really enjoyed playing with the dry erase board and dress up clothes. Next time, you could play with those again, or you can choose to do something different. I will also have an activity for you to do. I'll see you next Thursday at 4:00."

Really, we start our play therapy sessions with adolescents and adults pretty much the same way we start a play therapy session with a child client. You give the client an explanation of play therapy and why it can be helpful, you explain confidentiality and the limits of confidentiality, and you inquire about the client's perception of the presenting problem and what the client might think or believe about coming to therapy. You can also follow the guidelines of not asking questions to which you don't want the answer (so you would not say, "Are you ready to go to my office?"), you can point out something you notice about the client (e.g., his t-shirt, her purse, his haircut, etc.), and you can exude enthusiasm for meeting them and starting the play therapy experience (if you really feel that way—don't fake it if you don't because that can backfire on you). We do tend to simply walk to the play space with adults and adolescents because skipping or duck walking might also seem a bit weird to them—and we want to give the impression that play therapy is fun and age-appropriate rather than childish. It is also helpful to clarify that many of the activities we do in play therapy with this population were originally designed for working with adolescents and adults and have been adapted for use with children, rather than the other way around.

We usually tend to start our play therapy sessions with adolescents and adults by reviewing the various choices in our repertoire—we can do art, we can make sand trays, we can dance, we can play music, we can build things, we can play board games, we can do adventure techniques, and so forth. You will probably want to spend at least part of that first session exploring what interests your client in order to provide fun choices of activities that might be engaging to him or her. It is sometimes helpful to have your first session begin with an introductory bit of talk therapy, followed by giving the client a choice of several different structured play activities.

What to Do in Play Therapy Sessions

With children—play! (Sorry, we couldn't resist the obvious answer.) Seriously, as we have indicated, play is not a one-size-fits-all type of treatment. As you might have guessed, we conceptualize *play* to include telling stories and having adventures and dancing and hearing stories and making up songs and messing around in the sand and doing art and playing. The "doing" of play therapy has similarities and stark differences across play therapists' theoretical orientations, based on their beliefs about human nature and the change process. (We'll spend a considerable amount of time describing these differences in Chapter 2.) For now, it's important that you know that play has a wide range of permutations—from the play therapist never directing the play and always following the client's lead to the therapist always providing structured activities that happen in a session; from the play therapist being quite liberal in the toys allowed in the play space to the therapist having limited toys or no "toys" in the play space; and from the play therapist having no inclination to include parents (or other caring adults) in the play therapy process to the therapist being dependent on parents being willing to be active participants in the play space during sessions. Luckily for you, the rest of this book is dedicated to providing ideas about what to do in play therapy and rationales for why you would do them.

With adolescents and adults—play! The trick with adolescents and adults is getting them to buy into the idea that they can benefit from the activity and knowing how to propose they play in sessions. When you're working with older kids, teens, or adults, you can invite them to play by saying something like, "I have an activity that I'd like you to try. It's called sand tray play therapy." Then, you describe the process and gauge if the client wants to engage in the activity or play. If you're working with older clients in a "standard" playroom or a room with some toys, crafts, or other activities, you could notice where their attention is focused in the room and capitalize on their nonverbal interest, inviting them to try out a specific toy or material. For example, with a client who often gazes at the doll house, you can say, "You can rearrange the furniture if you'd like." This can get the client engaged in playing, and you can take it from there. The client who talks about memories of playing with siblings, cousins, or parents as a child could be engaged by first having discussions about the memories of play and then being invited to reenact those play experiences. Typically, older clients enjoy the process and are surprised at how the playful and creative activities can help to bring clarity to the presenting problem. In fact, many of our nonchild clients who do a play activity regularly ask to do others because they enjoyed the process and they believe it was helpful.

Regardless of how you engage them, you can do any number of activities. You can do nondirective play therapy, or you can direct the play therapy with adolescents and adults. With teenagers who tend to really enjoy doing different activities and can be most resistant to starting a creative activity, we sometimes start with more directed activities such as collages, sand trays, or drawing pictures. As they gain experience and trust the process of play therapy, we might introduce more fluid or symbolic play therapy such as drama or using clay. (In Chapters 4, 5, 6, and 7, we outline several different types of strategies and interventions to use in session that work toward different goals such as exploring clients' inter- and intrapersonal dynamics or helping the client to make changes.)

How to End a Play Therapy Session

In most approaches to play therapy, there are some common features to ending a session. When the end of the session is approaching, most play therapists say something like, "Bonita, we have 5 more minutes left in our session today." Young clients might not be able to read clocks or might be engrossed in their play and won't pay attention to the time. Either way, we want to give them warning that our time is nearing its end. Older clients are usually more attentive to time limits, so we don't usually have to give such warnings. However, if we are with an older client who is really engaged in the play process and might not be attentive to the time, it is sometimes helpful to provide the 5-minute warning to him or her as well. We also sometimes give a 1-minute warning. So, to be absolutely clear . . . we give a 5-minute *and* a 1-minute announcement that our time is nearing its end, so that clients can prepare themselves for the time to be over. It's excellent practice for clients who have a hard time transitioning (for instance, children who have a hard time going from play to bed, recess to class, or class to lunch; or adolescents or adults who have difficulty exiting from the video game they are playing). Here are some tricks of the trade:

1. Do not say "we have *about* 5 minutes," or any other tentative, wishy-washy announcement about the time ending. This is non-negotiable, people. We always want to be clear with our communication and our expectations.

2. Stick to your time limit. Not only is this a pragmatic approach, assuming you have other clients waiting, but it's practice for real life. Does your boss insist that you come to work for roughly 8 hours? Does school start around 9:00? No. We understand that clients sometimes have just a few finishing touches to complete their project and really want 2 more minutes to get it completed. However, the structure of the time is built in to help clients adapt to the time limits allowed. Clients have the choice to do the project differently, to finish it at home, to keep it in your office until the following appointment, or a slew of other options. This is why we give the time warning, so that clients can prepare. Usually after a few sessions of this happening, clients are better able to get themselves prepared to be done on time. Then, you can encourage their changed attitudes or behavior. "I remember that you used to have a hard time leaving the play session when it was time. This time, you made sure you were ready to go when it was time. Wow! That's really cool that you were able to do that."

3. You can choose to help the client prepare for ending the session with statements like

> "Remember, Knox, we have only 1 minute left. I wonder if you'll have enough time to finish playing with the clay in the way you'd like." You can do nothing or simply track the client's behavior: "You decided to get out the clay." You can decide that it is not practical for the client to play with a particular item because of the remaining time and help him or her with a different choice: "I know you'd like to use the clay, and we have only 1 minute left today. In the past, you've started activities right before the end of our session in order to stall leaving. I wonder if that's what you're thinking this time too. Since the clay will take longer than we have, what else could you do with the time remaining so that you'll be more comfortable leaving?"

You may be wondering how you decide what you do in times like this. Well, let us clear things up for you. It depends! (Ahhh . . . we kid . . . we kid. Or maybe we don't, because, well, actually it does depend.) It depends on the goals for therapy, what you know about this particular client, and what you believe is important in therapy. The degree of directedness inherent in your guiding theory will help you determine your responses.

Now for some differences between the various approaches to play therapy. Believe it or not, there is much discussion about clients cleaning the room following a play therapy session. Nondirective play therapists do not ask or expect clients to pick up their things after a session. This is rooted in a belief that cleaning up the room is symbolic for clients putting away their thoughts, feelings, and expressions. Nondirective play therapists also subscribe to the notion that if clients expect to have to clean up after a session, it may restrict what they're willing to express for not wanting to clean up a mess. If you follow this line of thinking, we recommend that you communicate this philosophy with parents (and teachers when appropriate). We can't count the number of parents who ask children if they helped pick up the play space after a session. If you don't expect clients to pick up, you don't want them to feel badly about not doing it. This could be a part of the initial discussion you have with parents.

Play therapists who are more directive may ask clients to help pick up the play space. When we say "pick up," we do not mean put everything back it its place and leave the play space in the exact way you found it. We mean contribute to the process of picking up the mess that was made during our time together. We clean up *with* children: *we* played, *we* clean up. For children who are more oppositional, we settle for small achievements like each of us picking up three items. (Of course, you'll be picking up the rest of the items when the child leaves.) Over time, we increase this to picking up the entire room together. The rationale for this practice is threefold: it makes a connection between what happens in the play space with what happens in the "real world," grounding the therapy in reality; it allows for a collaboration between clients and the play therapist so that they can deepen their relationship by cooperating with one another, policing the space they have shared; and it prevents therapist countertransference centering around having to clean up a mess created by clients who are intent on "trashing" the play space. (Believe us—it happens—we have had lots of clients who want to show us they are angry or don't have to follow the rules of the "real world" by knocking everything in the play space onto the floor and stomping on it.)

If you choose to engage in the cleaning up process with your play therapy clients, be careful to avoid getting hooked on clients returning the toys to the "right" places. You're not looking for perfection; you're looking for cooperation. We use this opportunity to encourage clients by noticing their pro-social behavior (something many kids we see don't get a lot at home or at school). "Hey Aaron, you're really being helpful today. I appreciate you picking up those toys and putting them on the shelf." With child clients, we may even rave to parents in the waiting room, in front of them, how helpful they were during time to pick up.

The Course of Treatment

The length of treatment and the number of play sessions will be determined by a number of factors, some of which can be roughly assessed prior to starting play therapy, and other factors that cannot be known until play therapy is underway. Some of the factors that influence the length of treatment are: severity of the presenting problem, support from others in clients' lives, clients' desire for things to be different, and clients' willingness and ability to engage in change. The more severe the presenting concern, the longer the treatment. The more support and the more willing clients (and family members) are to change, the quicker play therapy will be completed. (Certainly, this is a gross overgeneralization, but it is true in most situations.) Another important consideration that influences the number of sessions is the theoretical orientation used by the play therapist. Those who are more directive and base their session activities on cognitive and behavioral interventions reported the smallest number of sessions (three to twelve), and those who are more humanistic and nondirective reported a greater number of sessions (up to 100 sessions). To be most clear, this does not account for severe or complex cases, nor does it account for the longevity of play therapy treatment effects on clients. On average, and across theories, the optimal number of sessions was reported to be around thirty to thirty-four (Bratton et al., 2005; Kottman, 2011).

We recommend being clear with everyone involved that play therapy is not usually a quick treatment, nor is it a linear process. In our experience, we've found that many clients often follow a similar trajectory of change. We translate this to "sometimes things get better, then get worse, then get better again. So, don't be surprised if this happens." Adolescent and adult clients and parents (and teachers) of child clients frequently report positive results and almost magical changes immediately following the start of play therapy. We caution new clients and parents/teachers that this can be like a honeymoon period and is not likely to last more than a few weeks. We don't want clients to end therapy thinking that lasting change has been accomplished. With adolescent and adult clients, this honeymoon period may last from three to five sessions, with an expected escalation of the presenting problem after this that often lasts three or four sessions and then turns itself around. At about session three, with child clients, we notice that parents/teachers become more concerned again and may even fear that play therapy is creating problems (remember that they may be comparing this stage to the honeymoon stage, which, by comparison, seems problematic). We explain this in advance to normalize their experiences. At this point, we typically see a relatively steady improvement in the presenting concern from here on out. Once we decide that termination is the next step, we remind adolescent and adult clients and parents/teachers of child clients that the end of the relationship sometimes leads to a regression in clients' affect, cognitions, and behavior but the setback is typically temporary (about a week or two). All of this information is used to build trust and set appropriate expectations.

Termination

You begin the termination process when the client has reached the initial goal or goals of therapy. You will need to decide how you determine whether and when therapeutic goals are met. Because we frequently work with parents or teachers of child clients, we take their reports as evidence of change and readiness for them to be ready to terminate therapy. When you work with older clients such as adolescents and adults, you can use self-reports as evidence of their change. We also look for patterns in the playroom that have changed. An infinite number of changes can occur, but we'll list just a few that we see commonly. A client who was originally rather disorganized, impulsive, or inattentive becomes more intentional and focused. A client who originally played out themes of aggression and anger plays those themes much less frequently and displays more themes typical of the client's age and development. A client who was initially not able to self-regulate or follow the rules of the play space is now able to recognize triggers and make adjustments so that he or she can remain calm. These types of changes usually show us that clients are making progress and may be ready to stop play therapy. If the client is young (or an adolescent with whose parents or family members you are engaging), you will also want to consult with parents to see if they notice similar changes at home (or with teachers to see if they notice changes in the classroom).

Terminating play therapy is, in some ways, much like terminating other types of therapy. When we notice that client change is occurring, we have discussions with the client and, at times, the parents, teachers, or other adults in the client's life. We engage in conversations about the client's perceptions of change and any other goals the client (and/or adults) has for change. With child and many of our adolescent clients, we have joint sessions with the client and any significant adults involved in the process present so that everyone feels heard and understands the next steps of the process. Once it is determined that termination is nearing, we create a plan for moving toward the last session. While there is no "always" or "every time" way to terminate, we do have a few strategies we try to follow when we end a counseling relationship.

1. We start the play therapy relationship with the end in mind. Sometimes the end is not too far in the future; other times it is months and months away; and other times we have no idea how long we anticipate therapy will be necessary. Regardless, we communicate with the client or parents/teachers that, when termination comes, it is usually a semi-lengthy process and not a one-and-done type of session. We inform clients that we prefer to ease into termination because of the strong connections being built between client and play therapist and not wanting clients to feel abandoned or cut off by ending the relationship abruptly. Young children, particularly, often have a limited understanding of the nature of the therapeutic relationship and of counseling, so they might need more time to process termination. They tend to not understand that the therapy relationship is a temporary relationship and one in which the goal is to end the relationship. (Come to think of it, that is a really peculiar type of relationship, isn't it?)

2. In general, the longer we've worked with a client, the more sessions we give for the winding down process. For example, if we've worked with a client for a year or more, we might have three to five sessions of preparing to end therapy. If we've worked with a client for 2–3 months, we might have one to three sessions of preparing to end therapy.

3. The younger the client, the more time we give between introducing termination to actually concluding therapy. We would typically give more notice to a 6-year-old as compared to a 42-year-old, considering other dynamics such as length of counseling are similar.

4. We introduce the end of the relationship at the beginning of a session and count down each session thereafter. "We have four sessions left. We have today and three more sessions." At the end of this session, we'll say, "We have three more sessions together." At the beginning of the next session, "We have three sessions left. We have today and two more." We follow this type of script until termination.

5. For some clients, we start to reduce the frequency of our sessions as we near termination. We might start seeing them every other week or every third week to reduce their reliance on us and to help them practice their learned skills without weekly support.

6. It is possible to schedule follow-up sessions as a way to check in and assess the sustainability of the improvements made during therapy. Follow-up sessions could be in a month, 2 months, or any other length of time. You could do a brief follow-up call or a full-blown session. You'll determine this based on the needs of your clients and what you know about the likelihood they are going to be successful in sustaining the changes they have made in therapy.

7. We reinforce to clients that we can meet in the future if they run into other challenges. Termination (contrary to the typical use of the word) does not have to mean "forever." We give clients (even the really young ones, who can't really read) our business card with our name and number so that they will feel empowered and able to call us if they want to chat or need some support. Although the majority of our young clients never actually call us, they are happy to have a small token to take with them.

In practice, this works like the following example. Let's say I (Kristin) am working with a 7-year-old boy, termination has been agreed upon by the parent and me, and therapy will be concluded in four sessions. During the fourth to last session, I'd say:

"Grayson, I've noticed that in the past few weeks you have really improved, being able to stay calm when you are frustrated and to use your words to let people know when you need help. Your mom and your teacher have also noticed the same things. What are your thoughts? [Client shares, and we have a discussion.] Since you're doing so well, we have decided that you don't need to come in to see me every week. You and I are going to meet every other week for four more times. How does that sound to you? [More discussion.] So, we have four more play sessions together. We have today and three more. [At the conclusion of the session . . .] Our time is up for today. We will have three more sessions together. I'll see you in two weeks! [etc., etc., etc.]

During our last or one of our last sessions, we usually do some kind of a termination activity. As you've now grown accustomed to reading, not all play therapists do this type of activity. If you believe this would be important or helpful with a client, you can choose to do any number of activities. Some examples are a sand tray done independently or together to share how you feel about the client or what you've noticed about the client; a card or picture that shows what you've learned from the client; a dance party in which the two of you (or the client's entire family) celebrate the progress made by the client; a newscast, which can be recorded and given to the client, where you or the client is the anchorman (or anchorwoman) reporting on the history of the play therapy relationship or about the client's progress and future goals. You'll decide the type of intervention and the focus of the activity based on your history of interactions with the client, his or her preferred types of play, and the goals accomplished by the client.

MOVING ON . . .

We hope at this point that we have either piqued, or confirmed, your interest in play therapy. We have described some of the basic, fundamental principles of play therapy here (the who, what, where, why, and the beginnings of the how), and (hopefully) provided answers to some questions you might have had. In the following chapters, we delve a lot more into "how." We also invite and encourage you to seek out some of the references we provide throughout the chapters for you to deepen your own understanding and get other perspectives on play therapy.

Interlude 1

Show Up and Choose to Be Present

*W*e believe one of the most important things you can do in play therapy (or any other kind of therapy or any other kind of relationship, actually) is to show up and choose to be present and to be intentional with what you do. Showing up and choosing to be present with the client (Arrien, 1993) is essential for every aspect of play therapy—building a relationship, exploring the client's issues, helping the client learn to deal with issues—regardless of your theory or approach to play therapy. Showing up and choosing to be present allows you to give your complete attention to every aspect of the client and his or her behavior, communication, and energy. This means not making your grocery list as you sit with the client, not fretting about the call from your child's principal, not planning your next vacation—it really means focusing all of your energy and attention on the client and on what he or she is saying and doing in the session. By showing up and choosing to be present with the client, you convey your interest in and care for the client. The quality of the connection with the client is hugely enhanced when you choose to settle yourself in your body and to focus all of your awareness on what is happening with the client. Through choosing to be present, you let the client know that he or she is the most important person in the world to you during that session, which often increases the client's awareness of his or her worth. In choosing to be present with the client, you can also enhance your awareness of the client's subtle nonverbal reactions to the playroom and to you. Many of the client's responses to the materials in the playroom, the issues that emerge as the client plays, and the client's reactions to the comments or suggestions you make can be understated, even almost imperceptible. Choosing to be present will increase the likelihood that you can pick up on them, thus increasing the chances that you can use those responses therapeutically.

One of the main things we teach our play therapy students (well, really, all of our counseling students) in service of showing up and choosing to be present is a little thing we call (get ready for it) "Feel your butt." Now, just to clarify, this does not mean give yourself a squeeze on the posterior. It means making sure you are in your body and paying attention to where your body is right now in the physical world.

If you can actually feel your bottom . . . and use your mind to trace your body down through your hips . . . your thighs . . . your calves . . . your feet . . . your soles . . . your toes . . . down to where your feet are in solid connection to the earth—if you can feel all that, then if you can trace back up through your feet . . . your legs . . . your hips . . . your belly . . . your chest . . . your shoulders . . . down your arms . . . back up your arms . . . through your shoulders . . . your neck . . . your face . . . your skull . . . into your brain . . . and then back down again, you will really and truly be present—in this moment . . . and this moment . . . and this moment . . . and so on . . .

And if you do this at the beginning of every play therapy session, and then again in the midst of the session if you notice you are not feeling your butt, you will be present.

CHAPTER 2

Pick a Theory, Any Theory

There is nothing so practical as a good theory
—KURT LEWIN (1951, p. 169)

In this chapter, we are going to focus on the "systematic use of a theoretical model" part of the APT definition of play therapy in Chapter 1. (We hope everyone reading the book is interested, too, because we think it is important.) Not being part of the committee that developed that definition, we aren't exactly 100% sure why they included it. However, since we also think it is essential, we thought we should explain why we believe play therapists (and counselors who work with adults, teens, etc.) should have a consistent method for systematically conceptualizing clients and coming up with a "Big A agenda" (your long-term goals and objectives for your clients) and a "small a agenda" (a plan for specific sessions). We completely agree with Kevin O'Connor, co-founder of the APT, who in *Foundations of Play Therapy* (Schaefer, 2011) said that "therapists can be effective only when they consistently work from an organized theoretical framework" (p. 254). The simplest way for you to work from an organized theoretical framework (short of developing your own counseling theory, which is possible and lovely if you are willing to do the work to consider all of the following questions listed later and develop a consistent way to think about clients and their issues and how to help them) is to pick one of the established theoretical approaches to play therapy. In order to help you consider adopting a theoretical framework for your play therapy, we thought we would give you some information about how to go about exploring the various frameworks.

There are many different approaches to play therapy, some of which are based on major models of counseling and psychotherapy (i.e., Adlerian, person-centered, cognitive-behavioral, Gestalt, Jungian, narrative, and psychodynamic) and others that were developed specifically for play therapy (i.e., ecosystemic and Theraplay). We have chosen to consider Adlerian, child-centered, cognitive-behavioral, ecosystemic, Gestalt, Jungian, narrative, psychodynamic, and Theraplay because we feel comfortable enough with those approaches and their underlying philosophical assumptions to be able to explain them well enough to make a reasonable effort to give you a rounded picture of how and why their proponents believe they work. There are several other approaches to play therapy that we have not addressed: dynamic play therapy, experiential play therapy, existential play therapy, and object relations play therapy, to name a few. We didn't feel we were familiar enough with those models to be able to explain them adequately. There is another, currently popular, way to consider theory in connection with play therapy: prescriptive or integrative; we will deal with that ball of wax at the end of this chapter.

The process of finding a play therapy theory home (at least the way we believe it should be done) involves several steps. The first part of the procedure is to take the time to consider your stances/opinions on the philosophical assumptions that undergird each approach to counseling and/or play therapy and to think about your beliefs about how they work. The next step in the process is to investigate the various approaches to play therapy and decide how each of them would answer those same questions. (We know, we know—a counseling theory can't really answer questions, but we couldn't figure out another way to say it.) The third part of the quest for a theory is to look for the closest match possible between your personal beliefs, convictions, and opinions and a theoretical approach. And voila—you have picked a theory! (Cue the celebratory music!)

The first step in choosing a theory is to ponder your stance on the philosophical assumptions that underlie counseling and play therapy theories and your stance on how therapy works to help people make changes. Here are questions we think you need to consider:

1. What do you believe about the basic nature of people? Are people inherently good (positive, self-actualizing, etc.); bad (negative, irrational, evil, etc.); or neutral? Or some combination of these? If you believe people are some combination of good, bad, and neutral, how would you describe the configuration of these factors?

2. How are personalities formed/constructed?

   a. What factors influence the formation of personality?

   b. What combination of heredity/environment influences the formation of personality? Which do you believe is more important in the development of personality: nature or nurture? If you had to designate a percentage of each of them, what would you decide?

    c. In relationship to what you believe about free will and determinism in the formation of personality, do you believe that people exercise free will in the formation of their personalities, or do you believe that personal qualities are determined by outside factors without input from the person? Or some combination of free will and determinism? If you believe it is a combination, can you assign a percentage to each?

    d. What is the relationship between thinking, feeling, and behaving? Is there a linear, causal relationship between thoughts, emotions, and behavior? If so, what causes what? If not, what is the relationship between these factors?

    e. What is the basic motivation for people's behavior? What motivates people to do the things they do in their lives?

    f. What are the basic elements of a person's personality?

3. What is your stance on perception of reality—is it subjective or objective?

4. What do you believe is the role of the therapeutic relationship in counseling? Do you believe that the therapeutic relationship is necessary and *sufficient* (as in, it is the primary and only factor in clients moving toward healthy functioning)? Do you believe that the therapeutic relationship is necessary and that it serves as the foundation for helping clients through the creation of opportunities to entertain alternative perspectives, learn new coping skills, learn and practice socially appropriate behaviors, let go of destructive patterns, and so forth?

5. In counseling, do you think you need to help clients extensively explore the past, look at their current issues in the context of their past, or focus only on the here-and-now without considering anything about the past?

6. Do you believe it is important to help clients become more aware of their own motivation and patterns by helping them gain insight/become more conscious? Or do you believe clients will get better if they learn better coping skills without becoming more aware of their motivation and patterns? Or do you believe clients will get better if they experience certain conditions that activate their own self-actualizing tendencies without additional information, practice, or insight?

7. What do you believe should be the *primary* focus of counseling—creating a relationship with the client or helping the client make changes in personality, feelings, behaviors, attitudes, and/or

thoughts? If you believe it is important to help clients make changes, do you believe it is important to help clients make changes in only one of these factors or in some combination of these factors? If so, which would be the "firing order" you would prioritize?

8. How do you define psychological maladjustment?

9. What do you think should be the goals of counseling?

10. How can you tell if your clients are getting "better"? How will you judge whether or not clients are making progress?

11. Do you imagine your role as a counselor to be more directive or nondirective in your play therapy sessions?

    a. Would you prefer to create the space for the client to grow without making suggestions for in-session activities or homework (allowing the client to play without therapist intervention in play therapy)? Or are you more comfortable intervening by inviting clients to participate in structured techniques and assigning homework?

    b. How comfortable with participating in active interactions with the client [okay, what we mean is playing with them] are you? Do you believe it is never appropriate to play with the client in a session? Do you believe it is only appropriate to play with a client at the client's invitation? Do you believe it is acceptable to initiate playing with a client? If a client invites you to play something, do you think you must play even when you are not comfortable with what the client wants you to play?

12. If you are working with a child client, what is your stance on working with parents? teachers? Do you believe it is always necessary to involve parents and/or teachers? Do you believe it is not necessary to include these adults in counseling? If you believe it's necessary, to what degree do you think they should be included?

We recognize that these are difficult questions, and we want to acknowledge that there are no "right" answers—just the answers that feel right for you. We are asking you to take a stance by getting more clarity about your opinion around each of the questions. We also realize that, in many cases, we are asking you to overgeneralize by saying "people" rather than "some people." We know that there are always exceptions to the rule, and we ask that you consider the questions (which are *philosophical*, remember; not factual) seriously, talk them over with friends (and family if you want), dream about them, talk them over with your cat (if you think it would help), think about them again before you come up with your answers. Sometimes it helps to journal about them, do a sand tray or two about them, draw about them, make a collage about them—whatever works to help you ponder.

After you have answered each of the questions about your philosophical beliefs and how you believe counseling and play therapy can help people, the next step in discovering the theory with which you most closely align is to consider how each of these questions is answered by the various theoretical approaches to play therapy. We are only experts in Adlerian play therapy. We have done our best to research the answers for the other approaches, and we could have gotten them wrong. So, the ultimate method of doing this part of the quest is for you to do your own research and figure out for yourself how each approach to play therapy would answer the questions. (We know, you are probably thinking, "If I wanted to answer all this stuff for myself, I wouldn't have had to buy this book." Unless, of course, you had to buy it for a class.) Our ultimate goal is to pique your interest enough so that you will be willing to investigate further, and to help you narrow down the choices enough that it isn't completely overwhelming to seek out further depth to the two or three approaches that connect with your mind and your heart. We have provided a list of references for each of the approaches in Appendix A to give you a head start on the journey.

ADLERIAN PLAY THERAPY

In developing Adlerian play therapy, Terry used the concepts underlying Individual Psychology (a.k.a. Adlerian psychology) and combined them with the practices of play therapy. The Adlerian play therapist conceptualizes clients from an Adlerian perspective while strategically and systematically using a wide variety of directive and nondirective skills and techniques as vehicles for supporting clients' changing patterns of thinking, feeling, behaving, and interacting. For this section, we are going to give you information about the theory from Alfred Adler and contemporary Adlerians and about Adlerian play therapy from Terry and Kristin.

1. What do you believe about the basic nature of people? Good (positive, self-actualizing, etc.), bad (negative, irrational, evil, etc.), or neutral? Or some combination?

   Adlerians believe that people are basically positive and self-actualizing (Adler, 1931/1958; Ansbacher & Ansbacher, 1956; Carlson & Englar-Carlson, 2017; Maniacci, Sackett-Maniacci, & Mosak, 2014). Adlerian theory is a very optimistic approach to conceptualizing people. Adlerians believe that all people are born with the capacity to learn to connect with others (this is called "social interest" in Adlerian theory) and that parents, schools, and society must foster the full development of that connectedness in children as they grow.

2. How are personalities formed/constructed?

   a. What factors influence the formation of personality?

      Adlerians believe the members of a child's family, the personnel and peers in school, the neighbors, and society have an impact on the formation of personality. The experiences of the child's early development *and* what the child makes of those experiences all influence the establishment of the personality (Adler, 1931/1958; Carlson & Englar-Carlson, 2017: Kottman & Ashby, 2015; Kottman & Meany-Walen, 2016; Maniacci et al., 2014). Family constellation (psychological birth order) and family atmosphere (the general affective tone of the family) also influence the child's development of personality (Eckstein & Kern, 2009; Kottman & Meany-Walen, 2016).

   b. Nature/nurture?

      While Adlerians acknowledge that an element of heredity influences the formation of a person's personality in that everyone is born with a certain intellectual capacity and temperament, they tend to give more weight to nurture than to nature (Carlson & Englar-Carlson, 2017; Trippany-Simmons, Buckley, Meany-Walen, & Rush-Wilson, 2014). Over my career, I (Terry) have vacillated regarding the percentage of influence of heredity versus environment in the development of the personality. Most Adlerians would suggest the ratio would be 60% nurture with 40% nature, although some Adlerians might lean more toward 70% nurture and 30% nature.

   c. Free will or determinism?

      Adlerians are all about free will. Making choices about feelings, behavior, aspects of the personality, attitudes, and so forth is an important component of the formation of the personality and of living. One aim of Adlerian therapy is increasing clients' awareness that they always have choice. The idea that people are self-determining and creative is one of the basic premises of Adlerian therapy (Adler, 1931/1958; Carlson & Englar-Carlson, 2017; Kottman & Ashby, 2015; Kottman & Meany-Walen, 2016; Trippany-Simmons et al., 2014).

   d. Thinking, feeling, and behaving?

      Adlerians do not see the relationship between thinking, feeling, and behaving as linear or causal. It is more circular and influential. What we mean by that is that all three of these elements influence one another: thinking has an impact on feeling and behaving; feeling has an impact on thinking and behaving;

behaving has an impact on feeling and thinking. With certain people, one might have a bigger influence than the other two, and they are all interconnected in everyone.

e. Basic motivation for behavior?

According to Adler and other Adlerian theorists, there are several basic motivations for behavior. One motivation is to increase a sense of belonging and connection—all people are born with a need to find a place of belonging in the world, and they work to figure out how to find a way to gain significance within their family and with peers. They also strive to overcome the feelings of inferiority that haunt everyone stemming from childhood experiences in which they perceive they are "less than" others because they are not as competent as the older, more well-developed people in their world (Ansbacher & Ansbacher, 1956; Kottman & Heston, 2012; Mosak & Maniacci, 2010).

f. Basic elements of personality?

In thinking about personality, Adlerians consider clients' assets; functioning at life tasks (work, love/family, friendship, spirituality/meaning of existence, and self) (Mosak & Maniacci, 1999); goals of misbehavior (gaining attention, power, revenge, and proving inadequacy) (Dreikurs & Soltz, 1964); the Crucial Cs (courage, capable, connect, and count) (Lew & Bettner, 1998, 2000); and personality priorities (pleasing, comfort, superiority, and control) (Kfir, 1989, 2011). They use all of these elements when conceptualizing clients and developing treatment plans (Kottman & Meany-Walen, 2016; Maniacci et al., 2014).

3. Perception of reality—subjective or objective?

Adlerian theory is based on a phenomenological perspective, which lends itself to the idea that people make life choices based on their subjective interpretation of events, rather than on the facts of the experience (Adler, 1927/1954; Eckstein & Kern, 2009; Maniacci et al., 2014). Adlerians believe that reality is perceived subjectively and that what people make of what happens in their lives is more important than what actually happens.

4. Role of the therapeutic relationship?

Adlerians believe that, while it is helpful to have the right conditions to grow, children need to have others (sometimes professionals, like counselors and teachers, and sometimes other influential people like parents, grandparents, neighbors, and other important adults) provide active interventions in the form of information, guidance, structure, insight, alternative perspective, skills teaching practice, and so forth (Ansbacher & Ansbacher, 1956; Carlson & Englar-Carlson, 2017; Corey, 2017; Kottman & Meany-Walen, 2016; Maniacci et al., 2014). The relationship serves as the foundation for everything else that follows in the therapeutic process: exploring the client's lifestyle; helping the client gain insight into her or his lifestyle; and reorienting/reeducating the client by helping the client generate alternative, appropriate behavior; teaching skills (such as relationship skills, communication skills, self-regulation, problem solving, and so forth); and providing opportunities to practice skills. In Adlerian counseling (and play therapy), the relationship is a collaborative partnership in which the therapist and client share power and responsibility.

5. Focus on the past, the present in the context of the past, or only the present?

Adlerians believe it is important to explore clients' interpretation of situations and relationships from early childhood because the conclusions to which they came when they were very young inform how they see self, others, and the world (lifestyle). When an Adlerian play therapist explores the past, often using early recollections with clients 8 years old and up, it is always in service of helping clients understand what is happening in their thinking, feeling, and behaving in the here-and-now (Kottman & Meany-Walen, 2016; Maniacci et al., 2014; Watts, 2013).

6. Need insight/increased consciousness to make changes?

In Adlerian counseling, gaining insight is one of the key components of change (Carlson & Englar-Carlson, 2017; Eckstein & Kern, 2009; Watts, 2013). (It even has its own phase of the counseling/play therapy process.) Adlerians believe that it is important for clients to gain a sense of the patterns in their thinking, feeling, and behaving in order to change those patterns that are no longer working. As a vehicle for making shifts in their lifestyles, the aim is to help clients gain insight into their relationships, their problem-solving skills, their basic convictions about self, others, and the world, and how their behavior flows from those convictions. In play therapy, the counselor remains aware that clients' developmental level will determine the complexity and level of the insight that is possible (Kottman & Meany-Walen, 2016).

7. Primary focus in counseling?

While the relationship is foundational, Adlerians are always moving toward helping people make changes in how they are living their lives. The four phases in Adlerian therapy move through building a relationship with clients; exploring clients' lifestyles; helping clients gain insight into their lifestyles; and helping them make changes in thinking, feeling, and behaving. Shifts in thoughts, emotions, and behavior are all important, though the firing order changes from client to client, depending on their issues and underlying intrapersonal and interpersonal dynamics (Kottman & Meany-Walen, 2016; Maniacci et al., 2014). (In other words, "it depends.")

8. Psychological maladjustment?

Adlerians see maladjustment as discouragement (Corey, 2017). Discouraged clients are "acting as if" their self-defeating mistaken beliefs about self, others, and the world are true. They are stuck in feelings of inferiority—either giving up trying to feel better about themselves or overcompensating behaving in arrogant, socially useless ways.

9. Goals of counseling?

The general goals of Adlerian counseling are: fostering an increased sense of belonging and significance; helping clients learn to deal with feelings of discouragement and inferiority in healthier ways; assisting clients in changing their self-defeating beliefs, attitudes, and behaviors to more positive ones; helping clients gain a sense of equality with others; and helping people begin to make positive contributions to society and other people (Carlson & Englar-Carlson, 2017; Corey, 2017; Maniacci et al., 2014). For specific clients, the goals will depend on the presenting problem and the underlying dynamics of clients' interpersonal and intrapersonal struggles. (In other words, again "it depends.")

10. Measuring progress?

In Adlerian therapy, measuring progress depends on the goals of therapy and is measured by tracking whether clients are experiencing movement toward achieving these goals. When clients have developed more positive ways of belonging and gaining significance in their families, peer groups, and work/school; when they demonstrate adaptive ways of coping with feelings of discouragement and dealing with feelings of inferiority; when they manifest a shift from self-defeating attitudes, beliefs, and behaviors to more adaptive, prosocial ones; when clients begin to move away from feeling less than others toward feeling equal to others; and when they start positively contributing in their relationships with other people, the counselor can assume they are making progress. With individual clients, measuring progress again reflects what the counselor is working on with them, their parents, and/or their teachers.

11. Directive or nondirective?

   Both at different times and with different clients—it depends. . . .
Depending on the phase of therapy, the Adlerian play therapist might
be more or less directive. Depending on the presenting problem and
the personality of the client, they also adjust the level of directiveness
in sessions in order to best meet the needs of the client.

   a. Creating space or using structured techniques in play therapy?

      Adlerian play therapists combine nondirective interaction
   with directive intervention, depending on the phase of counseling
   and the needs of specific clients (Kottman & Meany-Walen, 2016).
   In the first phase of counseling, Adlerians might use a few directive techniques to build the relationship with clients, but they are
   usually more nondirective during that phase, though they do tell
   clients, "In here, sometimes you get to be the boss and sometimes
   I get to be the boss." During the second phase, they use observation of the client combined with questioning strategies and strategically planned activities to explore clients' lifestyles. The third
   phase unfolds with the counselor using intervention techniques
   along with metaphors and metacommunication to help clients gain
   insight. The fourth phase is the most directive phase in the process,
   with the counselor providing structured activities and assigning
   homework as a way to teach skills and help reorient and reeducate
   clients. There are some clients who are more amenable to directive
   techniques than other clients, so Adlerian play therapists tailor the
   degree of directiveness to the needs of clients. To be theoretically
   consistent, it is important to note that Adlerians cannot choose to
   be strictly nondirective in play therapy because it is impossible to
   teach, which is the primary intervention tool in the fourth phase,
   without being directive.

   b. Playing with the client in play therapy?

      In Adlerian play therapy, the therapist does play with the
   child—sometimes at the child's invitation and sometimes at the
   therapist's initiative. While we often wait to be invited by the child
   to play, we also may suggest and participate in play activities specifically designed to explore lifestyle, help the child gain insight, or
   teach or practice a skill.

12. Work with parents? teachers?

   In Adlerian play therapy, the therapist collaborates with the parents and, if the child is struggling in school, with the child's teacher.
One of the most distinctive features of Adlerian play therapy is the
strong emphasis on working directly with the important adults in

child clients' lives. The process of parent and/or teacher consultation is an essential, integral part of Adlerian play therapy. The consultation with parents and/or teachers follows the same progression as play therapy with clients. Adlerian play therapists also work with families in family play therapy and groups of school children with their teachers, when appropriate.

CHILD-CENTERED PLAY THERAPY (PERSON-CENTERED THERAPY AND THEORY)

Child-centered play therapy is based on person-centered therapy and person-centered theory (Axline, 1969; Landreth, 2012; Ray, 2011; Rogers, 1961). In this section, we are giving you information about the basic theory from Rogers and his work and information about the application to play therapy from historical and contemporary experts in child-centered play therapy like Virginia Axline, Garry Landreth, Dee Ray, and Rise VanFleet. Child-centered play therapy is based on the premise that the non-directive therapeutic relationship established in play therapy is necessary and sufficient to activate clients' self-actualizing tendency without any active or directive intervention from the therapist.

1. What do you believe about the basic nature of people? Good (positive, self-actualizing, etc.), bad (negative, irrational, evil, etc.), or neutral? Or some combination?

   Person-centered theory is optimistic. Person-centered therapists believe that people are born basically good; people are essentially positive and have an innate self-actualizing tendency (Corey, 2017; Raskin, Rogers, & Witty, 2014; Ray, 2011). "Rogers believed that at the core, humans tend toward development, individuality, and cooperative relationships" (Fall, Holden, & Marquis, 2010, p. 174).

2. How are personalities formed/constructed?

   a. What factors influence the formation of personality?

      According to person-centered therapy, when children are born, they use "organismic valuing" (their awareness of their sensory and visceral experiencing of their environment) to determine whether or not things are good for them (Fall et al., 2010; Raskin et al., 2014; Rogers, 1961). Children develop their original self-concept ("real self") based on this organismic valuing. As time passes, they get feedback from others in their environment, mostly from their primary caretaker, and they interpret the meaning of that feedback. Based on their perceptions of this feedback, they develop "conditions of worth," ideas about who they should be and how they should act in order to be worthy of acceptance and love. As this happens, children pay less attention to their organismic valuing and begin to give more weight to conditions of worth. While not all conditions of worth are in the conscious awareness of people, they constitute their "ideal self"—the self that all people are striving toward.

b. Nature/nurture?

Children are born with a tendency to self-actualize and with organismic valuing—these factors constitute the contribution of nature to the development of personality. The impact of the nurture component of development is determined primarily by the ability of parents and other caretakers to provide consistent unconditional positive regard to children (Fall et al., 2010). From our reading of person-centered theory, we believe the split between nature and nurture is 50/50. (We also spent an inordinate time discussing what we thought about this.)

c. Free will or determinism?

Rogers believed that free will was more important than determinism in the formation of personality. He believed that people were always making decisions about their lives and how they want to live. Sometimes these decisions are influenced by the judgments of other people that are introjected in the form of conditions of worth, which adds a small element of determinism in the formation of personality (Corey, 2017). It is also important to remember that conditions of worth are based on people's subjective interpretation of the input they get from other people and their environment. Our estimate of the percentages of free will/determinism on the evolution of the personality would be 80% free will/20% determinism.

d. Thinking, feeling, and behaving?

"The person is all that a child is: thoughts, behaviors, feelings, and physical being" (Sweeney & Landreth, 2009, p. 124). The relationship among thinking, feeling, and behaving was never a central focus in person-centered theory. According to Fall et al. (2010), thinking comes first, with children conceptualizing their needs and how to get them met. This is filtered through the organismic valuing in babies and then through conditions of worth as children get older. Feeling and behaving evolve from this process. (This has caused us some degree of cognitive dissonance since the therapy based on person-centered theory centers on reflection of feelings, and we always thought this meant that feelings caused thinking and behaving. We couldn't find any information that supported this idea though.)

e. Basic motivation for behavior?

The motivation for behavior according to Rogers (1951) is an attempt to satisfy the needs of the organism as they are experienced in the perceived field of life. Individuals are also trying to move toward their ideal self as a way to satisfy their conditions of worth (Raskin et al., 2010; Sweeney & Landreth, 2009).

f. Basic elements of personality?

Although Rogers (1951, 1961) did not divide the personality into components, the factors involved in the personality were the organismic valuing and conditions of worth, which form the basis of the real self and the ideal self.

3. Perception of reality—subjective or objective?

Rogers believed that human beings filter their experience of reality through their organismic valuing and their conditions of worth (Raskin et al., 2010; Ray & Landreth, 2015). He was so firmly convinced that individuals perceive reality subjectively that he even coined a word, "subceive," which is a conglomerate of subjectively and perceive. Clients' perception of their experience is their "reality," so it is essential for the child-centered play therapist to strive to understand clients' worlds from their perspective.

4. Role of therapeutic relationship?

"The relationship is the therapy; it is not the preparation for therapy or behavioral change" (Landreth, 2012, p. 82). Rogers outlined six core conditions for therapy to occur. The therapist and the client are in psychological contact, the client experiences incongruence, the therapist is congruent in the relationship, the therapist experiences unconditional positive regard for the client, the therapist experiences for and communicates empathy to the client, and the client perceives the therapist's unconditional positive regard and empathy (D. Ray, personal communication, January 13, 2018; Rogers, 1951). According to person-centered theory, clients' self-actualizing tendency leads them to grow in a positive direction if they experience unconditional positive regard, genuineness, and empathy (Fall et al., 2010; Rankin et al., 2014; Ray, 2011; VanFleet, Sywaluk, & Sniscak, 2010). In this theory, all six of these conditions are *necessary* and *sufficient* for change to occur. Genuineness, unconditional positive regard, and empathic understanding are often referred to as the "core conditions." In other words, if the child's parents, teachers, grandparents, play therapist (or other significant people in the child's life) provide the core conditions, the child will grow in a positive direction. Directive intervention is not necessary for change in a person-centered approach.

5. Focus on the past, the present in the context of the past, or only the present?

In person-centered counseling and child-centered play therapy, the therapist's attention is almost exclusively on the present, not the past (or even the future).

6. Need insight/increased consciousness to make changes?

In person-centered therapy and child-centered play therapy, increasing consciousness is not a direct goal of therapy. Rogers believed that clients' self-awareness grows as they experience the three core conditions. However, most child-centered play therapists do not feel the need to use structured directive activities expressly designed to increase consciousness (Landreth, 2012; Ray, 2011; VanFleet et al., 2010). They may, however, use some version of "soft" interpretation to help clients become more aware of their patterns.

7. Primary focus in counseling?

In person-centered counseling and child-centered play therapy, the primary focus is the relationship between the therapist and the client. As we have stated, child-centered play therapists believe that if they can create the three core conditions in therapy, the client's self-actualizing tendency will be activated and he or she will move toward healthy functioning.

8. Psychological maladjustment?

According to person-centered theory and child-centered play therapy, psychological maladjustment is the incongruence between the real self and the ideal self. The more incongruence between these two selves, the less well-adjusted the person is.

9. Goals of counseling?

The overarching goal of person-centered counseling is to create an environment in which there is psychological contact between the client and the counselor (Fall et al., 2010). Through this process, clients' actualizing tendency is activated, and they move toward greater self-acceptance and healthy functioning. Landreth (2012) suggested that when play therapists develop a relationship with clients that conveys unconditional positive regard, empathy, and genuineness, clients develop more positive self-concepts and internal locus of evaluation; assume greater responsibility; become more self-directing, self-accepting, self-reliant, and self-trusting; engage in self-determined decision making; and experience a greater sense of control in their lives.

10. Measuring progress?

In order to measure progress in person-centered therapy and child-centered play therapy, you would look for a reduction in anxiety, confusion, defensiveness, and other self-defeating emotions (Fall et al., 2010). It would be indicative of progress if clients demonstrated a more positive self-concept; an internal locus of evaluation; greater responsibility; more self-direction, self-acceptance, self-reliance, and self-trust; self-determined decision making; and a greater sense of control in their lives. In play therapy, the therapist would use observation of the child's behavior, the child's self-report, and reports from parents, teachers, and other significant adults to assess progress.

11. Directive or nondirective?

Child-centered play therapy is nondirective (Yasenik & Gardner, 2012).

a. Creating space or using structured techniques in play therapy?

Child-centered play therapists seldom, if ever, use structured or directive techniques in play therapy.

b. Playing with the client in play therapy?

Most child-centered play therapists rarely play with clients in sessions. If they do, they would assiduously avoid leading the client, relying on the client to initiate interactions and to take the lead in the play.

12. Work with parents? teachers?

Landreth (2012) and Ray and Landreth (2015) suggested that parents are important partners in the play therapy process. Because they are the most significant people in children's lives, it is essential that they feel accepted, understood, and safe with the play therapist. Every three to five sessions, many child-centered play therapists conduct consultation sessions with parents, providing support, teaching skills, imparting knowledge, and monitoring parental perceptions of children's progress. Some child-centered play therapists also consult with teachers. The other primary method for working with parents in this approach is filial therapy (Guerney, 2013; VanFleet, 2013). In filial therapy, the play therapist teaches parents basic play therapy skills and helps them learn to apply them in special play times with their children. Landreth and Bratton (2006) have a ten-session model of filial therapy called Child–Parent Relationship Therapy, and this model has been adapted for use with teachers. Although most child-centered play therapists believe that parental and teacher involvement is helpful, most do not believe it is required for play therapy to be effective.

COGNITIVE-BEHAVIORAL PLAY THERAPY

Cognitive-behavioral play therapy was developed by Susan Knell (1993, 2009). It is based on cognitive-behavioral theory and therapy, which was pioneered by Donald Meichenbaum (1986) and Albert Ellis (2000). In this section, we give you information about the basic theory as formulated by Meichenbaum and Ellis and information about the application to play therapy from historical and contemporary experts in cognitive-behavioral play therapy like Susan Knell and Angela Cavett. Cognitive-behavioral play therapists use interventions derived from the cognitive and behavioral schools of psychology related to how thinking and behaving form and how they can be altered with clients whose patterns are dysfunctional. It was difficult to answer some of these questions about the theory because, as Knell (2009) pointed out "there is no personality theory, per se, that underlies cognitive-behavioral theory" (p. 203). The focus in this approach has been on psychopathology rather than on personality development.

1. What do you believe about the basic nature of people? Good (positive, self-actualizing, etc.), bad (negative, irrational, evil, etc.), or neutral? Or some combination?

    According to cognitive-behavioral theory, people have the potential to be rational or irrational (Corey, 2017), which, because cognitive behaviorists believe that thinking constitutes the most important aspect of people's personalities, means that most therapists who subscribe to this approach tend to believe that the basic nature of people is both positive and negative. The positive slant can be attributed to the potential for individuals to be rational and behave accordingly; the negative slant derives from a tendency to think crookedly, emote inappropriately, and behave in self-defeating ways (Ellis, 2000; Fall et al., 2010).

2. How are personalities formed/constructed?

    a. What factors influence the formation of personality?

        Because the emphasis in cognitive-behavioral theory is on thinking, in this approach, the most important factor that influences the formation of personality is the development of the patterns of thinking (either rational or irrational) (Knell, 2009). While those patterns may begin with the cognitive patterns modeled by parents, people quickly become responsible for perpetuating them.

    b. Nature/nurture?

        Cognitive-behavioral therapists believe people are born with a potential for being rational or irrational and a predisposition toward happiness, love, communion with others, and growth (Corey, 2017).

As time passes, though, many people move toward the "dark side" of irrationality. Initially, individuals learn their irrational beliefs from their parents and other people in their environments. As folks grow older, they themselves repeat those early irrational thoughts until they become incorporated into their patterns of beliefs and influence their behaviors. If we had to give you a ratio of nature/nurture, we would estimate nature 20%/nurture 80%.

c. Free will or determinism?

According to cognitive-behavioral therapy, people always have a choice in how they interpret the events that happen, and it is that interpretation that determines how they react to those events. Ellis (2000) suggested that individuals always have a choice about how they think, feel, and behave; this clearly leads to the idea that in this theory, free will would be 100% with not a smidgen of determinism.

d. Thinking, feeling, and behaving?

In cognitive-behavioral theory and all of the different "flavors" of cognitive-behavioral therapy, there is a linear causal relationship between thinking, feeling, and behaving, with thinking leading to feeling and behaving (Knell, 2009).

e. Basic motivation for behavior?

For cognitive-behavioral therapists, the basic motivation for behavior is survival and pleasure (Fall et al., 2010). Behavior is designed to maximize survival and pleasure.

f. Basic elements of personality?

Because there really isn't a theory of personality in cognitive-behavioral theory, practitioners of this approach do not posit elements of personality.

3. Perception of reality—subjective or objective?

For cognitive-behavioral therapists, perception of reality is always subjective. Individuals filter their experiences through their perceptions and beliefs. Those perceptions and beliefs are much more important in this approach than the actual experience.

4. Role of therapeutic relationship?

The role of the therapeutic relationship varies depending on the brand of cognitive-behavioral therapy you practice. According to Ellis (2000), people do not need to be accepted or loved, so they don't need a therapist to care about them or convey positive regard. Burns (1999) and Beck (1976) both suggested that the relationship needs to be warm, empathic, and genuine. (You might recognize these as the three core conditions; however, while these experts believe they are necessary, in cognitive-behavioral therapy they are not sufficient.) Knell (2009) and Cavett (2015) would agree that the cognitive-behavioral play therapist must build a relationship that is based on positive regard, empathy, and genuineness; however, this relationship is not sufficient to lead to change.

5. Focus on the past, the present in the context of the past, or only the present?

In cognitive-behavioral therapy and play therapy, the focus is solely on the present. Therapists who subscribe to this approach do not believe that examining clients' past is productive.

6. Need insight/increased consciousness to make changes?

Insight in cognitive-behavioral therapy and play therapy is defined as an increased awareness of irrational beliefs and a willingness to shift to more rational beliefs (Corey, 2017). This is absolutely essential for change in this approach.

7. Primary focus in counseling?

This is a little tricky because in cognitive-behavioral therapy with adults, the primary focus is on helping clients change their pattern of thinking (Corey, 2017; Fall et al., 2010). In cognitive-behavioral play therapy, the focus is on feelings, thoughts, and behaviors as well as on the environment (Cavett, 2015). Cognitive-behavioral play therapy is problem-focused and goal-oriented. Goals are based on changing thinking and behaving in order to help reduce symptoms, and on improving functioning. If you were a cognitive-behavioral play therapist, you would work with clients using play to help them "identify and modify potentially maladaptive beliefs" (Knell, 1993, p. 170) and use play combined with behavior strategies to address the "issues of control, mastery, and responsibility for their own behavior change" (Knell, 1993, p. 70).

8. Psychological maladjustment?

For the cognitive-behavioral therapist, maladjustment is an exaggerated and persistent inappropriate response to stimuli based on faulty reasoning (Fall et al., 2010). When working with children, cognitive-behavioral play therapists look at inappropriate behaviors at home and school and dysfunctional patterns of feeling and thinking.

9. Goals of counseling?

The goals of counseling in cognitive-behavioral therapy are to help clients make shifts in their patterns of thinking, reduce negative ideation, and weaken the tendency toward irrational thoughts, which can lead to changes in emotions and behaviors (Knell, 2009). Knell

(1994, 2009) also suggested that in cognitive-behavioral play therapy it is important to work with children on changing their behavior, using behavioral techniques such as modeling. Another goal in this approach is to help clients learn to better understand and modulate their emotions, learn new and more appropriate behaviors, and develop the habit of reasonable thinking (Cavett, 2015). Play therapists, in conjunction with parents (and/or clients), develop individualized treatment plans with the end goal of teaching skills that are transferable to other relationships and settings outside the therapy room (resulting in doing themselves out of a job when it works).

10. Measuring progress?

In cognitive-behavioral play therapy, the therapist uses observation, reports from parents and teachers, and (sometimes) formal assessments to determine whether clients are moving toward their goals.

11. Directive or nondirective?

Cognitive-behavioral play therapy is usually directive, with the therapist using activities to actively teach clients new ways of thinking, feeling, and behaving and providing opportunities for clients to practice the more adaptive strategies for dealing with problems.

a. Creating space or using structured techniques in play therapy?

Cognitive-behavioral play therapists use many structured strategies, such as role-playing, modeling, imagery, journaling, relaxation, psychoeducation, systematic desensitization, development of trauma narratives, and bibliotherapy, as part of the play therapy process (Cavett, 2015; Knell, 2009).

b. Playing with the client in play therapy?

In cognitive-behavioral play therapy, the play therapist does indeed play with the client, at both the client's and the therapist's initiative. The play can be directed by the client or the therapist.

12. Work with parents? teachers?

Working with parents and teachers is usually part of cognitive-behavioral play therapy (Knell, 2009). In the first part of the process of therapy with a child client, the therapist interviews parents to obtain information about the child, the presenting problem, the child's development, and parenting strategies. As the therapeutic process proceeds, the play therapist may conduct consultation sessions in which he or she helps parents learn to modify their interactions with the child, provides support to them for reinforcing what the child is doing in therapy, and provides information to them about child development and the presenting problem.

ECOSYSTEMIC PLAY THERAPY

Ecosystemic play therapy was developed by Keven O'Connor (1993, 2000, 2009, 2011, 2016). It is not based on any one personality theory. "Ecosystemic play therapy does not presume that any one theoretical model is necessarily better than another. Therapists can be effective working from a psychodynamic, cognitive-behavioral, family system, or other theory as long as they use the theory consistently" (O'Connor, 2011, p. 254). Because of this factor, it was sometimes difficult to answer some of these questions.

1. What do you believe about the basic nature of people? Good (positive, self-actualizing, etc.), bad (negative, irrational, evil, etc.), or neutral? Or some combination?

    O'Connor (2009, 2011) suggested that, according to ecosystemic play therapy, people are basically neutral. Depending on the circumstances of their lives, they can develop in positive ways or negative ways.

2. How are personalities formed/constructed?

    a. What factors influence the formation of personality?

    O'Connor (2000, 2009, 2011) defines personality as the "sum of intra- and interpersonal characteristics, attributes, cognitions, beliefs, values, and so forth that make a person unique" (O'Connor, 2000, p. 90). He believes that the degree to which children's needs are met by the primary caretaker through the connection of attachment and the child's experiences in the world in which they live (the "ecosystems") are the most important influences on the development of personality. "The ecosystemic therapist views the child as being embedded in a series of nested systems, including family, school, peer, culture, legal, medical, and others" (O'Connor, 1993, p. 245). All of these systems may have an influence on the development of an individual's personality.

    b. Nature/nurture?

    In ecosystemic play therapy, the belief is that all people are born with a biological need to survive and avoid punishment. This belief is modified for a young child through socialization, first by getting his or her needs met by primary caretakers. The interactions with caretakers shape the child's expectations of how others will react to him or her. Later in life, the child learns that his or her needs can be met by working cooperatively with others. Based on our reading of O'Connor (1993, 2000, 2009, 2011), we would estimate the ratio of nature to nurture in this approach to play therapy is 30% nature and 70% nurture.

c. Free will or determinism?

Free will is extremely important in ecosystemic play therapy. All people have choices in their reaction to their circumstances. Their experiences and interactions with other people influence, but do not determine, the choices they make and the path they take through life.

d. Thinking, feeling, and behaving?

In ecosystemic terms, thinking influences feeling, behaving, and interpersonal relating. While O'Connor (2009) would pay attention to feeling and behaving, he puts cognitive functioning in a central role. He believes advances in cognitive development drive development in other areas. Ecosystemic play therapists use play interventions to work first on changing cognitive processes, followed by using the therapeutic power of play to shift clients' emotional processes and their interpersonal processes (O'Connor, 2011).

e. Basic motivation for behavior?

The basic motivation for behavior, according to ecosystemic play therapy, is getting needs met and avoiding punishment and pain (O'Connor, 2000, 2009, 2011).

f. Basic components of personality?

O'Connor (2000) incorporated many different theories of personality into his "personal theory," including psychoanalytic, humanistic, Theraplay, developmental therapy, and reality therapy (Kottman, 2011; O'Connor, 2000). Because he believes that each practitioner must develop his or her own personal theory of personality to explain the basic components of personality, the answer to this question would depend on which theory you choose to be the foundation of your work with clients.

3. Perception of reality—subjective or objective?

Ecosystemic play therapy is grounded in phenomenology, a philosophy that suggests that there are no absolutes, that all perceptions are subjective (O'Connor, 2000, 2009, 2011, 2016). This means the play therapist must give credence to all information gathered in the play therapy process and strive to understand each person in the context of the systems in which they live. (In other words, we filter everything through our own world view—no one's world view is better or more accurate than that of everyone else.)

4. Role of therapeutic relationship?

O'Connor (2011, 2016) acknowledged the importance of the therapeutic relationship as a vehicle for helping clients engage in problem solving, which ultimately leads to behavior changes and getting needs met in socially appropriate ways. However, he does not think the relationship is sufficient, in and of itself, to create the changes needed by the client.

Even before the work in the playroom begins in ecosystemic play therapy, an extensive assessment process takes place designed to investigate the presenting problem from the perspective of the client and the important people in the client's life; gather information about the developmental history of the client and the family; explore the client's past and present functioning in the various systems of the client's life; and examine the sociocultural and metasystemic influences that affect the client's experiences and functioning (Carmichael, 2006; O'Connor & Ammen, 1997). This process is facilitated by an interview with caretakers (obviously if you are working with an adult, which is rare in ecosystemic play therapy, you wouldn't do that part . . .), an interview with the client, an interview with the family, and standardized testing with the client using instruments designed to gather information about intelligence, personality, development, attention, and behavior. The therapist might also use projective instruments to measure the client's attitude and skills in interpersonal relationships and aspects of his or her intrapersonal dynamics. Based on the results of this assessment procedure, the therapist begins the establishment of the therapeutic relationship by meeting with caretakers (when there are some) and the client separately to develop a specific and explicit treatment contract (O'Connor, 2016). (Semi-obviously, if you practice in a state in which only psychologists are allowed to do this kind of assessment and you want to do ecosystemic play therapy, you will have to refer the client to a psychologist for the testing part and start building the relationship after reading the psychological evaluation.)

5. Focus on the past, the present in the context of the past, or only the present?

As you can see from the answer to Question 4, in ecosystemic play therapy, the past and the present are important, with the past providing clues for functioning in the here-and-now.

6. Need insight/increased consciousness to make changes?

(The answer to this question is, "It depends.") In some cases, ecosystemic play therapists believe it is important with certain clients to help them become more aware of their own motivation and patterns by using interpretation and feedback. For example, with a client who always says yes to other people even when she doesn't want to, it would be helpful to use interpretation and feedback to suggest to her that this is not an optimal way to get her needs met. With other clients, ecosystemic play therapists believe clients will get better if they learn better coping skills without becoming more aware of their motivation and patterns (O'Connor, 2009). For example, when working with a client who is afraid there are monsters under his bed, giving him a can of "Monster Repellent" can be adequate to help him alleviate this fear without any feedback or interpretation.

7. Primary focus in counseling?

The primary focus in ecosystemic play therapy is on helping the client maximize his or her ability to get his or her needs met effectively without interfering with the ability of others to get their needs met.

8. Psychological maladjustment?

Clients with psychological maladjustment (according to ecosystemic play therapy) manifest one or more of three factors: (a) they are unable to get their needs met without interfering with the rights of others; (b) they suffer from factors such as severe medical conditions, developmental delays, or mental health issues; and/or (c) they are "embedded in problematic systems or interpersonal relationships" (O'Connor, 2011, p. 260).

9. Goals of counseling?

The overarching goals of ecosystemic play therapy are to help clients learn to get their needs met without interfering with others' ability to get their needs met, to enhance attachment relationships, and to develop resources for reducing psychopathology and coping with interpersonal problems. Another goal is to bring clients' cognitive, emotional, and interpersonal developmental levels to their chronological age as close as possible, ensuring that the levels of these domains are relatively equal (O'Connor, 2011). Because each client's individualized goals are discussed in the preliminary session, there are also specific concrete goals for every client, related to making progress in the areas of cognitive, emotional, and interpersonal processes.

10. Measuring progress?

Measuring client progress in ecosystemic play therapy flows from the goals of the therapy. So, one level of tracking client progress monitors clients' general goals related to learning to get needs met without interfering with others' ability to get their needs met, enhancing attachment relationships, developing resources for reducing psychopathology and coping with interpersonal problems, and increasing and equalizing functioning in the areas of cognition, emotion, and interpersonal relationships. The other level of tracking checks in with individual clients to make sure they are moving toward attaining their personalized goals. Like practitioners of most approaches to play therapy, ecosystemic play therapists have several different ways of measuring progress: observation of client behavior in sessions, self-report from clients, and reports from parents and other adults for child clients. There is, perhaps, a stronger emphasis on client self-report in ecosystemic play therapy than there would be in other approaches because clients are more involved in setting treatment goals than they are in other approaches. In ecosystemic play, the therapist may also retest clients using psychometric instruments or may refer clients for retesting if they did not do the initial testing themselves.

11. Directive or nondirective?

Ecosystemic play therapy is directive and therapist-driven. It is actually the most directive approach to play therapy other than Theraplay.

a. Creating space or using structured techniques in play therapy?

Ecosystemic play therapists have an empty playroom, with a closet containing toys and other materials outside the room. At the beginning of the session, the therapist brings whatever materials into the playroom that he or she is going to use to work with the client on particular goals. Because each session is filled with activities designed specifically to help clients achieve their goals, the therapist plans all activities. At the beginning of a session, the therapist explains the activities they are going to do together that day (and sometimes, depending on clients' ability to understand, explains how the particular activities planned for that session will help clients move toward their goals).

b. Playing with the client in play therapy?

Since the activities are therapist-directed, the therapist usually participates in the experiences with the client. Obviously, this depends on the type of activity planned for the session, and overall, ecosystemic play therapists believe in playing with clients.

12. Work with parents? teachers?

Ecosystemic play therapists work with both parents and teachers; after all, these adults are important influences in the ecosystem of the child (or adolescent).

GESTALT PLAY THERAPY

Violet Oaklander (1992, 1993, 2003, 2011, 2015) developed Gestalt play therapy based on the work of Fritz and Laura Perls in Gestalt therapy. Oaklander described Gestalt therapy as a "humanistic, process-oriented form of therapy that is concerned with aspects of the person: senses, body, feelings, and the intellect" (Oaklander, 1993, p. 281). She believed that clients need to develop a sense of themselves that is differentiated from others and that the play therapist teaches clients how to set boundaries between themselves and others and how to recognize, define, and cultivate their own processes.

1. What do you believe about the basic nature of people? Good (positive, self-actualizing, etc.), bad (negative, irrational, evil, etc.), or neutral? Or some combination?

   In terms of Gestalt theory, the basic nature of human beings is neutral. People are believed to be born neither with an inclination toward positive thinking, feeling, or behaving nor with negative thinking, feeling, or behaving (Fall et al., 2010).

2. How are personalities formed/constructed?

   a. What factors influence the formation of personality?

      According to Gestalt theory, the factors that influence the formation of the personality are the striving toward need fulfillment and self-regulation, the individual's relationship with his or her environment and development of contact boundary disturbances (including faulty introjects from their parents), and the movement toward awareness of the environment and self-awareness (Fall et al., 2010; Oaklander, 2015; Perls, 1970).

   b. Nature/nurture?

      In Gestalt theory, personality is believed to be constructed from the combination of biology and environmental influences. All experiences contribute to the development of the personality. Each individual has a unique set of genetic blueprints that help to form how experiences are perceived and differentiated in the personality (Fall et al., 2010). "The emerging sense of self is affected by the biological predispositions of the child and interaction with the environment" (Carmichael, 2006, p. 122). We estimate the ratio of nature to nurture would be 40% nature to 60% nurture.

   c. Free will or determinism?

      Individuals are responsible for their actions and the choices they make (Naranjo, 1970), which means that Gestalt psychology comes down on the free will side of the argument (Carmichael, 2006; Fall et al., 2010).

d. Thinking, feeling, and behaving?

The emphasis in Gestalt therapy is on the whole person, which is defined as the senses, the body, the emotions, and the intellect (Oaklander, 2015). This implies that there is not a linear relationship between these aspects of self, which would lead us to believe that one is not more important than the other in terms of personality. Most Gestalt therapists tend to focus more on senses, the body, and the emotions and less on the intellect in therapy and play therapy.

e. Basic motivation for behavior?

Gestalt therapists believe that the basic motivation for behavior is reaching a homeostatic balance in one's life by getting one's needs met (Fall et al., 2010; Perls, Hefferline, & Goodman, 1951). Children realize that they cannot meet their own basic needs, and so they depend on the adults in their lives to help them survive. They often develop symptomology that involves restricting, inhibiting, and blocking different aspects of self in order to avoid rejection and abandonment and gain approval from the important adults in their lives (Oaklander, 1993). In many cases, just trying to avoid rejection and abandonment and to gain approval from these adults constitutes a large portion of the motivation for their behavior. This can extend into adulthood if clients do not deal with these issues when they are children or adolescents.

f. Basic components of personality?

Gestalt does not divide personality into component parts. Some important concepts go into understanding personality, however. These are organismic self-regulation (a balance between good health and need fulfillment); the development of a strong sense of self (one that is separate from other people, does not take responsibility for other people's behavior or feelings, and is able to recognize needs and works to get them met—even through the use of appropriate aggression); healthy contact boundaries (when all of the senses are engaged in the present, resulting in healthy mind, body, intellect, and a sense of security); and holism (whole greater than sum of parts and all aspects of the individual are important and worthy of consideration and support).

3. Perception of reality—subjective or objective?

Each person perceives the world through his or her own filter. Part of the Gestalt therapist's job is to psychologically step into the client's shoes to comprehend and appreciate the client's understanding of the immediate experience. The therapist respects the client's perception and works to understand *all* aspects of the client (Fall et al., 2010).

4. Role of therapeutic relationship?

In Gestalt therapy (and Gestalt play therapy), the role of the therapeutic relationship is central to the process of therapy. The therapist must establish a collaborative relationship with the client—an I–Thou relationship in which two people meet, are equal in power and entitlement, and are willing to bring their full selves to the relationship (Oaklander, 1994, 2003, 2015). It is a relationship of honor, respect, genuineness, and congruence in which the therapist encourages the client to take risks and experiment with new things (e.g., dialogue, mindfulness). This relationship depends on the therapist's willingness and ability to make and maintain "contact" with the client. It is a necessary component of the therapeutic process, but it is not sufficient, in and of itself, to bring about all of the changes many clients need to be healthy and to function optimally.

5. Focus on the past, the present in the context of the past, or only the present?

The focus in Gestalt therapy is on the present in the context of the past (Fall et al., 2010; Naranjo, 1970). Past interactions and experiences and self-acceptance influence how someone feels, thinks, and behaves in the present. The therapist helps the client deal with feelings in the present, recognizing (and at times acknowledging to the client) that many feelings are related to the past. The focus in many therapy sessions is on the senses and the body in the present, without reference to the past.

6. Need insight/increased consciousness to make changes?

In Gestalt therapy, clients must gain awareness of the present moment in addition to how the past is affecting the present moment in order to make healthy changes (Fall et al., 2010; Oaklander, 1992, 1994, 2003). The emphasis is on awareness of the environment, of personal process and feelings, of personal needs, of boundaries, and of the self. The Gestalt play therapist helps clients increase awareness through the various experiences and experiments presented through the play therapy techniques introduced by the play therapist in sessions. In Gestalt therapy, awareness is a holistic experience that involves the mind, the body, the emotions, and the senses.

7. Primary focus in counseling?

Because awareness is so integral to the client's ability to make changes, it is the primary focus in counseling (Fall et al., 2010;

Oaklander, 1992, 1994, 2003). The therapist works to direct the client's attention to the present moment so that the client gains awareness of the environment and self-awareness, which can help the client learn to appropriately fulfill his or her needs and allows the client to move toward optimal positive potential. In many Gestalt therapy sessions, the focus is on feelings and bodily sensations. The therapist may ask, "How does it feel?" and "Where do you feel it in your body right now?" Then the therapist can help the client make meaning about the feelings and work to accept that feeling or bring that feeling into a manageable experience (e.g., untying the knot in your tummy; pitching off the monkey on your back).

8. Psychological maladjustment?

Many times, psychological maladjustment involves contact boundary violations (which usually involve the inability to appropriately distinguish oneself from others and the environment, and a weak sense of self), faulty introjections from parents or society (which are almost always negative beliefs about the self), or the inability to meet one's own needs (Fall et al., 2010; Oaklander, 1992, 1994, 2003). With some adolescent and adult clients, maladjustment is often defined as "unfinished business," which commonly leads to anxiety and/or psychological discomfort.

9. Goals of counseling?

The main goal in Gestalt therapy is integration, which involves fulfilling one's needs or one's positive potential; reaching a balance or feeling of congruence in one's life; learning to self-regulate; enhancing one's self-awareness and self-acceptance; living in the here-and-now; and accepting previously unaccepted parts of self (Fall et al., 2010). "The disturbed child needs help to restore healthy organismic self-regulation, to awaken an awareness of internal and external events, and to be able to use the resources available in her environment to get her needs met" (Carroll & Oaklander, 1997, p. 188). The goals in Gestalt play therapy are to restore the child to a healthy sense of self, to learn to accept parts of the self that have been previously rejected, to learn ways to fully support the self, and to be willing and able to experience pain and discomfort (Carroll, 2009; Carroll & Oaklander, 1997).

10. Measuring progress?

In Gestalt play therapy, the therapist relies primarily on observation of the client to measure progress, with an occasional report from parents and teachers. The Gestalt play therapist monitors the following list of factors: (a) focus on the past and future and increased focus on the present moment; (b) increased skills for fulfilling needs; (c) increased willingness to experiment and try new things; (d) increased client willingness to take responsibility for actions; and (e) behavior that suggests the client's development of appropriate aggressive energy, contact boundaries, self-acceptance, and self-nurturance (Carroll, 2009; Carroll & Oaklander, 1997; Oaklander, 1994, 2003).

11. Directive or nondirective?

Gestalt play therapy is both directive (at times) and nondirective (at other times), depending on the needs of the client and the progression of therapy.

a. Creating space or using structured techniques in play therapy?

Creating a safe and caring space is important in Gestalt play therapy, but the main focus is on the experiences and experiments introduced by the therapist through strategies that include storytelling, music, art, dance/movement, photography, and so on. The key to the balance of directive and nondirective interactions in Gestalt play therapy is the therapist's awareness and respect for the child. The therapist may often have goals or plans for a session but hold no expectations of the child or the child's behaviors, working very hard to avoid pushing the client beyond the client's willingness to go (Oaklander, 1994, 2003, 2011, 2015).

b. Playing with the client in play therapy?

While the Gestalt play therapist may occasionally play with the client (usually at the client's behest), the main function of the therapist in Gestalt play therapy is to develop and introduce specific exercises or "experiments" and then scaffold the unfolding of the experience to facilitate the client gaining increased awareness. This scaffolding may involve questions about the product (if there was one—like an artistic creation or sand tray) and/or the process of doing whatever the experiment entailed. The Gestalt play therapist reflects many feelings but only uses "soft" interpretations in working to help the client understand the significance of his or her experience.

12. Work with parents? teachers?

Gestalt play therapists willingly work with both parents and teachers. They rely on these important adults in their child client's lives to provide information about the child's functioning and social supports. The therapist provides education, encouragement, and referrals to counseling if needed (Carroll & Oaklander, 1997).

JUNGIAN PLAY THERAPY

Jungian play therapy was originally developed by John Allan (1988) based on the work of Carl Jung, a contemporary of Freud. Jungian play therapy is built on the beliefs that "the psyche has a self-healing potential, that the archetypes assist in organizing the child's behavior, and that the creative processes of play, art, drama, and writing intervene and transform the child in the direction of healing" (Carmichael, 2006, p. 90). It is difficult to explain Jungian analytical psychotherapy simply because of the depth of the ideas that underlie the theory, and because Jung's concepts and language are sometimes difficult to understand. It is essential to understand, though, that

> this approach does not ascribe to the dictates of "treatment protocol," but rather receives every child into the therapeutic world as a unique individual who has and is processing his or her life in a unique and personally meaningful way . . . we seek to awaken the healer within them to ensure that their healing is genuine and authentic—not the product of an outside agent. Our goal is a true transformational healing, not an elimination of a cluster of symptoms. The reduction and elimination of symptoms are natural results of transformational healing. (Lilly, 2015, p. 49)

This means that, in some ways, the entire premise of this book (which is to provide a plethora of goal-directed play therapy skills and techniques) is contrary to the core purposes of Jungian play therapy. Jungian play therapy is almost always targeted at child clients rather than clients ranging across the lifespan. If you want to work with adults using play therapy, this may not be the optimal approach for you, unless you want to pioneer a new way of using Jungian play therapy (which we think would be supercool).

1. What do you believe about the basic nature of people? Good (positive, self-actualizing, etc.), bad (negative, irrational, evil, etc.), or neutral? or some combination?

   In Jungian theory, the basic nature of people would be considered to be neutral—neither good nor bad. The psyche (which consists of the conscious and unconscious structures of the personality) was developed for survival and leads individuals into both positive, self-actualizing behavior and negative behavior. In the process of growing up and developing their ego, humans unconsciously choose to cultivate some personality traits and reject others. Those others become the person's "shadow"—the traits the ego rejects as fitting into the Self that is being created (Jung, 1969; Netto, 2011). Jung also believed that people are born with all the answers to their problems (Allan, 1988, 1997).

2. How are personalities formed/constructed?

   a. What factors influence the formation of personality?

Multiple factors influence the formation of the personality in Jungian analytic psychotherapy (Allan, 1988, 1997; Green, 2009; Peery, 2003). One of these factors is children's relationships with their parents and their perception of whether their parents are meeting their needs. Young children develop psychological ego defenses, such as repression, projection, hallucinations, and the splitting of "good" and "bad" (Carmichael, 2006). The normal pressures of life (e.g., hunger, cold, pain, fatigue) can combine with the less-than-ideal responses from others (especially their parents) to these pressures and so can result in children's ego fragmenting. The process by which children and their parents deal with this fragmentation ("deintegration and reintegration") leads to the development of attachment patterns and adjustment or maladjustment in children. One of the other factors that influence the formation of the personality is archetypes, which are the "universal organizing principles that form the basic structural matrix of the human personality." (Peery, 2003, p. 23). Archetypes are images or symbols that have shared meaning across cultures and generations.

   b. Nature/nurture?

We believe that most Jungians would support the idea that influence on the formation of the personality is divided equally between nature and nurture. People are born with innate structures, like the psyche, which consists of the ego and the Self, and because the collective unconscious means that everyone inherits experiences and problems of the people before them. However, the relationship between children and their parent(s) shapes the differentiation of the ego from other psyche structures (Allan, 1997).

   c. Free will or determinism?

Jung did not believe much in either free will or determinism. From Jung's perspective everyone is capable of making their own conscious decisions but are influenced by the personal unconscious and collective unconscious.

   d. Thinking, feeling, and behaving?

In Jungian theory, the relationship between thinking, feeling, and behaving is not linear. Feelings can be attributed to persons' experiences or the archetypes with which they identify. These feelings contribute to how they think about themselves (Douglas, 2008). Behavior is in response to unfinished struggles of parents (in childhood and adulthood) or themselves. When people become more aware, balanced, and accepting of themselves, they have less need for the problem behaviors or their defense mechanisms (Allan, 1997).

e. Basic motivation for behavior?

Most motivation for behavior in Jungian theory comes from the unconscious—either the collective unconscious (the archetypal patterns that have evolved over time and across cultures) or the personal unconscious (repressed memories and instinctual drives) (Allan & Levin, 1993). The main drive in the psyche is for individuation. "To Jung, the individual is on a continually evolving journey that includes not only the self's past and future, but also a collective past and future, with some amount of interference from genetic and environmental influences" (James, 1997, p. 127).

f. Basic components of personality?

In Jungian theory, the psyche is made up of three parts: ego, the personal unconscious, and the collective unconscious. The ego is "a complex of representations at the center of the individual's consciousness providing identity and continuity" (Punnett, 2016, p. 70). The main functions of the ego are thinking, feeling, sensing, and intuiting. The ego cannot form the person's personality by itself—the other factor is the Self, which influences the ego, creating the "ego-Self axis" (Lilly, 2015). The personal unconscious is the repository of the memories or experiences that have been repressed or forgotten, and the collective unconscious is the repository of humanity's experiences across time that are revealed through archetypes, metaphors, symbols, fantasies, and dreams (Green, 2009; Lilly, 2015; Punnett, 2016).

3. Perception of reality—subjective or objective?

Jungians would agree with the idea that individuals perceive reality subjectively, but this is not a significant concept in Jungian theory.

4. Role of therapeutic relationship?

In Jungian play therapy, the therapeutic relationship is formed through authenticity, trust, and equality. It is the play therapist's job to create a space of *temanos,* "the sacred place where transformation can occur because it is safe" (J. P. Lilly, personal communication, February 2010).

5. Focus on the past, the present in the context of the past, or only the present?

Jung believed a person's past could influence his or her future, but future aspirations can also shape the way a person behaves. The focus in therapy is on the present. "It is our deeply founded belief that our job at the time the child enters our room is to assist him or her in safely engaging the overwhelming material, activating the self-healer from within and allowing the Self to make contact with the ego and express the healing process through the use of the symbols we have assembled in the play therapy room" (Lilly, 2015, p. 55).

6. Need insight/increased consciousness to make changes?

In Jungian therapy, an increase in consciousness is necessary for healing to occur. According to Lilly (2015; personal communication, February 2010), the Jungian play therapist uses "soft interpretations," giving feedback about clients' cognitive processes and identifying emotions for the client, as well as occasionally making a guess about the symbolic content of the play material or metaphor.

7. Primary focus in counseling?

The primary focus in Jungian analytical therapy is on helping the client to develop his or her unique identity and to overcome or come to terms with losses, and on adapting to demands of family, school, and society (Allan, 1997). In Jungian play therapy, the emphasis is on activating the individuation process, developing the ego, improving communication between the conscious and the unconscious, helping clients develop flexible defense mechanisms, and activating the self-healing mechanism so that reintegration of the personality can occur (Green, 2009; Lilly, 2015; Punnett, 2016).

8. Psychological maladjustment?

According to Jungian theory, psychological maladjustment occurs when disturbances in the ego–Self axis interfere with individuation process. Clients who do not have the ego strength to deal with materials or experiences that are disturbing to them have difficulty with reintegration, often using defense structures that are either too rigid or nonexistent to protect themselves from deintegration (Allan, 1988, 1997; Carmichael, 2006; Lilly, 2015). At times, maladjustment can result from an imbalance in synergy (the contrasexual aspects of the person) with roles and aspects of the anima (the "feminine" aspect of the identity) and the animus (the "male" aspect) (Carmichael, 2006; Evers-Fahey, 2016).

9. Goals of counseling?

The goals of counseling in Jungian analytical play therapy are to (a) activate the self-healing potential in the child's psyche, (b) strengthen the ego, (c) stimulate and develop the client's creativity and imagination, (d) heal and transcend the client's wounds, (e) help the client develop an interior life, (f) foster the client's development of a sense of competency and mastery, (g) help the client develop skills to cope with future problems, and (h) assist the client in gaining an understanding of the complexity of life and becoming open to change (Allan, 1997).

10. Measuring progress?

Jungian therapists monitor clients' progress toward achieving self-actualization and healing. The more they are healed, the more likely they are to display their true self (e.g., shadow aspects, anima/animus balance), and the more likely they are to have developed flexible defense structures. Becoming aware of unconscious wants and desires helps individuals reclaim their consciousness and begin to make important positive changes in their life (Douglas, 2008).

11. Directive or nondirective?

Jungian play therapy would be considered to be nondirective by most experts, and some Jungian play therapists are more directive than others.

a. Creating space or using structured techniques in play therapy?

While therapists' primary role in Jungian play therapy is to create the space they call temenos, they do ask questions for clarification and use some soft interpretations (Allan, 1988, 1997; Green, 2009; Lilly, 2015; Peery, 2003). They seldom use structured techniques, and when they do, they usually use the sand tray, art, or metaphoric storytelling. When Jungian play therapists do use a structured technique, they seldom guide or direct the activity beyond the initial prompt.

b. Playing with the client in play therapy?

Jungian play therapists will play with the client when invited by the client. The role of the therapist is participant–observer. By joining in the play, the therapist communicates acceptance of the client with no pressure for the client to change. This safety is part of the temenos, which is the sacred and safe place (Lilly, 2015; Peery, 2003).

12. Work with parents? teachers?

Jungian play therapists do work with parents. They usually meet with parents every three to four sessions, and they provide instruction about parenting strategies, gather information about the child's struggles or progress, and provide parent support or refer for counseling elsewhere (Peery, 2003). Allan (1997) suggested that the parents of children in Jungian play therapy should always be in Jungian analytical therapy themselves because the child needs to be freed from parental projections in order to be able to fully individuate.

NARRATIVE PLAY THERAPY

There are two very different approaches to narrative play therapy (Cattanach, 2008; Mills, 2015). Ann Cattanach (2006, 2008) used Michael White's narrative therapy model as the basis for an approach she called narrative play therapy. In this form of play therapy, the therapist asks the client questions as a means of developing vivid descriptions of life experiences. Joyce Mills (2015) developed StoryPlay, a separate way of using narratives as the foundation for the play therapy. Based on the work of Milton Erickson, in StoryPlay, the therapist uses both the client's symptoms and the client's story to "evoke behavioral and emotional transformational change" (Mills, 2015, p. 171). We are going to try answer the philosophical and practical questions from both of these perspectives, and these approaches may not provide easily accessible answers to several of the questions. We believe that, for the most part, the underlying philosophies about how people develop and psychopathology are similar, and that the primary differences are in their interactions with clients in the playroom.

1. What do you believe about the basic nature of people? Good (positive, self-actualizing, etc.), bad (negative, irrational, evil, etc.), or neutral? Or some combination?

    [Starting off with a bang!] We couldn't find any information related to this question in the literature on either approach to narrative therapy, so we are assuming that the issue of the basic nature of people is not an important construct for them. Cattanach (2006) suggested that "the self is relationally defined, and persons continuously construct their lives and identities" (p. 86). (So, we think the answer to whether the basic nature of people is good or bad is that people are neither good nor bad, but neutral.)

2. How are personalities formed/constructed?

    a. What factors influence the formation of personality?

    Both of these approaches to narrative therapy would suggest that the stories we hear (e.g., fairy tales, family stories, children's books, history lessons, television, movies) from the time we are born contribute to the formation of personality (Cattanach, 2006; Mills, 2015; Mills & Crowley, 2014; White, 2007; White & Epston, 1990; Taylor de Faoite, 2011). We obtain meaning from the stories we hear as we perceive them in the context of time and culture. For example, the stories Camilla (a 6-year-old little girl) hears about girls (capable girls, scared girls, smart girls, girls who give up, girls who persist) will influence how she perceives girls' roles and her view of herself as a girl. According to Aideen Taylor de Faoite (2011), who was a student of Cattanach, children are born with the natural disposition to play. Personal narratives are created during their natural developmental progression through embodiment play (learning and playing through the senses), projective play (developing language, symbols, and metaphor wherein they project experiences, wishes, feelings, and thoughts onto objects), and role play (trying out new roles, pretending to be a princess, super hero, teacher, parent, good guy, or bad guy, and developing social skills through taking turns and sharing). Both of these approaches would suggest that culture, family, perception, and interpretation are the key influences on the development of personality.

b. Nature/nurture?

Mills does not really address the question of nature versus nurture, and since she clearly believes that stories are pivotal in the development of personality, we suspect she would say that nurture is more important than nature. Our interpretation of Taylor de Faoite (2011) suggests that narrative play therapy would put the nature/nurture ratio at 30% nature (people are genetically disposed to particular difficulties such as depression, anxiety, bipolar disorder) and 70% nurture (stories told within families, environments, and cultures and the meaning individuals make from them).

c. Free will or determinism?

Free will is an important component of both narrative play therapies. Individuals have the freedom to choose different stories, change their interpretations of stories, and/or shift the meaning they make of stories.

d. Thinking, feeling, and behaving?

Again, this is not a central consideration in narrative play therapy. While neither approach to narrative play therapy seems to posit a linear, causal relationship between these three factors, both seem to focus primarily on thinking, with the focus on the meaning individuals make of the stories they hear and tell. Feelings and behavior seem to be secondary to thinking. Feelings appear to follow thinking because they stem from how individuals see themselves and behaviors are a response to who they think they are (Cattanach, 2006; Mills & Crowley, 2014; Taylor de Faoite, 2011).

e. Basic motivation for behavior?

This question is not answered in an obvious way by either approach to narrative play therapy (and we are guessing it has something to do with stories).

f. Basic components of personality?

Narrative therapy does not divide the personality into component parts, so this question isn't really relevant to this approach. According to both schools of narrative play therapy, the self is socially constructed in context of relationships and systems. Personality is developed through the stories people believe or tell themselves (Mills & Crowley, 2014; Taylor de Faoite, 2011; White, 2000; White & Epston, 1990; Zimmerman & Dickerson, 1996).

3. Perception of reality—subjective or objective?

Both Mills (2015) and Cattanach (2006) take a social constructivist stance on reality: although we might perceive an objective world through our senses, we are continually interpreting what we experience in our ongoing attempts to make meaning of our existence.

4. Role of therapeutic relationship?

In both approaches to narrative play therapy, the therapist works to create a safe and judgment-free zone in which clients are free to express feelings and co-create stories with another person (Cattanach, 2006; Mills, 2015; Mills & Crowley, 2014; Taylor de Faoite, 2011). The play therapist takes a curious but not-knowing stance, listening and telling stories, making suggestions of activities designed to shift clients' stories.

5. Focus on the past, the present in the context of the past, or only the present?

While narrative play therapists are willing to listen to stories from clients' past, the focus in the sessions is on the present. As Mills (2015) pointed out, she is focused on the present in the tradition of Ericksonian therapeutic principles, which are "not focused on analyzing the past or the pathology, but instead they are attentive to the present and to the utilization of hidden potentials and inner resources to facilitate positive change" (p. 173). Cattanach suggested that the therapist might ask a client to compare the old story with the new story being constructed in the session to see which direction suits the client better, but clearly she does not believe in dwelling in the past.

6. Need insight/increased consciousness to make changes?

While increased awareness and insight might be helpful for some clients in narrative play therapy, any shift in consciousness is almost always delivered through stories or metaphoric art, sand tray, or movement rather than in a direct or interpretive way.

7. Primary focus in counseling?

In narrative play therapy, clients come to counseling with a "problem-saturated" story, and the therapist's primary concern is to help clients separate problems from themselves. In both versions of narrative play therapy, clients are invited to create a narrative through a variety of options, including using toys, props, and sensory materials. The therapist and clients co-construct narratives through therapeutic activities, dialogue, and relationships (Cattanach, 2006; Mills, 2015). The play therapist may also create or adapt stories for clients that reprise their narrative themes.

8. Psychological maladjustment?

While the focus in narrative therapy is never on psychological maladjustment, cultural, interpersonal, and intrapersonal dynamics contribute to the development of stories that are problem-laden and/or stories in which the client is the problem. In many cases, the client's struggle derives from a lack of opportunity, capacity, or permission to develop stories in which he or she sees himself or herself as capable, competent, and of value (Cattanach, 2006; Mills, 2015; Taylor de Faoite, 2011; White, 2000; White & Epston, 1990; Zimmerman & Dickerson, 1996).

9. Goals of counseling?

The goal in both forms of narrative play therapy is to separate the problem from the person and to help clients transform their story over the course of counseling. Sometimes the goal is to make a new story, and other times it is to alter the current story in a way that will make a revised story that is healthier and gives power to the client. One way to do this is to externalize the problem (Cattanach, 2006; Taylor de Faoite, 2011), and another is to connect clients to their inner resources, hidden potential, transcultural wisdom and healing philosophies, the natural world, and their own creativity (Mills, 2015).

10. Measuring progress?

Progress is measured in narrative therapy by listening to clients' stories and observing their reaction to the stories that the play therapist brings into the sessions. An increase in positive or rational stories, stories with a more positive ending or an alternate ending to an originally negative ending, and stories that indicate that clients have been successful in separating their problem from themselves are all signs of progress in narrative play therapy (Mills & Crowley, 2014; Taylor de Faoite, 2011).

11. Directive or nondirective?

Directive and nondirective, depending on the therapist, the client, the presenting problem, and the unfolding process of the play therapy.

a. Creating space or using structured techniques in play therapy?

Therapists from both approaches to narrative play therapy believe that the first step in the therapeutic process is the creation of a safe, nonjudgmental space, and neither of these approaches considers that step to be sufficient. The narrative play therapist allows the client to direct many of the therapeutic interactions. In Cattanach's version, the therapist takes a curious and genuine stance, guiding the stories with questions designed to help clients develop their narrative and explore alternate endings (Cattanach, 2006). The therapist also asks clients to co-create stories with him or her and creates his or her own stories and delivers them to clients. The therapist can serve the role of recording clients' narratives as they emerge. Using sensory materials to aid clients in embodying stories and providing small figures and puppets, the narrative play therapist in Cattanach's tradition encourages role-playing and dramatization of stories. According to Mills (2015; Mills & Crowley, 2014), StoryPlay practitioners avoid questioning strategies and instead rely on metaphoric strategies designed to create "strength-based narratives in various forms that include storytelling, play, artistic metaphors, StoryCrafts, and therapeutic rituals and metaphors" (p. 178).

b. Playing with the client in play therapy?

The main form of playing with the client in narrative play therapy is the co-creation of stories. Most other times, the therapist serves primarily as the witness to clients' stories and play rather than as an active participant in the play.

12. Work with parents? teachers?

Most narrative play therapists consult with parents and teachers of child clients to gather information about the child and the stories he or she has heard (Mills & Crowley, 2014; Taylor de Faoite, 2011). This can help the play therapist to better understand and make meaning of the child's narratives. Sometimes parents are invited to consult with the play therapist for the purpose of teaching them to explore alternative stories with their children. Near the end of counseling, parents are encouraged to help children try out new stories, create safety for them to be different, and not stick to the same story/ways of being. Parents might be referred for their own counseling if this is deemed necessary.

PSYCHODYNAMIC PLAY THERAPY

One of the difficulties in writing about psychodynamic play therapy is that there are many different "flavors" of psychodynamic theory and therapy. Most people know that the psychodynamic approach to personality theory and therapy was founded by Sigmund Freud. Several of the therapists who studied with Freud or his students (e.g., Anna Freud, Hermine Hug-Hellmuth, Melanie Klein, and Margaret Lowenfeld) extended Freud's ideas and actually worked with child clients (Punnett, 2016). While much of the process of psychodynamic play therapy is nondirective (e.g., the therapist seldom initiates directed activities), the psychodynamic play therapist continually analyzes the underlying meaning of clients' play and verbalizations, waiting until the relationship is firmly established before using interpretations to share ideas about the unconscious process underneath behavior and motivation.

1. What do you believe about the basic nature of people? Good (positive, self-actualizing, etc.), bad (negative, irrational, evil, etc.), or neutral? Or some combination?

    Most psychodynamic theorists believe that people are born negative. According to this theory, humans selfishly try to satisfy their innate biological need—the death drive and the life drive (Fall et al., 2010; Freud, 1949). The death drive consists of the human tendency toward aggression and destructiveness, and the life layer consists of the movement toward seeking pleasure (often through sexuality) and avoiding pain (Fall et al., 2010; Mordock, 2015; Punnett, 2016).

2. How are personalities formed/constructed?

    a. What factors influence the formation of personality?

        In most applications of psychodynamic theory, humans pass through multiple psychosexual development stages: oral, anal, phallic, latency, and genital (Cangelosi, 1993; Fall et al., 2010; Punnett, 2016). The oral stage extends from birth until around 2, and the developmental task of that stage centers on survival and the formation of attachment. The anal stage is from age 2 to 4 (approximately), and the task is the development of bodily control and the start of a sense of autonomy. The phallic stage is approximately from 4 to 6, and the psychic energy is focused on the genital region. During this stage, the child must resolve the Oedipal/Electra complex that consists of the child wanting to "possess" the opposite-sex parent. In order to successfully negotiate through that stage, the child must begin to identify with the same-sex parent and give up the need to have the opposite-sex parent to himself or herself. During the latency stage, which lasts from the resolution of the

Oedipal/Electra complex to adolescence, the child rests and con-
solidates all that has happened up until that point and then moves
into the genital stage, which is the rest of life. The developmental
task of this final stage is the cultivation of the adult sexual relationship. As a person moves through the stages and is confronted with
conflicts at different times, personality is developed. The "how"
these stages are met influences personality, with fixations developing at stages that are not satisfactorily resolved (Cangelosi, 1993;
Fall et al., 2010; Freud, 1949; Mordock, 2015; Punnett, 2016).

b. Nature/nurture?

Because psychodynamic theory states that people are formed
by their innate drives toward sexual gratification and aggression,
most psychodynamic theorists believe that nature is the stronger
force in the formation of personality. However, the theory also supports the idea that childhood experiences and the passage through
the psychosexual stages influence the formation of the personality. We believe most psychodynamic play therapists would estimate
70% nature and 30% nurture.

c. Free will or determinism?

Because psychodynamic theory posits a direct cause and effect
relationship between biological drives/childhood experiences and
current behavior, without the mitigation of choice, psychodynamic
theory would be considered to be deterministic (Fall et al., 2010;
Safran & Kriss, 2014).

d. Thinking, feeling, and behaving?

This question does not really apply to psychodynamic theory.
People's behavior stems from unconscious urges, and they behave
before they really understand why they are behaving in a certain way.
After dysfunctional behavior is recognized, therapy is used to ana-
lyze the unconscious and resolve the issues leading to that behavior.
There is no emphasis on thinking, feeling, or behaving. The focus in
therapy that will help clients make changes is on bringing the unconscious motivation to consciousness and helping clients gain control
of their instinctive drives (Fall et al., 2010; Punnett, 2016).

e. Basic motivation for behavior?

According to psychodynamic theory, all behavior comes from
the two instinctual drives, Eros and Thanatos, both of which derive
from the id. Eros is the sex drive and life instinct, whereas Thanatos is the aggressive drive and death instinct. Therefore, the basic
motivation for behavior is to increase pleasure and avoid pain.
Because these drives have their roots in the id, psychodynamic

theory suggests that behavior originates in the unconscious (Carmichael, 2006; Fall et al., 2010; Freud, 1949; Safran & Kriss, 2014).

f. Basic components of personality?

In psychodynamic theory, there are three basic components of personality: the id, the ego, and the super-ego. The id, the sole component of the personality that is present from birth, is the source of a human being's instinctual drives, particularly our sexual and aggressive drives. The id moves people to act according to the pleasure principle, the instinct to avoid pain and maximize pleasure. The ego is the organized component of the personality that includes defensive, perceptual, intellectual-cognitive, and executive functions. It is the part of the personality that makes sense of the world—it makes realistic assessments about which of the id's demands and passions can be met with minimal negative impact on the person. The super-ego is the internalization of the rules set by society, which are usually taught to children by parents and family, and then are reinforced by schools. It is the component of the personality that deals with right and wrong—the seat of the conscience (Corey, 2017; Fall et al., 2010; Freud, 1949).

3. Perception of reality—subjective or objective?

Since so much is unconscious, according to psychodynamic theory, reality is perceived subjectively. However, this is not an important aspect of this theory.

4. Role of therapeutic relationship?

The psychodynamic counselor is a participant–observer who assumes responsibility for guidance and interpretation. Starting with Anna Freud, psychodynamic therapists who worked with children have used play to create alliance; then they shift from play to more verbal interaction to help the child gain insight (McCalla, 1994). The therapeutic relationship is considered to be necessary to create a space free of anxiety in which clients can access and freely express their unconscious. However, it is also thought to be important for the therapist to avoid self-disclosure in order to cultivate clients' transference (Carmichael, 2006; Cangelosi, 1993). The therapist must demonstrate three characteristics: empathy, intuition, and introspection (Fall et al., 2010).

5. Focus on the past, the present in the context of the past, or only the present?

The focus in psychodynamic theory is on the past—our adult feelings and behaviors are all rooted in our childhood experiences (Fall et al., 2010).

6. Need insight/increased consciousness to make changes?

Insight is extremely important in psychodynamic theory (Fall et al., 2010; Safran & Kriss, 2014). Usually, the therapist uses verbalizations to help clients gain insight and increased access to their consciousness. When working with children, play is the means to forming relationships and to revealing one's self to the clients. The play therapist interprets play and verbalizes these interpretations back to clients for insight (McCalla, 1994; Mordock, 2015). Working with adults, counselors use dream analysis and free association (talk, play, arts, etc.) to help therapists understand and interpret clients' issues and internal conflicts (Fall et al., 2010).

7. Primary focus in counseling?

The primary focus in counseling with adult clients is on free association through which "one reports one's stream of consciousness without interruption and without censorship" (Fall et al., 2004, p. 55). With children, the play is the free association, and the play therapist's task is to interpret the play to child clients (McCalla, 1994). Mordock (2015) contends that, rather than rely solely on interpretation, the psychodynamic play therapist works on enhancing children's "adaptive skills by helping them find better ways to express pent-up feelings and to develop more mature defenses against anxiety" (p. 75). Because there is an emphasis on helping children resolve internal conflicts, "the therapist is in the position to offer developmental assistance to the ego, to strengthen the ego and help children accomplish developmental reorganization, to address conflicts and defenses, and to make way for the emergence of the self" (Punnett, 2016, p. 76).

8. Psychological maladjustment?

"The ego is not up to the task of managing the demands of the id, the superego, and external reality" (Fall et al., 2004, p. 53). According to psychodynamic theory, the different structures of the personality are in constant conflict, which results in anxiety and maladjustment. Other sources of psychological maladjustment are fixations in specific psychosexual stages, lack of resolution of the Oedipal or Electra complex, and overuse or misuse of the defense mechanisms.

9. Goals of counseling?

The primary goal of psychodynamic therapy is insight. Clients must become aware of the internal unconscious conflicts underlying their self-defeating behavior and distress feelings for personality change to happen (McCalla, 1994; Fall et al., 2010). It is also helpful for clients to give up their overuse or misuse of primitive defense mechanisms and to move toward more mature defense mechanisms (Mordock, 2015).

10. Measuring progress?

Progress in psychodynamic play therapy is measured through observation of the play and reports from caretakers. Therapy is considered to have been effective when the presenting problem is no longer seen as a problem; when a child client has built the capacity for being appropriately aggressive, dependent, and adaptive; when he or she is able to deal with anxiety; and when he or she is using mature defense mechanisms (Carmichael, 2006; Fall et al., 2010; Mordock, 2015).

11. Directive or nondirective?

Psychodynamic play therapy is, at times, nondirective and at other times, directive (McCalla, 1994; Mordock, 2015; Punnett, 2016). It allows for directiveness (through specific interventions, interpretations, confrontations, and questioning strategies) and honors the disclosures that happen through nondirected play. Interpretations are usually given through metaphor with children who are playing in symbolic ways.

a. Creating space or using structured techniques in play therapy?

In psychodynamic play therapy, the therapist creates a space free from anxiety in which clients can freely express themselves. The play therapist will also introduce directed techniques in order to gather information about particular dynamics, help clients gain insight, and provide support for them to make changes in their use of defense mechanisms (McCalla, 1994; Mordock, 2015; Punnett, 2016).

b. Playing with the client in play therapy?

Because of their concern with transference, psychodynamic play therapists are very discerning about whether to actively play with clients in sessions. They may occasionally play "with" the child, and the primary role is as "participant–observer." Usually, if they choose to play with clients, the purpose is to gain information or to deliver an interpretation through a metaphor.

12. Work with parents? teachers?

Ideally, treatment would be several times a week and the psychodynamic play therapist would meet parents at least once each week (Lee, 2009). They usually work with parents on issues that have an impact on the emotional balance in the family and on issues connected to the child, with the goal of helping the parents gain a better understanding of the child's internal conflicts and a clearer picture of their impact on the child (Carmichael, 2006). They do not usually work with teachers because they would not think that teachers are as important as parents in developing the child's personality or as influential in helping the child proceed through his or her developmental process.

THERAPLAY

Theraplay was developed by Ann Jernberg (1979) when she was working with hundreds of Head Start children in Chicago, Illinois, and she noticed that many of them seemed to have deficits in the formation of their attachment to their parents. She adapted the works of Austin Des Lauriers (1962) and Viola Brody (1978, 1993) to develop Theraplay, which is a structured approach for working with children and their parents to establish or strengthen the parent–child attachment. Theraplay is an approach to play therapy, based on attachment theories, designed to help foster healthy interactions between parent(s) and child. It is intended to be an intensive and brief modality of play therapy. It is a playful, engaging, relationship-focused treatment model based on the necessity of a healthy, attuned relationship between child and parent (Bundy-Myrow & Booth, 2009).

Because Theraplay was designed specifically for work with families and is not based on a psychological theory of personality, some of the questions we would usually ask are simply not addressed in this approach. When there is a question that isn't relevant to Theraplay, we will note that in this section.

1. What do you believe about the basic nature of people? Good (positive, self-actualizing, etc.), bad (negative, irrational, evil, etc.), or neutral? Or some combination?

   Theraplay does not take a stand on the basic nature of people. Jernberg did emphasize that she felt there should be no blame or judgment when parents struggle with creating the connection of attachment with their children—that they were doing the best they could, given their life circumstances (Jernberg, 1979; Jernberg & Jernberg, 1993).

2. How are personalities formed/constructed?

   a. What factors influence the formation of personality?

   In Theraplay, "early interaction between parent and child is the crucible in which the self and personality develop" (Koller & Booth, 1997, p. 206). Positive, playful, fun, loving interactions between the parent and the child create a strong sense of self, feelings of worth, and secure attachment; negative, sporadic, inconsistent, neglect/abusive, flat interactions between the parent and the child lead to the development of intra- and interpersonal difficulties (Bundy-Myrow & Booth, 2009).

b. Nature/nurture?

This question is not directly addressed in this approach, but we would speculate that Theraplay practitioners would attribute 25% of the development of personality to nature because people are born with the need to connect and 75% of the development of personality to nurture because there is such a strong emphasis on the idea that people are shaped by getting or not getting the attuned, responsive care they need to develop in healthy ways (Bundy-Myrow & Booth, 2009).

c. Free will or determinism?

The idea of free will versus determinism is not addressed in the Theraplay literature. However, it seems that choice is important in this approach.

d. Thinking, feeling, and behaving?

This question is not addressed either. The emphasis in this approach is always on fostering attachment. Interventions focus on behavior rather than cognition or affect.

e. Basic motivation for behavior?

Theraplay is grounded in attachment theory, so basic motivation for behavior is explained in terms of parent–infant relationships, which are supported by two innate drives: the drive to stay close in order to be safe and the drive to share meaning and companionship (Booth & Winstead, 2015).

f. Basic components of personality?

The proponents of Theraplay are not concerned with the basic components of personality. Theraplay is "based on attachment research demonstrating that sensitive, responsive caregiving and playful interaction nourish a child's brain, from internal representations of self and others, and have a lifelong impact on behavior and feelings" (Booth & Jernberg, 2010, p. 4).

3. Perception of reality—subjective or objective?

Again, this question is not addressed in the Theraplay literature.

4. Role of therapeutic relationship?

In Theraplay, the focus is on the relationship between the caregiver and the child (or adolescent), with both the caregiver and the child participating in sessions. The parent or caregiver's therapeutic relationship with the child is critical, so the Theraplay therapist builds an attuned, supportive relationship with both the adult care-giver and the child, models expectations, and fully accepts both the adult and child (Munns, 2011). The therapist provides an interactive relationship-based experience designed to increase possibilities for the two of them to learn and practice ways of interacting that are filled with play, joy, safety, and security (Booth & Winstead, 2016).

5. Focus on the past, the present in the context of the past, or only the present?

The focus in Theraplay is on the present and the interactions that happen in the here-and-now (Booth & Winstead, 2016; Munns, 2011). The assumption is that the relationship between the adult caretaker and the child wasn't attuned in the past or that there had been a break somewhere in the attachment between them before they entered counseling. However, the past is not really addressed, nor is it considered important in treatment. The timing and circumstances of the break in attachment are only important in the context of the treatment plan for which parenting skills are taught to the caregiver. For example, an early break in the attachment might lead to the therapist modeling rocking, feeding, and other tasks typical of parent–child interactions during the age when the break occurred and then coach-ing the caregiver to reestablish the attachment through those actions (Munns, 2011).

6. Need insight/increased consciousness to make changes?

In Theraplay, for change to occur, there is no need for the child to gain insight. There might be times when it is helpful for the caregiver to have an increase in his or her consciousness as a means of being able to provide an organized, supportive, and coregulated experience for the child (Booth & Winstead, 2015, 2016). The caregiver needs to be able to reflect on his or her own internal state, along with the inter-nal state of the child. "A caregiver who has not been well parented finds it very hard to achieve the level of mindfulness necessary for sensitive responding. A major goal of our work with caregivers is to support the development of their capacity to reflect on their own and the child's experiences" (Booth & Winstead, 2016, p. 169).

7. Primary focus in counseling?

The primary focus in Theraplay is on the interaction between caregiver and child (Munns, 2011). The Theraplay therapist plans each session to incorporate the elements of healthy caregiver–infant inter-actions by modeling the actions and reactions of an attuned caregiver and coaching the caregiver so that he or she can replicate these actions and reactions both in session and outside the therapy setting. There are four dimensions of the attuned caregiver–child interaction, and the

Theraplay therapist might use all four in most sessions, but some are given more emphasis with certain families, based on the child's needs. The four dimensions are structure (making sure there are clear rules and boundaries and establishing a predictable routine—designed to meet the child's need for order, safety, and coregulation); engagement (connecting with the child in playful and joy-filled ways—designed to meet the child's need for attuned connection with activities such as mirroring, cotton ball fights, and body part sounds such as nose honks); nurture (providing physical comforting for the child—designed to meet the child's need for comfort, support, and soothing with activities such as feeding one another, lotioning/powdering hurts, rocking, and cradling); and challenge (helping the child enhance a sense of self-efficacy and self-confidence—designed to meet the child's need to take age-appropriate risks, master new skills, and increase confidence through activities designed to help the child cooperate with others and to learn new things like bubble catch and balloon tennis) (Booth & Jernberg, 2010; Booth & Winfield, 2016; Munns, 2011).

8. Psychological maladjustment?

Psychological maladjustment is the outcome of early and/or ongoing unresponsive, neglectful, or abusive care. The child views himself or herself as unlovable and regards others as uncaring and untrustworthy, and sees the world as unsafe (Bundy-Myrow & Booth, 2009).

9. Goals of counseling?

The goals of Theraplay are (a) to foster a positive and nurturing relationship between the caregiver and the child client, (b) to help the caregiver learn how to establish or reestablish secure attachment with the child; (c) to help the caregiver become attuned to the child's needs; (d) to help the caregiver learn to interact with the child in ways that change the child's perceptions of caregiving from negative to positive; (e) to help the caregivers learn to provide structure, engagement, nurture, and challenge to the child—both in session and outside session; and (f) to help the caregiver learn to reflect on his or her own emotional experiences and the child's emotional experiences in order to be able to coregulate with the child (Booth & Winstead, 2015; Bundy-Myrow & Booth, 2009; Munns, 2011).

10. Measuring progress?

In Theraplay, progress is measured primarily through observation and caregiver report. Since the primary goal in therapy is the improvement of the caregiver–child relationship, this is the center of the focus for measuring improvement, though at times the therapist might also monitor whether family interactions improve.

11. Directive or nondirective?

Undoubtedly directive! Theraplay is probably the most directive approach to play therapy, rivaled only by ecosystemic play therapy.

a. Creating space or using structured techniques in play therapy?

Theraplay is very directive, with every session filled to the brim with activities the therapist brings into the session. Theraplay is done in an uncluttered room, with a blanket or mat on the floor and pillows or cushions for participants to sit on. The therapist brings in selected materials and props (e.g., feathers, lotion, powder, cotton balls) for specific structured activities. The Theraplay therapist instructs caregivers on what to do to create a better relationship with the child, how to do it, and when to do it. Most of the session is taken up with the therapist modeling caregiving activities with the child, coaching the caregiver in ways of doing those caregiving activities with the child, and providing scaffolding, feedback, and encouragement for caregivers' efforts.

b. Playing with the client in play therapy?

Theraplay therapists play with children mostly to model attuned caregiver behavior for parents/caregivers. The ultimate goal is for the caregiver to do the "playing with" to practice this kind of behavior so that he or she can generalize, providing structure, nurturing, engagement, and challenge to the child.

12. Work with parents? teachers?

(This one should be totally obvious, and in service of being complete, we will still answer the question . . .) *Yes!* The Theraplay model absolutely requires the participation of at least one caregiver (usually a parent, but it could be a foster parent, grandparent, or guardian). Theraplay therapists work with teachers only on rare occasions.

INTEGRATIVE/PRESCRIPTIVE PLAY THERAPY

Prescriptive play therapy is a method of play therapy that uses a variety of theories and techniques as a way of creating a customized play therapy intervention designed to meet the specific needs of clients (Schaefer & Drewes, 2016). The proponents of integrative/prescriptive play therapy make the case that this approach has led to "exploration of change agents or competencies within psychotherapeutic models that cause positive therapy outcomes, as well as to the need for clinical flexibility in conducting comprehensive assessments that can identify treatment areas that can benefit from specific interventions" (Gil, Konrath, Shaw, Goldin, & Bryan, 2015, p. 111).

While many play therapists are beginning to apply this approach to play therapy (Kenney-Noziska, Schaefer, & Homeyer, 2012), we believe it can, at times, be the opposite of having a "systematic use of a theoretical model," which is where we started in this chapter. Prescriptive therapy can take two forms: systematic and intentional application of specific interventions designed to target selected problems or "kitchen sink" eclecticism (Norcross, 2005). Integrative/prescriptive play therapy can be a complex method of coming up with an organized way of thinking about clients and how to work with them by integrating several different approaches to play therapy. If you opt to do that, it is essential to explore whether the philosophical assumptions underlying the theories you want to integrate are congruent with one another. Otherwise, you wind up with "kitchen sink" eclecticism, in which you randomly apply techniques without understanding why you are choosing to do the things you are doing in the playroom.

1. What do you believe about the basic nature of people? Good (positive, self-actualizing, etc.), bad (negative, irrational, evil, etc.), or neutral? Or some combination?

   (You are going to love this . . . or maybe not . . . and the answer to every one of our questions for this approach to play therapy is, "It depends . . .") It depends on the play therapist and on the theoretical approach he or she has selected to use at that particular stage of therapy with that specific client who has that identifiable presenting problem.

2. How are personalities formed/constructed?

   a. What factors influence the formation of personality?

      It depends on the play therapist and on the theory he or she has selected to use at that particular stage of therapy with that specific client who has that identifiable presenting problem.

   b. Nature/nurture?

      It depends . . .

   c. Free will or determinism?

      It depends . . .

   d. Thinking, feeling, and behaving?

      It depends . . .

   e. Basic motivation for behavior?

      It depends . . .

   f. Basic components of personality?

      It depends . . .

3. Perception of reality—subjective or objective?

> It depends . . .

4. Role of therapeutic relationship?

> It depends . . .

5. Focus on the past, the present in the context of the past, or only the present?

> It depends . . .

6. Need insight/increased consciousness to make changes?

> It depends . . .

7. Primary focus in counseling?

> It depends . . .

8. Psychological maladjustment?

> It depends . . .

9. Goals of counseling?

> It depends . . .

10. Measuring progress?

> It depends . . .

11. Directive or nondirective?

> It depends . . .

> > a. Creating space or using structured techniques in play therapy?
> >
> > > It depends . . .
> >
> > b. Playing with the client in play therapy?
> >
> > > It depends . . .

12. Work with parents? teachers?

> It depends . . .

MOVING ON . . .

Wow! You *rock*! We are impressed and appreciative that you are still with us. Remember that at the beginning of this chapter we said that the ultimate goal in the quest to find a "play therapy home" is for you to ponder which of the available choices of theoretical approaches might be a close match with your personal beliefs, convictions, and inclinations. We also want to remind you that we have not covered every possible approach to play therapy, so if your answer is truly "none of the above," don't give up. Keep searching—use our questions and your researching skills to find answers for yourself among the other approaches to play therapy. And keep your answers to these questions and the possible approaches to play therapy in mind throughout the rest of the book because the how, when, and if you use the skills and techniques presented will flow from your theoretical orientation and how you think people grow, change, and become healthier.

Interlude 2
Showing Interest

*W*e know—we have kind of already mentioned the whole "showing interest" thing with our description of the Four-Fold Way, *and* we created this interlude because we want to emphasize showing interest as a play therapy tool because it is so important. We want to describe some specific methods for showing interest, and we want to identify some examples of particular topics you should know well enough to be able to credibly show interest. You can ask open questions; learn about topics that are significant to specific clients and be ready to talk about them in your sessions; match client affect with your voice and nonverbal communication; and use intonation and body language to convey enthusiasm.

- Ask open questions. Now, this is a tricky one because we want to remind you that we are not doing talk therapy in the playroom *and* we think it is helpful to give yourself permission to ask questions. While we believe it is okay to ask questions, we also think it is essential to make them count. So, limit yourself to four to six powerful questions per session. (We also want to acknowledge that some approaches to play therapy would hold asking questions to be inappropriate, even anathema.) Questions should focus on showing interest in (1) the people in clients' lives (i.e., who is important to the client, what makes those people important, who do clients find nurturing, who do clients find irritating, and so forth); (2) current events in clients' lives that are affecting them (the good, the bad, and the ugly); and (3) how clients spend their time (i.e., work, school, video games, sports, community theatre events, extracurricular activities, etc.).

• Learn about the things that are important to clients and be ready to talk about them in your sessions. (Even if you are not interested—if the clients are interested, you need to learn about them.) This might mean watching special television shows, learning about (and maybe even playing) video games, reading the books they are reading, going to the movies they mention, checking out comic books they like, and so forth. We want to acknowledge that this will take time (and maybe cost money). (We don't believe that just asking clients to teach you about these things is adequate. While it does set clients up as "expert," we believe this suggests to them that you don't care enough about them to make the effort to learn about the things that are important to them.)

• Match clients' affect with your voice and posture. (We are pretty sure this got covered in the training you have had up until this point, so we don't want to beat a dead aardvark.) Both of us have noticed that many play therapists struggle with matching their own nonverbal communication with client affect. In watching videotapes and live supervision with our students, we have observed that many play therapists tend to think they need to be perky and happy (or even sing-songy) when they interact with clients in play therapy, especially with younger children. In service of conveying interest, it is essential to match clients' affect with your voice and your posture, especially when they are sad, disappointed, irritated, and so forth—those feelings that tend to be labeled as "negative." This means that you also need to manage your own feelings—sometimes play therapists are uncomfortable with these feelings, and often they seem to think they need to rescue clients and not let them experience those emotions.

• Use nonverbals to convey enthusiasm. (We know you know these—the old leaning forward, making eye contact stuff. And we want you to do all that and to communicate enthusiasm about the things that are important to your clients through your voice and posture. Now, we know this could contradict what we just said . . . but we aren't talking about times when clients are sad, mad, depressed, and so forth.) When clients come to a session excited about something, it is important to jump on the enthusiasm bandwagon. Sometimes when clients act things out (or talk about things) that the play therapist finds uninteresting, some play therapists act bored or disconnected. We want to make clear that we aren't asking you to fake enthusiasm; we are suggesting you find it in yourself to connect with clients' positive energy. For instance, if you are working with a child who loves Shopkins™, you can get excited because she is excited; if you are working with a teen who is super-proud about a high kill/death ratio on *Call of Duty*, you need to get behind that accomplishment.

CHAPTER 3

Broad Play Therapy Strategies

In any of the stages of play therapy, play therapists have available to them several different broad play therapy strategies that they can use. With some of these strategies (sand tray and art especially), you will need specialized training to be competent using them with clients. We both use strategies borrowed from a wide variety of disciplines in our play therapy. Though we have specialized training in dance, art, adventure therapy, and sand tray, we are not art therapists, dance therapists, or music therapists; we are play therapists who use techniques that would fall into these realms. These broad strategies are atheoretical, so you will need to adapt them to your own theoretical orientation. The strategies we use generally fall into the following categories: adventure therapy, storytelling and therapeutic metaphors, movement/dance/music experiences, sand tray activities, art techniques, and structured play experiences. We provide you an overview of these strategies in this chapter, and then in every chapter that focuses on a particular stage of play therapy, we give you several techniques that fit into each strategy.

ADVENTURE THERAPY

Adventure therapy is "the use of games, activities, initiatives, and peak experiences to facilitate the development of group process, interpersonal relationships, personal growth, and therapeutic gain" (Ashby et al., 2008, p. 1). Adventure techniques can be conceptualized and explained from a variety of theoretical viewpoints. This is lovely from our perspective since we want you to think about how you would frame all of the methods we describe in this book filtered through your own theoretical orientation.

You can tailor how you introduce, facilitate, and process the activities depending on the objectives you want to accomplish, and depending on your clients and what you think will "grab" them. You can do adventure therapy activities with individuals, groups, families, children, teens, and adults. You can use adventure therapy techniques to give clients an experience that can lead to a discussion, or you can have the experience stand alone, with the learning coming from the doing (Kottman, Ashby, & DeGraaf, 2001). (After all, we *are* doing *play* therapy.) When using them with families and groups, in addition to being directed toward specific therapeutic goals, they also create collective good times that can help members experience shared fun (putting positive energy into their family/group energy bank). Adventure activities should always be used *both* as interventions and assessment for group members, family members, and individuals. At the same time you are conducting an activity aimed at achieving a specific goal with clients, you should also be paying attention to how clients act while doing the activity, which can tell you a huge amount about clients and how they solve problems, communicate, resolve conflict, and so on.

Adventure therapy activities can be grouped into four distinct broad categories (with some overlap) as identified by Schoel and Maizell (2002): ice-breakers, deinhibitizers, trust/empathy builders, and challenge initiatives/problem-solving activities. This is the order in which we usually sequence these activities if we are doing several in one session or across several sessions. If you have already made a connection and have built trust through other vehicles, you don't have to rely on adventure therapy to do that—you can jump to using challenge initiatives/problem-solving activities to help clients learn and/or practice making changes. Each adventure therapy activity can be done as a stand-alone method for accomplishing a specific goal or as part of a sequential process designed to move clients forward.

Ice-breakers are fun and success-oriented. The tasks can be easily accomplished with the minimal amount of frustration, and they require a minimal amount of verbal interaction and decision-making skills. With individual clients and in family play therapy, ice-breakers help clients to establish a connection with the play therapist in the relationship-building phase. With groups, ice-breakers are designed to provide opportunities for clients to get to know one another and begin feeling comfortable with one another. Usually, ice-breakers are some kind of name game, like taking turns saying your name along with an adjective that describes you that starts with the same sound as your name (e.g., Terrific Terry and Kapable Kristin). (We do know that capable doesn't start with a *k*, but we couldn't think of an adjective that starts with *k* that would describe Kristin.)

Deinhibitizer activities involve some emotional and physical risk, which may arouse discomfort and frustration in clients. If you frame them correctly, success and failure are less important than trying and making a good effort. These are fun activities that allow clients to view themselves as more capable and confident in front of at least one other person (that would be you). Deinhibitizer activities provide opportunities for clients to take some risks and increase commitment and willingness to appear inept in front of others (even if the "other" is only you—their play therapist). If you are doing them in a group or family, you will want to create a cooperative and supportive atmosphere to encourage participation and increase confidence for all members. For example, Pairs Tag (an activity in which you play tag with one other person—when the other person tags you, you are "it," and when you tag the other person, he or she is "it") gets everybody hopping, and you use it in a group, with a family, or an individual client. They can be used to build relationships or to explore dynamics. Every once in a while, if you have an inhibited client, you might use these activities to help a client gain insight or to facilitate changes in a client's behavior by giving the client a chance to practice new behavioral, cognitive, or emotional patterns.

Trust and empathy activities provide an opportunity for clients to trust their physical and emotional safety to others (this could be you in sessions with individual clients or other group/family members) by taking some physical and/or emotional risks. Generally, trust/empathy activities are fun, *and* they evoke anxiety at the same time. (We know—this is a tricky thing to achieve, and we promise it is possible.) They require that the client trust you or other group or family members in order for everyone to be safe and secure. They also help build empathy for others as you switch off being the person who is trusting and the person who is being trusted. Our favorite activity in this category is Safety Cars (an activity described in Chapter 5). These activities are often used for exploring dynamics or for helping clients gain insight.

Challenge initiatives/problem-solving activities provide an opportunity for clients to effectively communicate, cooperate, and compromise with one another solving a problem. These activities are usually done with families or groups, and, with some imagination, you can figure out how to adapt them for individuals. By listening, cooperating, and compromising, members can work together to discover how to attain the goal of solving a specific problem, like turning a table cloth over with the entire family or group standing on it, or carrying a balloon wedged between the bodies of the members without touching it with their hands and without dropping it. Often leadership roles evolve in the attempt to solve the stated problem or reach the stated goal. We describe several of these activities in Chapter 7; they are often used to help clients make changes.

When using adventure therapy techniques, it is helpful to remember the following guidelines (Ashby et al., 2008; Kottman et al., 2001; Rohnke, 2004):

1. Monitor safety considerations. Always be aware of clients' emotional and physical safety.
2. Don't just explain; involve yourself in the activity. Demonstrate games whenever possible. This is one way to make sure that clients understand the instructions before beginning the activity.
3. Understand and know the rules of the game. Keep the rules to a minimum. When in doubt, let the client or group decide how to play. Bend some rules occasionally or change them. Invite clients to initiate or suggest rule changes.
4. If there is equipment, set it up before you begin. This can help you avoid having clients wait for you to get ready—a sure way to sabotage your activity before you even start.
5. Keep games fresh and new. Use objects that are unfamiliar to players. Make the familiar unfamiliar by modifying activities.
6. Be involved and enthusiastic. With individuals and with groups and families, you can decide to *play* once in a while. (Well, with individual clients, you are probably going to have to play, so get used to being silly and taking risks. We happen to believe you should be willing to do everything you ask clients to do or you should not ask it.)
7. Bring closure to each activity. Always quit an activity at the height of its popularity, ensuring that clients will want to play the game again if you choose to use it. If an activity is not working, move on to something else.
8. In a group or family, challenge and involve clients as much as possible. Emphasize competition against self when competition is necessary. Challenge clients to play fair.
9. In a group or family, keep clients playing. Don't include rules that permanently eliminate players. Find creative ways to get participants back in when playing elimination-type games.

As clients participate in adventure therapy activities, you will want to observe the following elements (Rohnke, 1991)—partly to help you understand the interpersonal and intrapersonal dynamics and partly to guide you if you decide you want to verbally process what happened in the activity with members.

• *Leadership and followership.* Who took the lead and why? How was this decided? Under what circumstances would this have happened differently? How did clients handle being the "follower"? Were they willing to empower the leader when they were following? (We have observed that, while the answers to these questions might be clearer in groups and families, they can even be observed with individual clients.)

• *Support.* What is it? Where does it come from? In a group or family, how is support established? How does it shift from member to member?

How is it communicated? How would members like the communication to change or improve?

- *Pressure.* Does it have a helpful or harmful effect? When? What determines whether it is helpful or harmful? How is it conveyed? How is it perceived? In a group or family, where does it originate? Are there patterns in how it develops?

- *Negativism–hostility.* How does the client express it? Why is it there? How did you deal with it? What are the patterns that occur as to who expresses it, and who is the object of it? (Hopefully it won't be you radiating negativity or hostility—that would be bad.) How does negativism relate to what happens in the daily life of members?

- *Competition.* Does it occur against self, against you, another team, a nebulous group, or the record? What is the client's comfort level with each of these agents? How can you use competition in a helpful way?

- *Fear/anxiety.* What did the client fear? Were fears physical and/or psychological? How did the client deal with fears? How did you and/or other members help/hinder? What did the client need to help with fears and anxieties?

- *Joy and pleasure.* What was fun? How was joy/pleasure communicated? What made it fun? How could it have been more fun?

- *Carry over.* How are these fabricated problems related to real life? How can you make a bridge for clients so that they can think about applying what they learned in their lives outside the playroom?

STORYTELLING AND THERAPEUTIC METAPHORS

One of the broad directive play therapy strategies you can use to help clients gain insight and/or make changes is that of storytelling and therapeutic metaphors. (If you use your imagination, you might also be able to use this strategy to build a relationship and explore dynamics with clients.) By telling a story, reading a book, or helping the client shift a metaphor from a negative one to a positive one, you can allow the client to keep a safe distance from difficult material and still communicate important concepts or skills. That way the client can get the learning from a story even while continuing to pretend that the story is not about him or her. Rather than using generic stories, we believe it is helpful to custom-design your stories or therapeutic metaphors based on what you know about specific clients and their issues. In all forms of storytelling in play therapy, remember that you can have your characters be people, robots, bunnies and foxes, alien creatures, and so on and so forth—anything that will work with specific clients. We use several different types of storytelling and therapeutic metaphors: therapeutic stories (Kottman & Meany-Walen,

2016; Mills & Crowley, 2014), mutual storytelling (Gardner, 1993; Kottman & Meany-Walen, 2016), co-telling stories, specific change metaphors (Lankton & Lankton, 1989), Creative Characters (Brooks, 1981; Kottman & Meany-Walen, 2016), bibliotherapy (Malchiodi & Ginns-Gruenberg, 2008; Karges-Bone, 2015), and metaphor shifting. You would usually use co-telling stories for building the relationship with the client, listening to the client's story portion of mutual storytelling for exploring the client's interpersonal and intrapersonal dynamics. This broad strategy is most often used to help the client gain insight and make shifts in maladaptive patterns.

MOVEMENT, DANCE, AND MUSIC EXPERIENCES

Quite a few of the children, adolescents, and adults who come to play therapy are kinesthetic/tactile learners or are just people who like to move. We have noticed (yes, we have been paying attention) that many play therapy techniques that communicate using visual or auditory channels are not particularly effective with these clients. By incorporating dance and movement (and, with some folks, music—which quite frequently goes along with dance and movement but doesn't have to if you have clients who don't love music), you can help clients with sensory integration issues, ADHD, behavior problems, communication difficulties, learning disabilities, social skills deficits, and mood disorders. You can also use these strategies to work with clients who are uncomfortable with or in their bodies. Again, these strategies can be used as both assessment and intervention. You can use them to assess clients' capacity for relationships, body image, self-confidence, creativity, self-regulation, comfort with their bodies, and problem solving. As interventions, these dance, movement, and music techniques can help clients discover their feelings, attitudes, and patterns of behavior; access their body's wisdom; practice new ways of interacting with others; build trust; share control; increase cooperation, handle problem situations; and enhance their relationships with others (Devereux, 2014; LeFeber, 2014).

It is important to remember that some clients will freak out if you ask them to move using the word "dance," just like some clients will have a pretty significantly negative reaction if you ask them to write poetry, even though asking those same clients to move some magnetic words around on a metal background (yes—magnetic poetry, one of our favorite play therapy tactics with teens) doesn't faze them. So, you just need to remember to call what you want them to do "moving" instead of "dancing."

Depending on specific clients and their inclinations, you can use music with your movements/dances, or you can do them without music. We find that many older children, teens, and adults like to bring music into sessions or request that we get specific music for them. Sometimes we also use a drum in our playrooms to lay down rhythms for clients to have a beat for dancing, or we invite clients to lay down rhythms for us.

You will want to tailor whether you participate in the dancing to the individual client. (As you know, the answer to every question that starts with "Should I . . ." is "It depends . . .") There are some clients who are self-conscious or hesitant who would benefit from your modeling, allowing yourself to be in your body and freely expressing yourself with movement. (We also want to point out that you might not be comfortable being in your body and freely expressing yourself with movement—work on that.) There are other clients who would compare themselves to you, and if you are an accomplished dancer, they might decide they can't meet your dancing standards and won't want to take that risk. There are yet other clients who enjoy dancing with others but do not like to dance alone, and other clients who only like to dance by themselves. It is helpful to examine both the product (the dance or movement) and the process (the act of generating the movement) to help clients understand what there is to learn from participating in these activities.

We see the dance and movement strategies that you can incorporate into your play therapy as being-with dances, releasing dances, celebrating dances, invoking dances, connecting dances, practicing dances, and storytelling dances. (We made these labels up; they are not official categories from any discipline.) Connecting dances are described in Chapter 4 since they are used as a vehicle for building the relationship with clients, and storytelling dances are described in Chapter 5 because they can be a way to explore clients' dynamics. We describe the being-with, releasing, celebrating, invoking, and practicing dances in Chapter 7 because we use them mainly for helping clients make changes. You can use them anywhere in the process where they work best for you and your clients.

SAND TRAY PLAY THERAPY

Our name for what we do with this broad strategy is sand tray play therapy—it is a method of using small toys and a sand tray as a vehicle for exploration and expression in play therapy. We think of this process as clients choosing figures from a collection of miniatures and putting them into a tray of sand. (We recognize that this is a bit less formal than many approaches to sand tray and acknowledge that, depending on your theoretical orientation, you might be more formal about this process than we are.) Sand tray play therapy works well with clients who think symbolically (since the figures are meant to represent people, events, ideas, relationships, and so forth from clients' lives). We often think of it as an activity similar to art therapy for folks who prefer choosing and placing objects in the sand rather than generating some kind of artistic creation. You can do sand tray play therapy with just a few figures to represent important categories (people, animals, vegetation, buildings, vehicles, household objects, fences and signs, natural objects, fantasy characters, spiritual or mythical creatures, and outside structures) (see Homeyer & Sweeney, 2017, for lists of things you could include), or you can have many, many, many, many figures to represent each category. (If you decided to go this route, remember: we cannot be held responsible for creating or feeding your new addiction.) There are many different ways of arranging your figures on shelves—you should explore the suggestions made by a variety of experts and decide on the one that works for you (for examples, see Boik & Goodwin, 2000; Carey, 2008; DeDomenico, 1995; Turner, 2005).

When we work with clients using sand tray play therapy, we use the following steps adapted from *Sandtray: A Practical Manual* (Homeyer & Sweeney, 2017): (1) you prepare the room/prepare yourself for the process, (2) you introduce the sand tray to the client, (3) the client creates the sand tray, (4) you guide the client in experiencing and rearranging the tray, (5) the client gives a tour of the tray, (6) you help the client process (and potentially rearrange) the tray, (7) you or the client document the tray, and (8) you and/or the client dismantle the tray. To prepare the room/prepare yourself for the process of creating the sand tray, you will want to look through your collection of miniature figures, making sure that the figures are in their usual places. To prepare yourself, you will want to make sure you are calm and centered—your role in the sand tray creation is usually weighted toward being a witness to the client and his or her process, rather than being an active participant like you would be in many of the adventure therapy, dance and movement, and storytelling activities.

By introducing the sand tray to the client, we mean that you are going to suggest topics for this particular tray. You can be nondirective in your introduction (e.g., "Create your world," "Pick whatever you want to include in the tray and put it in the tray," or "Pick figures that attract you and/or figures that repel you, and put them in the tray." Or you can be much more specific and directive (e.g., "Pick figures to be each of the people in your family, and put them into the tray," or "Pick figures to represent your boss, several co-workers, and yourself at work," "Pick figures to show me how you feel about math and your math teacher."). Depending on how we think clients will respond, we usually give them a couple of choices of topics. Sometimes we limit the degree of directiveness to just asking clients to do a tray, and we let them pick the topic. [Of course, we always use developmentally appropriate language they will understand—if you are working with Aki, a 6-year-old, he might not understand "attract and/or repel," and you will have to make your directive simpler.]

Next you step aside and let the client "have at it" as in "the client creates the sand tray" stage. (We're not sure what else to say about this; they pick the figures and place them in the tray . . . you watch them to observe how they do it—which figures they treat gently, which they pick up and put back down, what their body language conveys as they choose, and so forth.)

After they have done the picking and placing, you will want to guide them to "experience" the tray, by which we mean you ask them to sit with the tray for a little while, just taking it in, and then you would suggest that they move around the tray, looking at it from all the sides so that they can see what is in the tray from different vantage points. After they have done this, we ask them whether they would like to rearrange the tray by asking, "Sometimes at this place in the process clients like to move things around in the tray, take some things out or put other things into the tray. Would you like to do that?" (We say it this way to avoid implying that we see something wrong with the tray and they should fix it by rearranging things.)

When they have completed this process, you will want to move them on to the "touring" of the tray. (When I [Terry] first learned sand tray, I was taught to ask clients to "give me a tour" of the tray—while my adolescent and adult clients quickly complied with this, my child clients looked at me with blank faces, so now I tell them to "tell me about what is in the tray." That works much better for me.)

In some cases, clients will process the tray (talk about what it means) while they give you a tour, but this does not always happen, so sometimes you need to scaffold the processing. If clients need a jumpstart, we usually use what we call the "I notice . . ." technique, which is when you simply verbalize that you are noticing things in the tray. (While it might take some self-restraint not to be interpretive, we like to start off simple and give clients a chance to come up with meaning before we jump in and make interpretations.) The "I notice" technique involves pointing out things like (1) spacing (e.g., how far apart are the figures? are there patterns in the placement of figures? which figures are closer together? are there figures that are separate from the majority of the figures?); (2) relative size of items; (3) an item being moved by the client from one place to another; (4) buried items; (5) a figure or figures that stand out in some way (e.g., is one of them different from the other figures? does it seem that there is an unexpected placement of one or more figures in the tray?); (6) orientation of figures (e.g., who/what is facing toward the outside of the tray? who/what is facing some other figure? who/what is facing away from some other figure? are some of the figures upright, and are others placed flat in the tray?); (7) grouping of figures (e.g., are there clear groupings of figures? which figures are placed in each group? what do the figures in the group have in common? how are the groups different from one another?); (8) patterns of the chosen figures or the arrangement of the figures in the tray; and (9) the affective tone of the tray—what sets that tone? You can do this processing directly or metaphorically.

Directly means labeling the person or relationship the figure is representing, whereas metaphorically means using the name of the figure rather than the name of what the figure is representing.

If, at the end of the "I notice" part of the processing, you have questions that haven't been answered by clients' responses to your noticing, depending on your theoretical orientation, you can ask questions about the process of doing the tray and/or what is in the tray. Those questions tend to be guided by the same kinds of things you look at when you are using "I notice." In addition, if you have observations you want to share with clients, you can move to the interpretation section by using tentative hypotheses or "soft" interpretations about the meaning of these various elements of the tray. Your interpretations are going to depend on your theoretical orientation because each approach to play therapy has distinctly different ideas about what is important to help clients understand through the sand tray process. This can often lead to a lively give-and-take with clients, which looks a little like talk therapy. You can take care of these parts of the processing either directly or metaphorically. When you are done with the verbal processing, you can again ask clients if they want to rearrange the tray now in the context of what they have discovered. More processing might evolve if clients want to rearrange things. (We also want to acknowledge that you will have clients who don't want or need to explore the meaning of the tray or what they have put in it. There's no need to get your knickers in a knot about this—many people get exactly what they need from the tray simply through the process of creating it.)

In the "olden days," we used a Polaroid camera to take a photograph of trays (well, I [Terry] did). Documenting trays has become a bit easier with the advent of cell phones with cameras. Our older clients often just take a picture with their cell phones for their personal use, and we usually take a digital picture if we want an image of the tray for their files. When it comes to dismantling the tray, there are again many different choices as to how to proceed, depending on your theoretical orientation. Jungians generally wait to dismantle the tray after clients have left the session. As Adlerians, we give clients the choice of dismantling the tray themselves, working together as a team to dismantle the tray, or having us dismantle it while they are still in the playroom or dismantle it after they have left.

ART STRATEGIES

Most play therapists use some art strategies in the playroom. Many clients spontaneously fashion artistic creations, and others need to be invited to create. There are a bazillion resources describing art techniques you can use with clients to explore feelings, relationships, and cognitions; understand interpersonal or intrapersonal dynamics; gain insight into their patterns; set up a way for them to practice new behaviors or attitudes; and so forth (e.g., Brooke, 2004; Buchalter, 2009; Malchiodi, 2007, 2015). Strangely enough, art techniques seem to work better with clients who like to do art. We always invite clients to create something artistic in one of our early sessions to assess their willingness to participate in artistic projects. It is often helpful to give clients several different choices of modality as part of this assessment because different forms of art appeal to different people. We tend to think of the categories of artistic expression that work best in the playroom as drawing or painting, creating images with stickers, constructing, sculpting, collaging, and making puppets or masks. (We decided we couldn't get away with calling creating images with stickers "stickering.")

You can use many different materials in setting up drawing or painting with clients. For drawing, you can use just regular pencils, fat markers, skinny markers, colored pencils, pastels or charcoal, and oil pastels. For painting, you can use tempera paints, acrylic paints, watercolors, and finger paints. We like to give clients choices of materials for doing the art. While the significance of the clients' choice is more the purview of specialists in art therapy who have the training to discern the meaning of material choice, we like to notice whether clients choose a medium that is messy or neat, precise or inexact. We are always looking for patterns that can tell us something about how clients tend to express themselves.

If you are directive in your approach to play therapy, this is another area in which you can be directive in a broad way (i.e., "It's time to paint a picture. You can choose what you want to paint.") or directive in a more specific way by giving your clients a choice of subjects (i.e., "You can choose whether you are going to draw everyone in your family or just draw your favorite person in your family and your least favorite person in your family," or "Pretend you are a princess. Paint the castle you would want for the place where you live or the carriage that would drive you to places where you would want to go," or "You are a mad scientist. Draw or paint a picture of the creature you would create."). When we set up the creating, we usually suggest that clients get to choose whether they want to be representational (i.e., "The thing you are drawing can look like you think that thing looks in real life.") or nonrepresentational ("The thing you are drawing doesn't have to look like you think that thing looks in real life—you can just use colors, shapes, and textures if you want to show it.").

With clients who like to verbally process, the conversation after the art project is completed can focus on either the process of the creating or the product that was created, or both—depending on the inclination of specific clients and on your own theoretical orientation. We tend to invite clients to talk about both the process and the product, and we usually start the processing by doing the "I notice" thing we do with sand trays, then moving into any questions we have and interpretations we might want to share. (We tend to be pretty sparse with interpretation because we don't believe in universal symbolism, so we think that each person is going to attribute his or her own meaning to the artistic creation.)

We have recently noticed (okay, really over the past 10 years we have noticed) that many clients are reluctant to draw or paint, so we have started letting folks use stickers, which seems to feel safer/less risky for them. We just give them a selection of stickers, an assignment of what we want them to make or represent, and let them choose stickers and put them on a piece of paper. Then we do the same procedure that we would do with a sand tray, drawing, or painting. (We know you are not going to believe this, but that is all we have to say about this subject—we just wanted to offer this format as a possibility.)

Actually, both of us love constructing things and find it is a strategy that is especially effective with that hard-to-engage population: boys between the ages of 10 and 14. It also works particularly well with clients who have ADHD. We find that those two groups of clients (and lots of other clients, including teens and adults, so don't avoid using this strategy with others) like to build things. We use a variety of commercially available construction materials that are specifically meant for building (Legos, Tinker Toys, Lincoln Logs) and stuff that you can find around your house, like recyclables (recycled egg cartons, Styrofoam take-out cartons and boxes, pill containers), toothpicks, pipe cleaners, popsicle sticks, straws, tongue depressors, and so forth.

For sculpting, we make papier mache from flour and water, and we buy clay, Model Magic, Play-Doh, Sculpey, and other similar materials. Again, we either give clients a general directive (e.g., "Make something with this") or a specific directive (e.g., "Build a snow man that is melting because she is sad," "Make a bridge that could take you from your current feelings of depression to the joy that you say you want to feel," or "Build a robot who would do whatever you wanted."). We might try a generic directive first and see how that goes, then shift to a more targeted directive that would depend heavily on whatever we are trying to accomplish with specific clients.

Collaging works better with adolescents and adults than it does with younger children, partly because it requires specialized motor skills. (Yes, by "specialized motor skills" we mean cutting with scissors and gluing.) Also, the amount of time required to go through magazines, cutting out words and images, means you cannot usually complete a collage in one session, which is difficult for young children who frequently do not deal well with having projects extend across several sessions. One way we get around the extended time problem is having a folder full of already-cut-out photographs from magazines in our offices, which can cut down on the time requirements of collaging. (And we want to acknowledge that we have "lots" of spare time for cutting images and words out of magazines, and you might not.) Again, you can ask clients to make collages that are general (i.e., "Go through and pick images that attract and/or repel you.") or targeted (i.e., "Choose one of these animal photographs for each person in your family," "Choose words that might tell me something about your personality," or "Choose photographs that show what you want in a friend."). You would process collages the same way you would process sand trays, paintings, or drawings.

Making puppets and/or masks is an art strategy that works well with all populations of clients who come to play therapy. You can invite clients to do really simple puppets or masks, using materials like paper plates, paper bags, and markers or crayons. You can up the complexity by adding other materials such as glitter, glitter glue, jewels, and beads, along with paper plates, paper bags, foam sheets, old (clean, of course) socks (for puppets), or commercially available masks. With older clients, you can make puppets on a base of a wooden spoon decorated with yarn, ribbon, glitter, jewels, beads, and material.

You can ask clients to make puppets that represent themselves or other people in their lives; you can ask them to make puppets that represent their past selves, their future selves, their best selves, their worst selves, their ideal best friend, their least favorite person in the world, and so on and so forth. You are only limited by your own imagination in this process.

When working with older clients (ages 10 and up), you can make more complex masks by putting plaster gauze like they used to make casts for broken arms onto a wig head and either painting it or decorating it when it is dried. (If you have a microwave in your office, you can even dry it and decorate it in a single session—just don't blow the wig head up. First, cover the wig head with petroleum jelly. Then, dip the plaster gauze into some water, squeeze the excess water off the gauze, and layer the gauze on the wig head. Put the wig head into the microwave, run it on high for 4 minutes, take it out, and wave it around for a minute to cool it off, then repeat once or twice.) (We recognize that some clinicians actually put the plaster gauze directly on clients' faces and make a mask with their actual features, but I (Terry) was once in a therapy group in which the counselor was guiding the members through this process and one of the members had a panic attack. Ever since then, wig heads seem like a good idea to me.) We know you are not going to be surprised at this, and you can do a more general directive (e.g., "Make a mask.") or a more targeted directive (e.g., "On the outside, depict the face you show the world and on the inside, depict the face you keep to yourself," "On the outside use a Sharpie to write the things you tell yourself when you are feeling optimistic and on the inside, write the things you tell yourself when you are feeling discouraged," or "Make a mask that shows what your brother looks like when he is doing things that hurt your feelings."). Again, you can do your verbal processing (with clients who respond well to this procedure) about the act of making the puppet or mask and/or the product; this processing can be direct or metaphoric.

STRUCTURED PLAY EXPERIENCES

Structured play experiences are pretty much exactly what that label implies—play experiences that you introduce and structure, as opposed to free play. You can do these activities with individual clients (usually children or teens), groups, or families. With individual clients, you can use structured play activities as an assessment process designed to help you understand clients' intrapersonal or interpersonal dynamics, as a vehicle for helping clients gain insight, or as a way to help clients make changes. Structured play experiences can be simple things like playing pitch and catch or blowing bubbles up to more elaborate activities like puppet shows, role-plays, tabletop games, and scenarios done in the doll house or kitchen area.

MOVING ON . . .

You might want to ponder which of these broad strategies appeal to you.

- Which ones might fit into the theoretical orientation that best fits your own beliefs and interactional style?
- Which ones sound like they might be fun to do with clients?
- Which ones sound as though they might be helpful to the clients with whom you want to work?
- Which ones sound like interventions you would like to further explore?

In order to make it easier for you to find the types of activities that most interest you, we have organized the following chapters to highlight each of these strategies—all of the techniques described for each of the four phases of play therapy are arranged under the heading of one of the broad strategies. So, for example, if you are particularly drawn to adventure therapy, you can find several different adventurous techniques for building the relationship with clients, several for exploring clients' dynamics, several for helping clients gain insight, and several for helping clients make changes.

Enjoy . . .

Interlude 3

Being Intentional with Your Interventions and Making "Stuff" Up

$\mathcal{B}$eing intentional with your interventions in your work in the playroom is incredibly important. For many nondirective play therapists, this is relatively easy to do because they are basically going to do the same thing with every client—they are going to use the basic skills of play therapy (tracking, restating content, reflecting feelings, returning responsibility to the client, limiting) to build a relationship and create a space that will activate the client's natural tendency toward positive growth and change. For more directive play therapists, this becomes more difficult because they use techniques and activities in their play therapy sessions in addition to (or instead of) these basic skills. We believe it is essential to choose those techniques and activities carefully, based on where play therapists want to go with the client. We want to encourage play therapists to really think about what they want to accomplish in a particular session and in their overall work with specific clients. Many times, directive play therapists fall into a pattern of using the same activity or technique with every client—the "I learned this at this workshop last weekend, and I am going to do it with every client," or the "let's throw it against the wall and see what sticks" approach to play therapy.

We want to encourage you to avoid doing this and to use what you observe about the client and what is important to the client to choose specific activities to try with him or her and to adapt activities to meet his or her needs. By attending to whether this particular client likes to do art and how (painting? drawing? using stickers? building things? doing crafts?); the topics the client brings up to discuss (video games? sports? robotics? board games? skate boarding?); the ways the client expresses him- or herself (dancing? doing puppet shows? making sand trays? playing with figures or the doll house? drumming and making music?), you can be intentional in designing and delivering your play therapy interventions.

Big A agenda, small a agenda . . . is a phrase I (Terry) learned in a co-active leadership program created by the Coaches Training Institute. Your Big A agenda for therapy is made up of your long-range goals and objectives toward which you are constantly moving with your clients—it involves you keeping in mind (over many sessions) where you are trying to take the client. Your small a agenda is your tentative plan for what you want to do in your session. Since it is essential to meet clients where they are when they come to a session, you will need to be flexible and unattached to following your small a agenda—it is a tentative plan, based on what you know before the session begins. Depending on what is happening in your clients' lives, you may have to discard your exact plan, adjusting what you want to do according to what clients need in the moment. You should be locked in to moving toward your Big A agenda (with, of course, an understanding that the Big A agenda might need to change as clients and their circumstances change), and your commitment to your small a agenda should be much more fluid.

We think part of what makes a really good play therapist is the willingness and ability to "make stuff up." One of our discoveries as we have taught play therapy and have supervised play therapists over the years is that many very creative, inventive, fun people who get trained as play therapists stop being very creative, inventive, and (sometimes even) fun after they are trained. We have also noticed that play therapy interventions really are never "one size fits all." This means that, in addition to originating new interventions, you may also need to customize other ones you already know. And it means that it is also super important to custom-design the ones you are making up for that client you have in today's play therapy session.

We want to invite you to (nay, exhort you to) let go of your old, restrictive ideas (rules even) about what play therapy is and let your imagination lead you into inventing activities and stories and dances and adventures for using with your clients in your playroom. So, to provide support for your ingenuity (in case all this freedom kind of freaks you out), we want to suggest some possibilities that can help structure your thoughts as you take the leap of faith involved in thinking you can invent stuff (or adapt it) to do that will meet your clients' needs. As you think about designing new interventions (or adapting ones you learned in other places, including in this book), ask yourself:

1. What is my understanding of how this client goes about connecting with others (including me)?
2. What do I know about what is important to this client?
3. What do I know about the interpersonal and intrapersonal dynamics of this client?
4. What am I trying to accomplish with this client? In this session (small a agenda)? What are my overall goals with this client (Big A agenda)?
5. What do I think is important for this client to learn in order to be successful in life (whatever that means with this particular client)?
6. What do I think is important for this client to practice in order to be successful in life (whatever that means with the particular client)?
7. How can I prioritize your treatment goals for the client? What will give me (and the client) the biggest bang for therapeutic buck at this time with this client?
8. What is going on with this client today, in this hour of therapy?
9. How does this client usually communicate? In metaphor or directly?
10. What are this client's rules about communicating about feelings?
11. What does this client do in the playroom (drawing, painting, other art strategies, puppets, figures, sand tray, stories, movement, music, projects, games, books)?
12. What are this client's usual thinking patterns? Abstract or concrete? Linear or tangential?

13. What is this client's best learning modality (or modalities)? Listening? Seeing? Doing? Moving? Some combination of the above?
14. What are the client's interests outside the playroom?

After you know the answers to some (or maybe all) of these questions (and you have asked other questions that come up for you that might also be important in customizing play therapy interventions), you can begin to make stuff up and try it out with clients. Remember, as long as you are being intentional with your interventions and paying attention to the impact your interventions are having on your client, it is unlikely that what you try will do anything harmful. And sometimes you have to exercise the courage to be imperfect and try something new.

CHAPTER 4

Building a Relationship

Despite theory-related differences in understanding human development and personality, and differences in the application of play therapy skills and techniques, play therapists across theoretical orientations pretty much all agree that a therapeutic relationship is a necessary component for the therapeutic process to be successful. The development of that therapeutic relationship is hard to define and describe, as many play therapists would attest that "doing" relationships is a part of who they are and not a cloak of skills they put on in order to meet a therapeutic objective. For many play therapists, relationship is a way of being.

We agree. Both of us naturally build relationships with others. (You might say it's one of our superpowers. We think there's a good chance that it is one of your superpowers too.) There are play therapists who have many innate skills and superpowers, *and* they still sometimes need a bit of guidance (which can just be specific play therapy skills, strategies, and techniques) to help them build relationships with clients (and to proceed through the other parts of the process as well). That's what this chapter is all about. . . .

USING THE FOUR-FOLD WAY IN PLAY THERAPY

Regardless of a person's inborn and/or learned relationship-building skills, we believe the following attitudes are necessary to foster a genuine, therapeutic relationship with clients. The Four-Fold Way is a set of principles developed by Arrien (1993) to describe the process of healing ourselves and living in harmony with others and the environment. Arrien believed that throughout the existence of humanity, all people (not just therapists) are connected and responsible for healing each other. The Four-Fold Way consists of four guidelines:

1. Show up and choose to be present.
2. Pay attention to what has heart and meaning.
3. Tell the truth without blame or judgment.
4. Be open to outcome, not attached to outcome.

Arrien is not a therapist, so her writing is not about being in a therapeutic relationship. It is about a way of life. When I (Terry) first read her book on the Four-Fold Way, I thought "I want to apply these principles in my family and friendships." As time passed and the principles permeated my nonwork life, I realized I was using them in my work relationships as well (with my colleagues and in my counseling, teaching, and supervision), and that they were super-helpful in those relationships. I teach them to all my play therapy students, so now we are teaching them to you.

Choose to Be Present

You have a choice. You can be completely attentive, involved, focused, and interested in the relationship between you and the client and all that your client is expressing; or you can check out, mentally tending to other interests or obligations (such as what you're fixing for dinner, who's going to win the game, or how you're going to take care of your ailing brother). To follow this guideline, it is essential to consider what you can control in the moment, and intentionally (remember our emphasis on being intentional?) make the choice to be present with your clients during your sessions.

We are not suggesting that other areas of your life are not important. In fact, we believe that to function optimally you must tend to all areas of your life. We also know from experience that when other things are pressing (i.e. personal or family illness, stress, and obligations) it is difficult to be present with clients. A strategy that I (Kristin) have found that works for me is making a list of areas in my life that demand my attention. Using Covey's (2013) matrix of urgent and important, I then prioritize and make plans on how to address each area. This helps me to put aside my other responsibilities and make the choice to be present with my clients. On the other hand, I (Kristin) am not quite so organized. I just decide that I am going to put all my personal concerns and thoughts away during my sessions so that I can focus on the client. You will need to find what works for you to be able to choose to be present with your clients.

Pay Attention to What Has Heart and Meaning

Play therapists listen with their ears, their eyes, their "guts," and their hearts. We notice what matters to clients. They might tell us or they might show us. Attuned play therapists also *feel* what the clients are sharing. We focus our attention on what is at the heart of clients' disclosures and expressions. Often, there will be obvious and directly stated points of importance such as parents' divorce, death of a pet, or being bullied at school, and there may also be a subtle, underlying current of emotions, attitudes, or beliefs that emerge from clients. Perhaps clients fear not belonging, being rejected, or being unimportant. Many clients, especially children, might not express these directly, mostly because it is out of their awareness or too abstract. It's the job of the play therapist to be attuned to these messages.

While we cannot give you specific ways of knowing exactly how the client is feeling or what has meaning to the client, we can give you some strategies that might help in noticing what has heart and meaning to your client. Pay attention to (1) recurrent themes or play patterns, (2) play disruptions (when a client abruptly stops doing some activity and moves to do something else), (3) consistent use of the same object in the playroom, (4) avoidance or attraction to particular activities or toys, and (5) how clients touch and hold objects. Probably the most important instrument you have for assessing what's important to your client is your own feelings and gut reactions. This comes with practice and taking the risk of trusting yourself. (Warning: be aware of your own "stuff" in order to differentiate your reaction from that of your client. Quite often, we have to do a self-check before we make the leap into believing whatever is going on is the client's, not ours.)

Tell the Truth without Blame or Judgment

Imagine for a moment that you are a child. How often do you hear information or get feedback without feeling blamed or judged? Wait! Even as an adult, how often do you get feedback without feeling blamed or judged? Probably not as frequently as you'd like. The play therapist's job in the relationship with a client is to notice. It's not our job to blame or judge. Blame or judgment could inhibit the client from expressing him- or herself in ways that disclose heart and meaning. We work intentionally to communicate empathy through our body language and verbal language.

"How do you do this?" you might ask. First, be sure that your voice tone and facial expressions are neutral. Try practicing with a friend who will give you honest feedback (without blame or judgment). You've heard of "counselor face." That is the nonjudgmental, unsurprised facial expression. Use that face frequently at the same time that you are careful to not appear disinterested or bored. (Easier said than done, right?) You also want the rest of your body language to be neutral because it is pretty easy to have body language that conveys disapproval.

Another suggestion is to make comments that start with sentence stems such as "I noticed . . ." This implies that you are really paying attention to what the client is doing without judgment. Statements like "I noticed you like to play with the elephant family." "I noticed you smiled when I came to the waiting room to get you," communicate that you are watching and not judging.

Sometimes it is also necessary to give honest feedback to clients. You can be truthful and impart your own reactions and feelings, your thoughts about how other people might be reacting to them, and your guesses about the possible consequences of their behavior without having an undertone of censure in your comments. For example, when you make comments such as "It's not fun for me to play games when I don't get to make any decisions. I wonder if there is a way for us to share in making decisions about how we play," "When you yell at the other students at the high school, they don't want to hang out with you." or "When you show up for work late, it is probably difficult for your boss to keep you working there," you can give feedback to clients. Again, you'll want to be sure to be nonjudgmental in your words, voice, facial expressions, and body language

Be Open to Outcome, not Attached to Outcome

As with many dimensions of therapy, being open to outcome is not as easy as it sounds. It can be quite difficult for therapists to trust the process and be okay when things do not turn out the way that they wished or had planned. This gets easier with time. This applies to what happens in a single session and what happens in the entire process. For those of you who are nondirective, you may sometimes go into sessions with ideas about how clients are going to be or act, and they may disappoint you. If you are following the guideline to be open to the unfolding, you will let go of that disappointment and work on letting go of your expectations. If you are a directive play therapist, you will probably go into sessions with an agenda. It is important to avoid getting attached to your planned activities and how they will work. Sometimes clients won't like the activities you have planned; many times clients won't react the way you expect or the techniques you have planned don't work the way you envisioned. It is essential to be open to the learning in whatever happens in your sessions. You always learn about clients, no matter how they react—you just might not learn what you thought you were going to learn. (And you always learn about yourself . . . just letting whatever unfolds unfold instead of rigidly insisting that you can control how others react or how activities work. So, chill.)

It is also important to be open to the unfolding of the entire play therapy process. It is a slow process and you cannot get impatient or judge your competence based on whether clients get better in the ways you want them to get better. In our experience, when we are fully open to trusting the process and being a witness and co-companion with the client, therapy is more fun! It is a journey in which we don't know what we will discover. We trust that whatever treasure emerges will be important and meaningful. Being attached to a particular set of outcomes interferes with the therapy process and stifles client and therapist creativity. Trust yourself, your clients, and the process.

PLAY THERAPY SKILLS

We've described our foundational guidelines for building therapeutic relationships with clients, so now we want to turn toward specific basic play therapy skills to use with clients in order to build and strengthen the relationship. According to Kottman (2011), most approaches to play therapy, whether they are directive or nondirective, use tracking, restating content, reflecting feelings, returning responsibility to the client, and setting limits to establish a relationship with clients. Some other approaches to play therapy also use encouraging clients, cleaning the room together, and playing with clients as a way to build the relationship with them.

Tracking

Tracking is a skill in which the play therapist describes what the client is doing (Kottman, 2011; Landreth, 2012; Ray, 2011; VanFleet et al., 2010). The goal of this skill is to communicate to the client that you are paying attention and you notice. This is similar to paraphrasing or using minimal encouragers in talk therapy. Beginning play therapists often state that they feel awkward and stiff when they use this skill. Rest assured, this becomes more natural over time. To use this skill, you describe what the client is doing and/or how the client is doing it. For example, "You moved it over there." "You used a lot of colors on that." "You moved that swiftly." You can also track from the perspective of the toys. "That moved over there" (tracking the behavior of the lion) or "He moved quickly." It is important to avoid labeling nouns so that the client can decide what he or she thinks the toy is, rather than you imposing your ideas about the identity of the toy on the client.

Restating Content

Restating content is the equivalent of paraphrasing in talk therapy (Glover & Landreth, 2016; Kottman, 2011; Landreth, 2012; Ray, 2011; VanFleet et al., 2010). You restate to the client what the client said. Avoid parroting (saying exactly what the client said), and attempt to reiterate in your own words what the client shared with you. If a client says, "I get to go to my dad's house tonight." You might say, "You get to go stay with your dad" or "You don't usually stay at your dad's house." You can also restate the content of the statements of the toys. If a wizard puppet says to the police officer puppet, "Go to jail. You have been a bad boy." the play therapist could restate content with, "He's in trouble for doing something against the rules." As with tracking, the goal of restating content is to convey to the client that you are paying attention and working to understand the content of the client's communication.

Reflecting Feelings

You guessed it! Reflecting feelings in play sessions is for the same purpose as reflecting feelings in talk therapy sessions (Glover & Landreth, 2016; Goodyear-Brown, 2010; Kottman, 2011; Landreth, 2012; Ray, 2011; VanFleet et al., 2010). The counselor reflects the overt feelings expressed by the client and/or the covert feelings communicated by the client. Play therapists make guesses about how a client feels if the client doesn't use a feeling word to describe him- or herself. Much like tracking or restating content, the play therapist can reflect either the client's feelings or the feelings of the toys. To a client who is smiling when you see her in the waiting room, you might say, "You're happy to be here." Or "You're looking forward to our time together." To a child who aggressively throws the trucks into the sandbox, you could say, "You're frustrated with that." Or "You don't like when things don't go your way." You could also reflect the feelings of the toys. If the baby elephant is snuggling with the big elephant you could say, "Awe, she really loves her mom." "The little one feels safe with that big one."

Returning Responsibility

Returning responsibility is a skill used to empower clients (Kottman, 2011; Kottman & Meany-Walen, 2016; Landreth, 2012; Ray, 2011). The play therapist believes clients are capable of making decisions and/or attempting tasks. This skill gently pushes clients to use and experience their own agency. It is important to avoid taking responsibility for making decisions for clients, and probably the best way to handle this is to return responsibility to them. An example would be a child who picks up a toy and says, "What is this?" The therapist empowers this child by saying, "In here, you can decide." or "You can decide what that is." If a teen client asks whether she should throw away a painting she made, the therapy could return responsibility by saying, "Seems like you're wondering what to do with that." By choosing not to do things for clients what they can do for themselves and returning responsibility to them, you can also empower them. For example, an adult client doesn't attempt to open the glitter glue and immediately hands it to the therapist, saying, "Will you open this?" A play therapist who is returning responsibility would say something like, "I think that is something you can do for yourself." If the therapist is not sure whether clients are capable of doing something, he or she might say, "Show me how you think this works." This way, the therapist still encourages clients to attempt the task and assesses their ability at that skill. In many cases, it would be easier for the therapist if he or she would give information or do something for clients, but this would not teach or empower them. We want to avoid reinforcing the idea that "others will do things for me." "I am helpless and unknowing." "It is better to ask for help than to make mistakes." Returning responsibility provides clients with the experience of making decisions and attempting the things for themselves.

Encouraging

Encouraging is a skill intended to help build internal locus of evaluation and motivation for clients (Kottman, 2011; Kottman & Meany-Walen, 2016; Nelsen, Nelsen, Tamborski, & Ainge, 2016). It takes the place of praise and other evaluative words and phrases. In praise, the therapist says things such as, "That's wonderful." "Great job!" "You did that just right." Praise focuses on the outcome and product of an activity or task. Encouragement focuses on the effort (e.g., "You worked really hard on that." "You put forth a lot of effort." "You didn't give up."), progress (e.g., "Yesterday you gave up and today you figured it out." "Last week that puzzle was too hard for you, and today you got it all put together."), client feelings about accomplishments (e.g., "You are really proud of doing well on that test." "You are happy that you tried jumping on the trampoline even though you were scared."), and the personal assets of clients (e.g., "You are a woman who knows how to get what you want." "You know how to paint pictures."). While several different approaches to play therapy use this skill, it particularly important in Adlerian play therapy. Other approaches, such as cognitive-behavioral play therapy, might use praise as a technique for changing or reinforcing children's desirable behaviors.

Setting Limits

One way of deepening the play therapy relationship is to use limit setting to establish predictability, safety, and boundaries. While there are different strategies for setting limits, play therapist experts agree that limits should be introduced only when they are needed, not delivered as a litany of rules outlined at the beginning of therapy (Bixler, 1949; Glover & Landreth, 2016; Kottman, 2011; Ray, 2011; VanFleet et al., 2010). Play therapists should set limits when they believe the client's behaviors risk hurting (1) the client, (2) the therapist, (3) the room or materials, or (4) the relationship between the child and therapist. Two popular approaches to setting limits are the Adlerian play therapy model (Kottman & Meany-Walen, 2016) and the child-centered play therapy model (Landreth, 2012; Ray, 2011). The Adlerian play therapist (1) communicates the limit by saying, "It's against the playroom rules to _____, (2) reflects the client's feelings and/or metacommunicates about the goal of the client's behavior, (3) invites the client to cooperate in generating acceptable alternatives, (only if this one is necessary—otherwise, rest on your laurels if the client complies with the behaviors you brainstormed as acceptable), and (4) helps the client to decide on potential consequences for continuing to break the playroom rules (only if the client has chosen not to follow through with the acceptable alternatives generated in the third step). In child-centered play therapy, the therapist (1) acknowledges the client's feelings, (2) communicates the limit, and (3) suggests an appropriate alternative.

Here's how they would work in a session. Let's say a child is about to pour glue on the puppets. We think most therapists would agree that this would not be an acceptable behavior because it violates the rule of not damaging the room or materials. The Adlerian play therapist would say, "(child's name), it's against the playroom rules to pour glue on the puppets. I'm guessing you're trying to show me that you have creative ideas and you're wondering what I would say if you pour glue on the puppets. What are some things you could pour glue on that would not be against the playroom rules? Let's think of some together." The child-centered play therapist would say, "(child's name), you think it would be fun to pour glue on the puppet, but the puppet is not for pouring glue on. You could pour glue on the paper." Importantly, both options respect the client and acknowledge the client's wishes, motivations, or feelings. The aim in both approaches is to help the client find acceptable avenues of expression. The difference between the two approaches is that the Adlerian version uses active voice, clearly states the rule, and engages the client in coming up with alternatives (and, if necessary, consequences), and the child-centered version uses passive voice and redirects the client to appropriate behaviors.

Playing with Children

To play or not to play . . . that is the question! (Or at least something to consider, we think. Not everyone who teaches play therapy would agree with us though, so you need to know that.) Your personality and beliefs about what clients need will "play" a role (see what we did there?) in how you interact with clients in play therapy. Some play therapists operate in the playroom much like a sportscaster operates during an athletic game.

They report on the client's behaviors, thoughts, and emotions as the client plays independently. Other play therapists engage collaboratively with the client, actively playing with the client. Even within the group of therapists who choose to play with clients, another decision must be made: to wait for the client to ask you to play or to initiate play with the client. One way is not necessarily better than the other, but you should choose the path you follow with intentionality and genuineness. As Adlerians, both of us tend to play actively with clients, sometimes asking them to play and sometimes waiting for them to ask us. I (Kristin) have been known to roll on the floor hiding from "bad guys" and being an ally with my client to protect ourselves from danger. I (Kristin) play hide-and-seek with my child clients and engage my adolescent and adult clients in board games and adventure therapy techniques on a regular basis. There are also occasions when our intuition tells us that a client needs space to work independently, so we leave them alone.

Cleaning the Room

How the room gets cleaned is also an opportunity for decisions based on how you think about the play therapy process and how it unfolds. Believe it or not, if and how a play therapist decides to clean up with clients is embedded in theory.

According to some play therapy approaches (e.g., child-centered, Jungian, psychodynamic), the ways in which toys are used, including the way the room is left, is an integral part of the therapeutic process (Axline, 1969; Landreth, 2012; Ray & Landreth, 2015). In this line of thinking, having clients clean up at the end of the session is synonymous with asking them to take back what they've shared in the playroom.

Other play therapy approaches (e.g., Adlerian, Gestalt, integrative, Theraplay) use the clean-up process as a way to ground the therapy in reality and to strengthen the relationship through a collaborative enterprise (Booth & Jernberg, 2010; Kottman, 2011; Kottman & Meany-Walen, 2016). Few social situations would allow for a child (or adult for that matter) to leave a mess for another person to pick up. Therapists who subscribe to this line of thinking collaborate with the client to clean the room together. (Now remember, clean is a subjective term.) I've (Kristin) often engaged very young children, clients with defiant behaviors, or clients new to therapy in picking up only three toys or figures. The idea is to create opportunities for clients to practice collaboration and social responsibility, and to provide opportunities for me to encourage their helpful behaviors. There are also a few occasions when we might not ask a client to help clean up. Such might be the case with a client who has a history of trauma, is a perfectionist, or is so discouraged that the interaction would be futile or potentially damaging to the therapeutic relationship.

TECHNIQUES FOR BUILDING RELATIONSHIPS

In addition to play therapy skills, you can use techniques from the broad play therapy strategies for building a relationship with a client: adventure therapy, storytelling and therapeutic metaphors, movement/dance experiences, sand tray activities, art techniques, and structured play experiences. All of these techniques can be adapted for use with different ages, populations, and presenting problems. They can be employed in a variety of different theoretical approaches to play therapy. If you are willing to use your imagination, most of these same techniques can be applied as tools in other phases of the play therapy process as well. Notice that we have described a variety of goals for each activity. Though we use all of the techniques in this section primarily to build relationships, we also use them for other purposes, which we have tried to describe. Don't be limited by the ways we have used them; be free with inventing other ways to use them. You have our permission.

It is important to remember that most of these techniques are directive in nature—most of them would not just "happen" in a play therapy session. You would need to set the activities up by giving clients several ways to participate or by inviting them to engage in several different techniques as part of the play therapy process. We always give clients a menu of numerous directive techniques, with one of the options being to decline to participate in any of the choices. In other words, we do not advocate "making" clients do any of the techniques we employ. Not every approach to play therapy presents directive techniques this way. In ecosystemic play therapy and Theraplay, the therapist does not blatantly present directive activities as a choice. However, every theoretical approach to play therapy that employs directive techniques would support making the activities capitalize on client interests. Remember that we advocate custom-designing all of the directive techniques you introduce to clients.

Adventure Therapy Techniques

Paint Your Name

The main goal for this activity is to build relationships—it is a fun way to get folks laughing with you, which is, of course, a great way to build connection. It can also be used to build self-confidence and positive feelings toward self, to help enhance skills necessary for cooperating in group activities, and to serve as a vehicle for gently inviting clients to take a (small) interpersonal risk.

This is an ice-breaker game that works well with clients who are able to spell their own names (Ashby et al., 2008). You can do it in a group or a family or with an individual client. If you are doing it in a group or family, first have the participants form a circle (even if it is a small circle for some groups or families). If you are doing it with an individual client, you can just make a two-person line. Using an imaginary paintbrush in their right hand (even if they are left-handed), explain to the members (or the client) that the task is to paint their name in the air as big as they possibly can. You can model reaching high into the air (up on tiptoes) and down to your knees to form the first part of your name. If you are doing it in a group or with a family, explain that, as they write, they will be moving around in the circle so that the letters in the air are next to each other rather than on top of each other. If you are doing this activity with a single client, you would both move in a straight line, side-by-side painting your names. (This makes sure you and the client or the members of the group or the family have to coordinate their movements, which also builds connection and cooperation.) After you finish with the right-handed painting, repeat the activity holding the imaginary paintbrush in their left hands, followed by holding it in their teeth, and (if you are feeling frisky) in their belly buttons.

Mirror Game

The goal for this activity depends on the needs of specific clients. For clients who struggle with connecting with others, this activity could be a vehicle for building connection. For clients who need practice in taking turns, sharing power, and cooperating and for clients with ADHD, this can be a chance to practice taking turns, sharing power, and cooperating. For clients who have ADHD, it can also be a chance to work on reducing impulsivity, inattentive behavior, and noncompliance. With clients who engage in power struggles (which can include clients with ADHD), the cooperation required to do this activity can give them a chance to be in a relationship without trying to overpower the other person. Because the modification requires you to do the opposite action, which is frequently stressful, you can build in stress-inoculation practice for clients who need to learn strategies for coping with stress. It can be done with individual clients, families, and groups.

With individual clients, you are the client's partner; with families and groups, have members choose a partner. (Watch how the choosing happens; you might want to comment on it or just use it to guide a future activity.) Stand facing the client. (With groups and families, tell the partners to stand facing one another.) With individual clients, have a conversation with the client and decide who will "go first." With groups and families, have the partners determine who will "go first." Explain that this person will be the initial "Leader" and the other person will be the "Follower" in the activity. Explain that the "Leader" will engage in some physical movement (that he or she knows the other person will be able to copy) and that the "Follower" is to mimic that movement so that it looks like the mirror image of the Leader's actions. (It is not necessary to give this explanation to the clients, and we think it will help you with Modification #1 later. This really means that facing one another, when the "Leader" raises her right hand, in order to mirror that, the "Follower" actually lifts his left hand, and so forth.) *Stress that this is a cooperative activity and the goal is to observe, communicate, and cooperate–all in silence.* After about 4 or 5 minutes (shorter with younger kids, longer with older clients), have the partners stop and switch roles. Let this Leader be in charge for about the same amount of time as the first Leader was. You can switch back and forth and do this several times with clients who are engaged in the activity. With clients who are not engaged in the activity, you can just do it once.

MODIFICATION 1

Instead of being a "mirror" for the partner, have the Follower do the opposite (so, when the Leader lifts her left hand into the air, the Follower will actually lift his left hand too, which makes them look like they are doing opposite things.) This variation is much more difficult than the mirroring in the previous activity, requiring the partner who is following to translate what he or she is seeing to make sure to do the opposite, which makes it more stressful. Again, take turns leading and following. Afterward, you can process if, how, and why this was more difficult and inquire about whether it was more stressful. If it was, this can become a teachable moment to describe some anxiety-management strategies (getting grounded, remembering to breathe, paying attention to where stress lives in the body and relaxing those places, etc.) and repeat the activity, with both of you practicing these strategies. (Okay, you are modeling and the client is practicing.)

MODIFICATION 2

In this Follow-the-Leader variation (which is super-helpful for clients with ADHD and clients who engage in power struggles), both partners face the same direction, one behind the other. In this activity, you want to repeat that the person leading needs to be sure that the person following can do the movements and that this is a cooperative venture. Then tell the Leader to move around the room (lifting arms, skipping, nodding heads, wiggling bottoms, etc.) and the Follower to do the same thing the Leader is doing. After about 3–5 minutes, have them switch. You can do this in silence; you can use it as a way to practice giving feedback, with the follower telling the leader the movements he or she likes and dislikes; you can do it to music; and so on. With a family or group, instead of having the members divide into two-person partnerships, you can do it with all the members in a line, with everyone facing the same way. The first person in line leads around the room and everyone else follows mimicking his or her movements.

Storytelling and Creating Therapeutic Metaphors

Co-Tell Stories

The goal of co-telling stories is to build connection and provide a chance to practice cooperation (which is why it is in this chapter). You can also use it for setting up a situation in which clients practice taking the affective and/or cognitive perspectives of others, recognizing and interpreting social information, sharing power with others, taking turns and sharing, actively listening to others, and maintaining and forwarding the appropriate content of conversations. It works particularly well with clients with ADHD, learning disabilities, and social skills deficits. You can use it with individual clients, groups, and families.

First of all, just to be clear, co-telling a story is when you take turns with a client (or with the members of a family or group) telling a story. There are many different ways to co-tell a story. You can set up the topic and the first part of the story by choosing the title and telling the first segment of the story and passing the telling to the client when you have established the setup of the story. Or you can ask the client to choose the topic for the story and to start the story, with you taking over after the first part of the story, then passing the telling back to the client. It is sometimes fun to have a conversation with the client, deciding together what the story is going to be about and choosing the characters and the setting in collaboration with the client, and then deciding who is going to start the story. You can each tell a sentence at a time, alternating sentences; you can tell a paragraph at a time, switching off at the end of each paragraph; or you can have no set formula for how the story gets told. You can have a puppet or a figure operated by one person who comes in like a reporter and interviews the various characters (played by the other person) in the story about emotions, thoughts, and motivations (like Creative Characters) (Brooks, 1981; Kottman & Meany-Walen, 2016). You can also co-tell a story in a family or group by going around the circle and having the next person in the circle tell the next part of the story or letting anyone in the family or group who thinks he or she knows what happens next in the story take over the telling.

Tell Me/Us a Story

The primary goal in asking clients to tell you a story is to build a sense of connectedness between the storyteller and the audience. Other goals would be to assess clients' self-image, willingness to take risks, ability to communicate with others, attention span, anxiety level, and ability to actively listen to others. The story can also be used to help clients practice active listening, take interpersonal risks, and maintain and forward the appropriate content of conversations. The stories can serve as a springboard for mutual storytelling when you get to that part of the therapeutic process. This can be an excellent intervention with clients who believe that no one listens to them, those who struggle with anxiety or shyness, and those who believe they don't count or are not capable. It can be appropriate for individuals, groups, or families.

The description of the technique is embarrassingly simple—you ask the client to tell you a story, with a beginning, a middle, and an end. Pay attention to what the client likes doing (painting, puppets, animal figures, etc.) and set up the modality for the telling, using that information so that the client is comfortable with the telling of the story. Then you listen to the story. If you think it would have a positive impact on the client, you can summarize the story or even act it out to let the client know that you have really been listening. If the client likes to answer questions (and you should probably know this before you introduce the activity to the client), you can ask some questions about the story. If it is a "true life" story (something that happened to the client), you can pose "real-life" questions; if it is a "made-up" story, even if you think there are some components of the client's real life, stay in the metaphor of the story for your questions. If you are working with a group or a family, you can give each person a certain amount of time (like 5 minutes for most elementary children, 7 to 10 minutes for teens and adults) to tell his or her story. The "task" for the other members is for them to listen to the story without asking any questions. Afterward, if you want, you can ask for volunteers to summarize the contents of the story. Only do this, though, if you think the person who attempts the summary can actually understand most of the content correctly because if the person gets a bunch of things wrong, you will have defeated the goal of conveying the idea that the teller counts with other members.

Cave Painting

We learned this technique from John Young (personal communication, November 2016), who created cave paintings to build relationships with clients, help clients shift negative feelings and beliefs, and/or provide a vehicle for clients to use art and storytelling to process their experiences. Cave paintings combine storytelling and drawing to help clients express themselves and try on more positive ways of feeling, thinking, and/or behaving. Because cave paintings are of stick figures and made-up symbols, the focus is not on the actual drawing but rather on what the drawing represents, which invites clients to just relax and have fun in the process, contributing to a sense of connection with the play therapist, especially if you decided to collaborate in the cave painting process. This intervention is particularly helpful for clients who believe that they are not good enough, that they can't do things correctly, and that they are not valuable. For these clients, the goal would be to begin recognizing negative, self-defeating self-talk and substituting positive self-talk. To achieve this goal, clients would create a story along with the cave painting, and you could make additions or edits to the story designed to combat negative thinking or negative self-evaluation. Using retelling, you could provide alternative explanations or gently challenge clients' perspectives. Cave painting can also be helpful for clients who have short attention spans or are careless about details because the nature of cave painting is that it is choppy and nondetailed. For these clients, the goal can be to decrease impulsivity and off-task behaviors by inviting them to tell a story from start to finish or to complete a project. This intervention works for children of all ages, adults, groups, and families. You will need acrylic paints, tempera paints, or finger paints; large sheets of newsprint or white paper; poster board; or some other type of drawing surface. (For clients who are reluctant to get dirty, you can also use dry erase markers and a dry erase board.)

As you introduce this technique, inquire about your clients' knowledge of cave paintings/drawings. If they have never heard of this before, you can explain to them that cave people used to write stories or messages on the walls of their caves by using symbols or stick-type figures to communicate to others in their tribes or future travelers who might come across their caves. You might even show a picture of cave paintings to emphasize the importance of communication, not a dependence on art ability. (Of course, we play therapists value all sorts of artistic expressions without judgment about the quality of the art work, *and* many people believe that art work should look a certain way in order to be "good." We want to help clients move past the "goodness" of the art and pay attention to the story of the art—cave paintings are one way to do that.) We often invite clients to use finger painting, rather than brushes to get that primitive cave painting ambiance.

The way you set up and introduce the activity depends on your goal for using this intervention. For example, if you want to learn about Sally's family, you could ask her to draw a picture of her tribe. If you want to learn about how D'Mani views himself or another person, you could ask him to draw a cave painting of that. You can ask clients to draw their fears, goals, what gets them in trouble, what they wish other people knew about them, and so on. You could have a client tell a story about a time when his or her tribe had to move to a different city or when the tribe's leader (grandfather) died. You can guide the story and have alternate endings (e.g., what happened, what the client wishes had happened, how the client handles the situation, what the client needs in order to cope with the situation better).

With clients who enjoy this technique, you can ask them to extend the story illustrated in the cave painting. For example, you could ask the client to paint what happens next or what happened before the picture he or she created. Maybe you want to know how the client (or someone else in the client's life) contributes to the problem or the solution, who supports or takes care of the characters in the painting, or the strengths of the people in the drawing or tribe. Maybe the client drew a warning to cave people who come in the future. What was the warning, and how will future people know how to keep themselves safe? One of the things we like best about this activity is that the "cave painting modality" can replace any art/drawing technique if you believe clients might be more likely to do an art project if it is in the form of a cave painting.

Movement/Dance/Music Experiences

Choreograph Collaboratively

For clients who like to dance or move, the primary goal would be to give them a safe and fun way to connect with you (or other members of the family or group). It can also be used as an assessment tool for exploring clients' self-image; willingness to take risks; ability to communicate with others; self-regulation; cooperation skills; willingness to take others' cognitive perspectives, recognize their own needs, recognize and interpret social information; begin and end social interactions smoothly, and take turns and share. When you are in the making changes phase of therapy, this technique can give clients a chance to practice communicating with others, self-control, cooperation, taking someone else's cognitive perspective, being aware of their own needs, recognizing and interpreting social information, beginning and ending social interactions smoothly, and taking turns. This is another activity you can do with individual clients, families, and groups.

For this strategy, you can either provide the music or invite clients to bring in music they like and then plan a dance together, with steps you both make up (or with steps either one of you already knows and are willing to teach one another). It is often helpful to decide together whether there are parts to the dance (my [Terry] dances are usually pretty unsophisticated—they have a beginning, a middle, and an end) and who is going to design each of them. Alternatively, you can take turns just like you would with co-telling a story—you are really just co-creating a dance . . . so you might start, come up with a step or two, then turn it over to the client who would come up with a step or two, and so on until the end of the dance. Then you would "perform" the dance together, either taking turns or doing the whole thing together. With younger children, you can also spontaneously have a dance party together rather than actually plan the movements you are going to do together. With groups and families, you would either put one member in charge of coming up with the steps and the other members executing them, or you could have all of the members contribute ideas for how the dance could go.

Make a Machine

In the relationship-building phase of therapy, the goal of this technique is to solidify the collaborative relationship with clients. We don't usually use it as an assessment or insight-creating strategy, though we often use it as a way to help clients work on recognizing and interpreting social cues, accepting responsibility in interpersonal interactions, setting appropriate limits and boundaries, sharing power with others, recognizing familial roles, and cooperating with others. This is an improv technique usually done in a group or with a family, though you can do it with an individual client.

To start, one person goes to the middle of the room and makes a noise and a movement. The second person joins the first person, adding another noise and a different movement. This continues until the last person has joined as part of the machine. With an individual client, the machine can have moving parts—with you making a noise and a movement, then the client joining you with another noise and movement, followed by you changing your noise and movement, and then the client changing the noise and movement he or she is making, and so forth until one or both of you declares a finish to the activity. After the machine is completed, you can (if you want to—not turning this into talk therapy, so you can just stop there) work together to figure out what the purpose of the machine was and how each person's contribution made it more likely that the machine would succeed in its purpose (whatever that was). The way you set up the activity is, as always, dependent on your goal for doing the activity. For example, if you are working with a group of clients on recognizing and interpreting social cues, you would want to have one person be the person who indicates to the rest of the members that it is time to stop, but without actually saying, "Stop!" That way, the other members can pay attention to the nonverbal social cues that might indicate it is time to stop. If you are working with a client on setting boundaries, you could have her tell you how far away you need to be when you join the machine as another component of the action. If your goal is to work with family members on family roles, you can have them each have their part of the machine reflect their role in the family. (And so forth—you get the idea.)

Connecting Dance

Connecting dances are all about relationships (we know, this is a Captain Obvious name)—relationships clients want to initiate, relationships clients want to sever, relationships clients want to repair, and so forth. When you ask clients to participate in a connecting dance, you are suggesting co-creating a movement to represent how they want to connect with someone else. Since the dance is about connection, you will usually need to participate in the movement to represent the other person, though clients can use a puppet or some other toy to represent the other person. First of all, you would ask clients to describe how they want to connect to the other person. The next part of designing a connecting dance is to ask them how they imagine they would move if they wanted to connect with someone in that way. If clients want you to represent the other person, this is followed by them coaching you in how you would move if you were the other person. Next, you act out both movements with the clients—with them playing themselves and you playing the other person. After you do this, you might want to ask them if there is anything they want to change and then redo the movement with those changes. Sometimes it is helpful to also have clients switch with you, so that they play the other person and you play them. This works well with all ages of clients, though you will want to make sure you use developmentally appropriate language with clients to explain who you want to do.

Sand Tray Activities

In Chapter 3, you were given an overview of the steps involved in doing a sand tray and how to process a sand tray. For each of the four phases, we will give you a list of possible topics you could use to set up a directive sand tray if you are comfortable with being directive in the play therapy process. Here is a list of trays that you could use for establishing a connection with the client:

1. A tray to introduce himself or herself to you—a tray you could introduce as a "Me Tray"
2. A general "my world" tray
3. A tray by the client on what he or she knows/has been told about coming to counseling
4. A tray about the people (creatures) who share his or her world
5. A tray about "things that bug me" or "the problem(s) in my life"
6. A tray about "things I like about my life"
7. A tray about his or her assets or accomplishments
8. A tray about his or her contributions to home, school, or work

Unlike many approaches to sand tray play therapy, we also occasionally do a tray for a client to show the client what we think about certain people, situations, patterns, or relationships. This models doing trays and invites the client to try a procedure that might normally be rather intimidating. If you are comfortable doing a tray for a client, as part of building the relationship you could do any of the following trays:

1. You could do a tray to introduce yourself to the client
2. You could do a tray on what you know/have been told about the presenting problem
3. You could do a tray on how play therapy (or sand tray) works

Art Techniques

Sticker World

Stickers are part of an activity that is appropriate with all clients. Little kids, teens, and adults all seem to get excited when presented with an envelope or drawer filled with stickers. You can actually use this technique with any client, with any presenting problem, at any phase of play therapy, depending on how you set up the activity. The only kind of client with which you might not want to use stickers would be a client who actually prefers drawing and/or painting activities. With this particular configuration of a sticker activity, your primary goal would be working to build a relationship with clients, and your secondary goal would be assessing a "sense" of how they feel about their lives and the people in their lives and the situations in which they live. You can do this with individual clients, groups, and families.

For this technique, you will need some materials: stickers—we prefer a wide variety of stickers—animals, people, super heroes, trees, signs, butterflies and other bugs, princesses, professional wrestlers, sports equipment, and so forth and so on. We tend to avoid stickers with words on them because it becomes tempting (especially for teens and adults) to turn things into talk therapy. You can find stickers everywhere. Because stickers can be expensive, we tend to go for stickers on sale or for stickers in less expensive venues like Dollar Tree or Family Dollar or we may look for stickers on sale at places like Michael's and Hobby Lobby. We like to use card stock paper for the background for the sticking of the stickers because it is sturdier than just regular copy paper.

So, to start, give the client a piece of card stock paper and a selection of stickers, then ask the client to select stickers that represent his or her world—people, activities, objects, and so on. With younger clients, you might need to be more specific, asking for them to choose stickers to represent friends, family, school, play, and the like. With older clients, you can let them decide what they want to include in the portrait of their world. Ask the client to describe what he or she has included in this portrait of his or her world. If you think clients would be open to this, you can make observations of things you notice about the stickers' placement, relative size, orientation, symbols, and so forth. We usually do this by saying, "I notice that . . ." without any judgment or interpretation of what any of this means. This strategy opens up the possibility that clients will elaborate on the portrait they have created. Ask any questions you might have about the placement, relative size, orientation, and the like. When the client has finished with the description and you have completed making your observations, you can ask if there is anything that he or she would like to add, take off, or move around on the paper. Give the client another chance to process what is there now and what prompted any changes he or she wanted to make.

Build Construction Projects

Construction projects are fun, interactive ways of building relationships with clients. They can also be used to explore clients' intrapersonal dynamics such as self-image, willingness to take risks, willingness to "own" personal assets, attitudes toward and skills for solving problems, and willingness to take responsibility for problems. They can also be used as a tool to assess interpersonal dynamics, including family dynamics (if you are working with a family), friendship skills (if you are working with a group), and communication skills. During the gaining insight phase, you can make interpretive comments or use the metaphor of the process of building as a way to help clients get clarity about what is going on with them. You can also use construction projects to help clients decrease impulsivity, bossiness, power struggles, and blaming others for a problem, and increase compliance with requests, cooperation, taking appropriate risks, negotiation skills, problem-solving skills, ability to self-scaffold, self-control, willingness to take responsibility, and willingness to reset after a problem occurs. Construction projects seem to work especially well with clients with ADHD, anger management, social skills deficits, and struggles with problem-solving and taking responsibility for their own behavior. This activity is appropriate with individual clients, families, and groups.

There are lots of different ways to use construction activities to develop or deepen a relationship with clients. You can collaborate with clients in building structures with Legos, blocks, Tinker Toys, and other construction toys. It is also fun to build things or make long lines with dominoes and (our child clients love this part) knock them down. My (Terry's) personal favorite, though, is building stuff with recycled materials. I save clean recyclables like Styrofoam containers, toilet paper rolls, plastic cartons, pill bottles, and plastic straws and invite clients to work with me to build things. Depending on clients' interests and situations, we might build Mine Craft structures, mazes for a mouse to run through, a track for racing cars, a house for dolls, a robot created by a mad scientist, a model that shows the relationships between a teen friend group, and so on. You can use masking tape, Scotch tape, pipe cleaners, and (for older elementary children, teens, and adults) hot glue to make connections as you are constructing. Lots of times, I ask clients to create the connections while I hold the construction materials, or I create the connections while they hold the materials. This way, we work as a team, which facilitates relationship-building (and in later sessions, problem-solving and collaboration skills). This is often used as a homework assignment for families when we want to give them activities they can do to store positive energy in the family "positive energy bank."

Create a Mural

There are many different ways to build a relationship through co-creating art with clients, and one fun method is to co-create a mural. You can also use this technique to build cooperation skills, communication skills, negotiation skills, and problem-solving skills with clients who need to work on these. You can make murals with individual clients, groups, and families.

The first step in this activity is taping a big piece of white paper or newsprint on the wall and getting out markers, crayons, paints, and/or oil pastels (whatever you think will be most appealing to your particular client). You can have the activity be structured, with you and the client (or the members of a group or family) taking turns adding something to the design, or you can have the process be relatively unstructured, with you and the client (or all the members of the group or family) adding things at the same time. You can spontaneously draw together without a theme or topic, collaboratively coming up with a title for the creation when you are done. You can also reverse that order, having a conversation about the title or topic before you start creating to give yourself a theme for your creation. Remember to tell clients that the important thing is the process, not the product. Otherwise clients may get anxious about their ability to draw or paint. If this happens and your admonishment that the focus should be on the fun of the process fails to calm clients' fears, you can always invite them to use stickers rather than actually drawing or painting. And you can reflect their fears related to wanting to be perfect or their performance anxiety.

Have Drawing Conversations

One way to engage clients who are nonverbal or who have something to say that they don't actually want to say out loud is to have a drawing conversation. The main goal of this technique is to engage a client who does not want to have a verbal conversation in an exchange of ideas and information. (Remember, we have said, just a few times, that it is okay for clients not to talk, so this activity isn't designed to pressure clients to talk—it just gives them a chance to communicate more directly than some forms of playing might.) For clients in the phase focused on helping them make changes, this activity can give clients a vehicle for communicating about feelings, recognizing the feelings of others, considering other people's emotional perspective, and practicing frustration tolerance. It is a blast to do this with groups and families as well as individuals. We have done it with clients from 4 years of age to 80, so it works with a wide range of ages.

Though you can do this activity on paper, we find it works best with a white board because then you can quickly erase or move things around to change or amplify your meaning. So, here is how it goes: you draw something, then the client draws something, then you draw something, then the client draws something, and so forth. For example, I (Terry) might draw a week calendar and a question mark to indicate I would like to know how Valentina's week went, and Valentina could draw a frowny face, then I could draw either another question mark or a taller figure looking concerned at a smaller figure; then the client could draw a picture of two people with one of them punching the other one. You can continue this conversation until you reach some kind of conclusion or until one of you decides you want to be done with the discussion. After you are done, if the client is inclined, you can talk about the process or about the meaning of a certain drawing if something was not all clear. Or you can just let the experience and the product stand, without the need for verbal discussion.

Structured Play Experiences

Invent Mini Sporting Events

This is a rather generic technique with specific applications that vary depending on the interests of specific clients. It seems to work best for connecting with clients who are interested in sports; clients who struggle with being capable; clients who need practice with frustration tolerance, cooperating, taking turns, taking responsibility for their own behavior, learning to reset after a problem, and/or winning and losing gracefully. With clients diagnosed with ADHD, you can also use it as a way for them to practice being more attentive, less impulsive, and more able to listen to and comply with requests. These activities seem to work better with individual clients because in families and groups, they might bring out too much competition or a sense of being just like interactions outside the playroom. They also seem to work better with children and teens than with adult clients.

You can make any sport work here if it can be played in a small way and would be engaging to clients. We play pitch and catch, basketball, bowling, and track and field events. For pitch and catch (we know this seems simple, because it is), we use a soft ball like a Nerf ball, a stress ball, or sock ball. You can make a sock ball by taking a soft athletic sock and, starting with the top, rolling it in on itself until you run out of sock, which results in a ball. It helps if you start with a clean sock because clients are sure to ask if you washed the sock before you made the sock ball. (We always tell them we washed it—wink, wink, nudge, nudge.) You can either throw a ball back and forth with clients or, with clients who might be too rough with the throwing, roll it back and forth. In order to make this work, eye contact needs to happen. Cooperation pretty much ensues because if you don't collaborate with one another, you can't pitch the ball in a way that the other person will catch it and/or you won't be able to catch the ball when the other person throws it. (Which can hurt even when you are using a soft ball, which we always do. We know this from personal experience.)

The Nerf basketball is super fun, and it combines both collaboration (retrieving the ball, bringing it back, resetting the net if it gets knocked down), and a bit of friendly (usually) competition. Bowling (with those plastic pins and balls everybody had when they were kids) is also entertaining and can build connection through collaboration and competition; setting pins up and taking turns knocking them, you can work with one another. I (Terry) also do these weird track and field events, like slow-motion races, sock balls discus throwing, hurdling over pieces of paper folded in half, and fake Tai Chi or karate to engage athletic clients. (It helps to build clients' self-confidence when they play with me (Terry because I am decidedly not a jock; when they play this type of game with Kristin, it might be more likely to help them stay humble because she is quite accomplished at sports.]

Blow Bubbles

Blowing bubbles with clients is an enjoyable way to connect without any pressure to talk. You can take turns blowing the bubbles, with the other person either trying to pop them, blow them around, or keep them up in the air by waving arms. (There might be other choices here, but we can't think of any. Don't be limited by our lack of creativity—make up your own procedures.) There is no sophisticated meaning or highfaluting goal here, just some fun. While you can do this with groups and families, we especially like to do this activity with individual teens or adults who are "too tight" to loosen them up. You can also assign it as a homework activity for families when you are trying to work on fun things and connections between members.

Figure Introductions

We use this technique pretty exclusively in the building of the relationship phase for (drum-roll . . . you got it) building the relationship. We seldom use it for anything else, so we don't have a list of other goals for you. We have used this activity with clients from very young children to older adults, and we have used it with individual clients, families, and groups—it is super-adaptable.

Figure introductions is one of the only techniques in the book that requires very specific materials. (We are sorry . . . and we think this one is worth it.) You will need twenty or thirty small plastic figures—we usually use an assortment of animals (wild, farm, pets, bugs, sea creatures) and aliens. Every once in a while, we also include weird creature figures, soldiers, astronauts, and super-heroes. You can get assortments of inexpensive figures from U.S. Toy (*www.ustoy.com*) and Constructive Playthings (*http://products.constructiveplaythings.com*). We use small plastic figures because we let clients keep them at the end of the activity to remind them of what happened in the activity, but you don't have to do that part. You can also use plush animals, finger puppets or foam shapes instead if that would work better in your setting.

When you are ready to begin the activity, lay your figures (or plush animals, finger puppets, or foam shapes) out on a table. Tell the client to choose one that he or she likes or feels connected to. (We even sometimes say something that "resonates with you," and that is a pretty fancy word and concept unless you are working with adults or pretty savvy teens.) Ask the client to pretend to be that animal (or person, alien, or creature), imagine the figure can talk, and introduce himself or herself by answering some questions. (You can choose from the following questions or make up your own.)

"What's your name?"
"Describe a typical day for you."
"What is your birth order [oldest, second, etc.]? What do you like about that being your position in your family?"
"What do you do for fun?"
"How do you connect with others?"
"What gives you joy/happiness? How do you show other people/ animals/creatures you are feeling joyful/happy?"
"What do you get angry about? How do you show others you are angry?"
"What do you do when you are angry?"
"How can others tell when you are angry?"
"How do you react when you don't get your own way?"
"What are some things that are challenging for you?"
"How do you handle it when things are challenging for you?"
"What kinds of things are disappointing to you?"
"What do you do when you are disappointed?"
"What do you get sad about? What happens when you feel sad?"

"What worries you? How can someone else tell when you are worried?"

"What do you do when you want attention?"

"What do you do when you feel powerless?"

"What do others like about you?"

"What do you like about yourself?"

"When do you feel that you are not valuable/special/important?"

"What is your proudest accomplishment?"

"What are your favorite things to do?"

"When and where do you feel the most relaxed?"

"What are things you do when you are happy?"

"How do others know when you are happy?"

"What are your passions?"

"What are the things you like best about your life/world/existence?"

"If you could change anything about yourself, what would you change?"

"If you could change anything about your life/your world, what would you change?"

"What impact do you think you have on the world?"

"What impact would you like to have on the world?"

Remember to make sure the questions you ask the figure/puppet are developmentally appropriate and remember to limit the number of questions you ask in a single session, lest you fall into the talk-therapy-in-the-playroom trap. We suggest no more than five or six questions in a single session. Also keep in mind that it is important to tell your clients that they can pass on any of the questions they don't want to answer.

Play Tabletop Games

We are currently into playing tabletop games as a way of connecting with clients. (And we think how the connection happens is pretty obvious, so we aren't going to go on and on about how you can use playing games to break the ice with clients.) Playing tabletop games combines elements of play therapy (yes, there's playing involved) and talk therapy (usually when you play a game with a client, you both wind up having some conversation about what is happening in the game, and sometimes about other aspects of the client's life). Depending on the game and the client, you can also use tabletop games for assessing clients' issues and patterns, helping clients gain insight into their issues and patterns, as well as helping them learn and practice more effective patterns of thoughts, emotions, and behaviors. We can't be more specific here because tabletop games are so versatile—again, you are only limited by your own imagination—so, imagine we are waving a magic wand and giving you permission to be creative—go for it! Tabletop games can be useful for individual clients, groups, and families, from young children to older adults.

For younger elementary students, our current favorite tabletop games are *Blink, UNO, Don't Break the Ice, Jenga*, and *Race to the Treasure*. For older elementary students, the games are *UNO Attack, Mancala, Quidler, Connect 4*, and *Farkle*. With clients who are 10 years of age and older, some great games to play in therapy are *Ticket to Ride, Settlers of Catan, Forbidden Island, Forbidden Desert, Pandemic, King of Tokyo, Dixit*, and *Munchkin*. Several games that can work with younger children, older children, teens, and adults are *Tsuro, Chicken Flickin', Oh Snap*, and *Stormy Seas*. (Thanks to my [Terry's] friend Neal Petersen for help with expanding our horizons with suggestions of games he plays with kids, teens, and families.)

THEORETICAL CONSIDERATIONS IN BUILDING RELATIONSHIPS WITH CLIENTS IN PLAY THERAPY

I (Terry) surveyed experts in specific theories applied to play therapy to find out which of the approaches were more likely to use which skills in working with clients (Kottman, 2011). According to the experts surveyed, play therapists who adhere to cognitive-behavioral play therapy, ecosystemic play therapy, Gestalt play therapy, and Theraplay would not usually use tracking or restating in their sessions. All of the approaches to play therapy support reflecting feelings in interactions with clients. While all of the approaches advocate setting limits, there are as many different approaches to limit-setting as there are approaches, and there is quite a variety in what is deemed necessary to limit. Returning responsibility to the client is reportedly used in Adlerian play therapy, child-centered play therapy, Jungian play therapy, Gestalt play therapy, and psychodynamic play therapy, but is not usually used in narrative play therapy or Theraplay.

Of the three nondirective approaches to play therapy we have addressed, child-centered play therapists would be the least inclined to use strategies or techniques in their interactions with clients because they (1) believe the core elements of a therapeutic relationship (empathy, genuineness, and warmth) can be created through use of play therapy skills and (2) avoid doing anything that might be construed as leading the client (Ray & Landreth, 2015). Most Jungian play therapists use the client's metaphors (though at the client's initiation rather than the therapist's), sand tray, and art techniques—usually in a nondirective, unstructured way (Lilly, 2015). Many psychodynamic play therapists use metaphors, sand tray, and art as modalities of expression for clients—usually in an unstructured way; they may also introduce structured play experiences as a vehicle for achieving specific therapeutic goals (Mordock, 2015).

Practitioners of Adlerian play therapy, cognitive-behavioral play therapy, Gestalt play therapy, and integrative play therapy are all likely to use strategies and techniques from adventure therapy, storytelling and therapeutic metaphors, movement/dance/music experiences, sand tray activities, art techniques, and structured play experiences for building the relationship with clients, depending on the client and the play therapist's level of comfort and training. Not surprisingly, given the name of the approach, narrative play therapy usually focuses on storytelling and therapeutic metaphors, with the occasional application of art techniques and structured play experiences. Ecosystemic play therapists tend to focus primarily on structured play experiences, as does Theraplay, though both may also use movement/dance/music activities.

MOVING ON . . .

So, you say, "Okay, I have a good start on building a relationship with my play therapy client . . . now what?" Lucky you—it just so happens that the next chapter is your guide for where you go moving forward.

Interlude 4

Take a Breath

*T*ake a breath.
Now take another one.
Now take another one . . .

Remember that one of the most important parts of being a play thera-pist is taking care of yourself. We are pretty sure you have heard folks use the metaphor of being on an airplane and the flight attendant saying "In the event that the cabin loses air pressure, be sure to put your own oxygen mask on before you help others put on their oxygen masks." This is super important because it is critical that you do what it takes to keep yourself healthy and well grounded so that you will have the energy to help others.

We are shoveling lots of information your way and are inviting you to exercise your brain in ways that you might not have ever done in your life before now. So, take time to breathe. Go outside. Have a bubble bath. Take a walk. Smile at people, make eye contact with them—really see them, and let them really see you. Take a breath. Watch the sun set, or watch the sun rise (if that is your inclination [shudder]). Feel your body. Take a walk. Get a treat for yourself. (You deserve it.) Stretch. Go out and play (however that looks to you). Read a book just for fun. Take a breath. And another . . .

Okay . . . now you can go on with the book. Next time, when you feel like your brain is bursting, take another breath and do the whole thing over again. Remember, you deserve care too.

CHAPTER 5

Exploring Intrapersonal and Interpersonal Dynamics

Just in case you thought you were the only ones who have ever wandered in the wilderness of "Okay, I have got a theory, I have started building a relationship with my client. Where do I go now?"; here is a story about our development as play therapists we want to share with you. Early in graduate school, as part of defining and understanding who we were as counselors, we took practicum, which meant seeing "real clients" (as opposed to practicing on our fellow student guinea pigs). The beginning of the work with clients went pretty well because both of us are pretty good at building relationships. We supplemented our natural abilities for connection with the relationship skills we had learned in our classes to create trust and communicate genuineness and positive regard. After a while with our clients, though, both of us started feeling frustrated and aimless. We both found ourselves asking, "Now what?" Coming into practicum, Kristin thought she was person-centered, and Terry believed she had found a home in existential theory. So, technically, all we had to do was lean into creating and deepening the therapeutic relationship (because that is the main tool in both person-centered and existential counseling), and yet we felt that wasn't enough for us (or for our clients). We wondered (a bit obsessively), "Where do I go next with my clients, and what do we do to get there?" Both of us decided (not together—we were in school years and years and years apart) we needed to look further into the different theories of counseling because, while we thought the relationship is important, we didn't feel it was enough—we felt as though we needed more—we needed more direction for determining where to go next with our clients and how to get there.

If you have found resonance with child-centered play therapy or if you are trying to apply existential theory to play therapy, you basically already have the answers to those two questions—you are going to continue to deepen the connection with your clients, radiating empathic, genuine, and unconditional positive regard, being supportive, and believing that clients' actualizing tendency is going to be activated by the relationship with you and move them toward health. If, however, you are still wondering "now what?" you might want to keep reading to find some tools you can use to answer that question.

First of all, your goals for your client and your theory can actually deliver many of the answers to the questions of where you are going and how you are going to get there. In broad strokes, your theory will provide some guidance to help you figure out where you are going with the client and the goals you (and the client and, in many cases, the client's parents) should set up. Your theory should serve figuratively like a neon sign saying "You are going here!" Your theory, the client's interests and inclinations, as well as your training and experience, should give you the vague outline of a road map showing you how to get there. Hopefully, the strategies and techniques presented in this book will provide some of the vehicles that will move you down that road, and your imagination and reading, combined with the client's willingness and motivation to change, will provide the rest of the vehicles.

In most approaches to play therapy, the client's presenting problem will provide some clues about therapeutic goals for the client. With child and teen clients, discussions with their parents (and teachers), supplemented by conversations (or sand trays, drawings, puppet shows, etc.) with clients, are some of the ways to establish what they want to work on (along with giving you an idea about what the important adults in the clients' life want to change). However, the presenting problem is often just the surface "itch" that needs to be scratched. It is therefore almost always helpful to look "underneath" the presenting problem—at the intrapersonal and interpersonal dynamics of clients and of significant other people in their lives to discover more specific details about the road map showing where you and clients are going and how to get there.

INTRAPERSONAL AND INTERPERSONAL DYNAMICS: WHAT ARE THEY? (AND WHY MIGHT THEY BE IMPORTANT TO YOU?)

Before exploring dynamics, we thought it would be good to define what they are. We tried to find definitions that would fit what we wanted to describe in this chapter; once we found that impossible, we decided to give you our definitions. (This does not mean you have to be confined to our definitions; ours will simply give you a "feel" for what we mean by intrapersonal and interpersonal dynamics. You can add anything else you believe should go into the dynamics mix. As we wrote this chapter, we kept thinking of more things to add to our list.)

By our definition, *intrapersonal dynamics* concerns the "stuff" that goes on within a person's mind, heart, and spirit—in fancier language, the psychological dynamics that occur inside the mind without reference to the person's exchanges with other people. As part of the intrapersonal dynamics, we look at emotional patterns (e.g., depression, anxiety, anger, despair, discouragement); cognitive patterns (e.g., faulty convictions, irrational beliefs, tangential, abstract, concrete); behavioral patterns (e.g., avoidance, isolated, uncooperative, impulsive, aggressive); body patterns (e.g., hunched shoulders, butterflies in stomach, dizziness); and attitudinal patterns (e.g., giving up easily, getting into power struggles, insisting "it's not my fault").

We think the following areas are also important aspects of clients' intrapersonal dynamics: self-image, character traits, recognition of personal strengths and weaknesses, emotional self-awareness, ability to self-regulate, capacity for making decisions, skill in setting and monitoring progress toward goals, willingness to assess and take appropriate risks, and movement on the path toward self-actualization. Your self-image includes your beliefs about yourself as a person; your sense of yourself in the various roles you play in your life; and your self-confidence, self-efficacy, and self-responsibility. Character traits include qualities such as creativity, imagination, playfulness, sense of humor, resiliency, honesty, courage, responsibility, independence, decisiveness, adaptability, determination, generosity, loyalty, tolerance, discernment, patience, kindness, and optimism. (The list of character traits is endless—insert the traits you think are important and the traits the client and [when appropriate] the client's parents/teachers think are important.) Recognition of personal strengths includes being able to "own" your strengths and being realistic about your assets; recognition of weaknesses consists of being willing to take responsibility for times when you are struggling and being realistic about your limitations. Emotional self-awareness involves your being able to recognize your feelings, as well as your triggers, the places in your body where you experience certain emotions, the patterns of emotions you experience on a regular basis, and the intensity of your feelings. The ability to self-regulate involves your ability to monitor and control your emotions, thoughts, and behaviors; it also affects whether you are "too loose" or "too tight" (Kissel, 1990). For you to be able to make decisions and become proficient in setting and monitoring progress toward goals, (you guessed it) you must have the capacity to make and take responsibility for your choices and be willing to set short-term and long-term goals, in addition to being competent in assessing movement toward goals. The willingness to assess and take appropriate risks (physical, intellectual, emotional, interpersonal) includes the aptitude for assessing which risks are "real" and which risks make sense for you to take. The path toward self-actualization involves combining a desire to grow, to become, to change in positive ways with actual positive momentum toward becoming your best self.

To us, *interpersonal* dynamics are how a person interacts with other people. We think the important areas to explore under this banner are family dynamics, relationships at school (for children and teens) and at work (for adults), the ability to make and maintain friendships, the capacity to communicate with others, the ability to recognize and solve interpersonal problems, and the willingness and skill in taking responsibility for personal behavior and the impact it has on others. When you are doing play therapy with children and adolescents, it is especially helpful to consider the intrapersonal and interpersonal dynamics of the significant others in their lives, especially their parents and other family members (and, with regard to clients who are struggling in school, their teachers—we will get to that in Chapter 8).

Now that we have explained what we mean by intrapersonal and interpersonal dynamics, it is your turn to think about what you mean by those terms. (We'll now pause to give you time to think about what you would include in your consideration of intrapersonal and interpersonal dynamics.) When you have figured that out, your next step is to consider whether you believe it is necessary for you to understand clients' dynamics in order to accompany them on their journey toward health and healing. Do you believe that understanding how the client thinks, feels, and acts can help you get "underneath" the presenting problem to the underlying issues? Do you think that exploring these dynamics will help you set meaningful and achievable goals for clients? If you don't, you can skip this chapter. If you do, read on . . . this chapter is for you.

You will also need to decide if you would want to consider any other factors as you explore dynamics. Your theoretical orientation will provide some guidance with this decision, as will your own beliefs about people and your ideas about what is important to understand that might aid the unfolding of the therapeutic process. For instance, in addition to all of the elements laid out so far, as Adlerians we also seek to understand (1) the goals of the client's behavior, (2) the Crucial Cs (courage, connect, capable, and count) of the client and how well each of the c's has developed in the client, (3) the personality priorities (comfort, control, pleasing, and superiority) of the client and how the client manifests the strengths and the liabilities of his or her personality priorities, and (4) how the client deals with his or her feelings of inferiority (Kottman & Meany-Walen, 2016). We also pay close attention to birth order and how the client's perception of his or her psychological position and the family atmosphere of the client's family-of-origin impacts the client's behaviors, attitudes, emotions, and thoughts. (We will include more information about what practitioners of each of the theoretical approaches would want to explore in the last section of this chapter.)

In addition to the factors that your theoretical orientation deem important to explore, you might also have other things you believe are important to find out. For example, we care about the ways the client learns best (e.g., visual, auditory, tactile/kinesthetic) and the way the client prefers to express himself or herself (e.g., through stories, art, movement, music, playing). We also pay attention to whether the client is more comfortable communicating directly or through metaphor. And it is important to us to notice the client's pace—of speech, of processing, of action, and so on. You will need to begin thinking about which factors are important to you to know about the client so that you can better help the client proceed through the therapy process and work on finding ways to gather information about these factors. (Don't worry if you don't have a complete list in a couple of weeks of consideration. Keep in mind that I [Terry] have been doing play therapy for 30 years and Kristin for 10 years, and we are still adding things to our list of things we want to discover with and for our clients.)

You're still reading. We assume that (1) you believe knowing this information is important, (2) you're not sure if this information is important, so you want to know more, (3) you're mindlessly reading the words on the page without really paying attention to what you're reading just because this chapter is a class assignment, or (4) you're an insomniac who's trying to go to bed and you're reading anything in an attempt to make you sleepy. Whatever your reason, we hope to help.

SKILLS FOR EXPLORING DYNAMICS

So, once, again, we are going to start with skills, and then we will move into techniques. There are fewer skills for exploring dynamics than there were for building the relationship. The two main skills for exploring dynamics are questioning and observing.

Questioning

The first order of business about asking questions is for you to decide whether you believe it is okay to ask questions in play therapy. There are several approaches to play therapy (e.g., child-centered and Jungian) that deem questions inappropriate in the playroom, so if you subscribe to either of those approaches, you might want to skip this section.

If you believe it is acceptable to ask questions in the playroom, here are some guidelines designed to help you use this skill to get useful information from asking questions.

• Think about what you want information about. Depending on your theory and your personal curiosities, you will put weight on different kinds of information. For instance, cognitive-behavioral play therapists want to know about clients' thinking patterns (e.g., which ones are self-defeating? which ones are working for them?) and about their behaviors (e.g., what is the secondary gain of specific behaviors? what are reinforcing specific behaviors?). Adlerian play therapists want to know whether the course of therapy has had an impact on the original presenting problem (e.g., what is happening with the behaviors that led to the referral to therapy? what is the impact on relationships of shifts in behavior or attitude?). They also want to know information about clients' lifestyles (e.g., what are the family rules and how do they affect clients? how do clients gain a sense of significance in their lives?). You may also put weight on some things that your theory doesn't emphasize and are still important for you to know. You need to be familiar enough with your theory and with what you want to find out about clients so that you can choose important questions designed to acquire the information you need to be able to understand your client and make plans for where to go next with clients and how to help them get there.

• Be sure that asking a question is the best way to get the information you want to gather. There may be better ways to find the answers you want about your clients' patterns—perhaps just observing, asking them to do a sand tray or a drawing, setting up a structured play activity, or something else that would appeal to a particular client. Also, consider whether you already actually know the information you were trying to get—sometimes this happens, and it is important to avoid asking a question you have already answered.

• Make your questions count. You want to avoid turning your interactions with clients into interrogations. Especially working with children and teens, you want your exchanges with them to be different from many contacts between children (and teens) and adults—those conversations in which the majority of the interchanges are the adult asking a question and the child is required to respond. Be sure the questions you decide to ask are powerful and will be most likely to elicit the information you desire. Limit the number of questions you ask so that clients don't feel inundated or badgered. When I (Terry) was in my doctoral program, one of my mentors, Dr. Byron Medler, told me that before I asked a question I should always ask myself, "How will the answer to this question either help me better understand the client or help the client better understand himself or herself better?" He suggested that if the question would not do either of those things, I should refrain from asking it. I follow that advice. . . . since I am also unusually curious, I limit myself to six questions a session, and I try to ask fewer than that.

- Ask open-ended questions. Lots of people are in the habit of asking closed questions . . . even people who have counseling training who should know better. So, remember to open those questions up—you will get lots more answers if you start questions with "what" instead of "did" (e.g., "What happened after that?" as opposed to "Did you call the police after that?"); "how" instead of "are" (e.g., "How did you feel when that happened?" as opposed to "Are you angry about what happened?"); and so on. (You can use your imagination—we know you have already covered this in your skills classes. And we are kind of taken aback that we have to reteach it to many of our play therapy students, so we thought it merited repeating here.)

- Avoid asking "why?" questions. (This is another bit of advice you probably have been given more than once, and it's a hugely important one, so we are willing to say it again.) We think "why?" questions should be banned from the lexicon of possible queries. For one thing, "why?" sounds like an accusation. When someone asks you a why question, often the subtext appears to be something like "What were you thinking!?!?" Even when what you really mean is "What was behind your decision to do _____?" a why question seldom yields actual understanding of the motivation for a particular decision or behavior. The other primary drawback of a why question is that people seldom really know why they made a decision or did some action—most of the time, without help in exploring the underlying dynamics, clients (especially child clients) do not have conscious access to the why of their choices or behaviors.

- Ask "The Question." One way to use questioning with older child clients, teens, and adults is to ask what Adlerians call "The Question" and what solution-focused therapists call "The Miracle Question." In the Adlerian version, you would ask something like, "How would your life be different if you did not have _____ (the symptom)?" (Griffith & Powers, 2007, p. 87). The solution-focused therapy version would be something like, "Suppose that tonight while you sleep, a miracle happens and all of your problems are solved. When you wake up tomorrow morning, how are you going to know that miracle happened? What will you see yourself doing, thinking, or believing about yourself that will tell you that a miracle has happened in your life, your relationships, school, or your work?" (Metcalf, 2006). Obviously, in play therapy, you can ask the question paired with a drawing, a puppet show, a sand tray, or whatever form you think will appeal to the specific client. The answer to this question can help you understand how the client perceives the problem and will guide you in developing goals for the therapeutic process.

- Be okay with clients answering you without words. Remember that, in play therapy, clients' actions, rather than their words, are the important mode of communication. So, keep in mind that, many times, clients will answer your questions—just not with words. You need to pay close attention to what clients (especially those who are in the habit of not using their words to answer you) do in response to your questioning. Sometimes the answer in the actions is obvious. For instance, when you ask 7-year-old Shyanne about what her father did to her mother when her mother was drinking, she puts the bigger doll into the tub in the bathroom of the dollhouse. In cases like this, the answer to your question is pretty clear. Other times, the answer embedded in the action is more obscure. For instance, when you ask 17-year-old Elijah what happened over the weekend with his girlfriend, he slams the book he is holding shut. In these situations, you might not understand what the client's behavior signifies. When that happens, quite often, rather than asking another question, your best course of action is often to simply track the behavior. So in this latter case, you might say something like, "When I asked you the question about what happened with Cassie over the weekend, you slammed the book shut." Then, (*here is the key*) you have to be quiet and let the client fill in the gap by filling you in.

• Be okay with clients not answering you. Remember that, in play therapy, freedom and safety are essential elements of the relationship. It is important that clients do not feel coerced in any way to respond to your questions—they need to be in charge of themselves and their own behavior to a greater degree than they are in other situations and relationships. Play therapy clients should get to ignore you; they should get to turn their backs on you; they should get to change the subject; they should get to tell you that they would rather not answer the question. Whether they verbalize their desire to avoid answering your questions or whether they use a nonverbal method of not answering you, they need to have your permission to have the power not to answer—unless, of course, you need the client's answer to a question related to the client's safety or the safety of others. In those circumstances, the rules change, and you will need to rescind your permission for the client to avoid answering questions and insist that he or she give you verbal answers.

• Make sure your questions fit into your clients' method of expressing themselves. So, with clients who express themselves in metaphor, ask your questions in the metaphor—ask the tiger about what she is angry about; ask the client how the little boy figure who is hiding in the dollhouse can get himself to safety; ask the client what is going on between his "friend" and his "friend's girlfriend;" ask the client how the bug that hits the windshield reacts; and so forth. With clients who speak directly about their problems, you can ask questions directly—ask "What happened after your mom hit your dad?" "How did you feel when your teacher yelled at you?" "How did you react when your girlfriend told you she was breaking up with you?" "What are some ways to change the path you are taking with your boss?" and so forth. With clients who slip back and forth between speaking through a metaphor and speaking about their situation directly, work on matching whatever form their expression is taking when you want to ask your question.

 • Decide who you want to ask what. Some of the questions you have might be better answered by a parent, a grandparent, a teacher, a doctor, or some other person in the client's life. Obviously, you will need to consider confidentiality, and if you need permission to talk to someone other than the client and a legal guardian of the client, you will have to obtain signed consent.

 • Answer a question . . . get an answer to a question. Although some theoretical approaches do not support the therapist answering clients' questions because it can lead the client in a certain direction (e.g., child-centered) or undermine the countertransference (e.g., psychodynamic), sometimes answering questions clients ask you can lead to getting information about them. For one thing, the types of questions clients ask you can give you information about them (Kottman, 2011). Also, clients' reactions to your answers to their questions can often supply clues to their thoughts, feelings, and attitudes.

Observing

The other skill involved in exploring dynamics is paying attention—to the client's behavior in the session, to the things the client says in sessions, to the client's emotional expression, to the client's self-descriptions, to the way the client acts in your waiting area, to the interaction between the client and other people in his or her family, to the parenting skills of a child client's parents, to the classroom management style of his or her teacher, to the client's facial expressions and body language when he or she describes the behavior and attitudes of his or her boss and co-workers, and so on. What we're trying to say is that your job is to notice everything! Everything is relevant; everything is meaningful. (Okay, we admit this might be consistent with how we see counseling and might not be true for all counseling theories. Like we've said, your theory is really a part of how you see the world; it's a natural extension of who you are.)

Your own ideas about what is important and the basic tenets of your theoretical orientation will give you guidelines for what to focus on in your observation. For instance, if you are a cognitive-behavioral play therapist, you will probably pay a lot of attention to your clients' cognitive and behavioral patterns (we know, you could have guessed that without reading this book) and to their interpersonal dynamics connected to their ability to recognize and solve interpersonal problems and their willingness and skill in taking responsibility for their behavior. If you are a Gestalt play therapist, you will most likely focus on your clients' emotional and body/physical patterns, their emotional self-awareness, and their ability to self-regulate. For narrative play therapists, the important elements to observe would be the cognitive patterns involved in the stories clients tell themselves and others, their self-image, their ability to make and maintain friendships, and their capacity to communicate with others.

TECHNIQUES FOR EXPLORING INTRAPERSONAL AND INTERPERSONAL DYNAMICS

The techniques you choose for gathering information during this phase will also depend on your theoretical orientation and personal inclinations. There is, of course, some overlap in the information you can get about intrapersonal and interpersonal dynamics from the very same technique. We have tried to outline the goals for each of the techniques we provide and the ways these techniques could be used in the other phases of play therapy. And remember, you can invent new ways to use the techniques we describe and new techniques altogether. We have also given you the population and contexts in which we think these techniques will work best, and (you guessed it) don't be confined by our suggestions: use your own clinical judgment and experience.

Adventure Therapy Techniques

Circles of Comfort

Circles of Comfort (Ashby et al., 2008) is a fun way to explore clients' emotional patterns and to help them gain a sense of the patterns of their feelings and reactions. It will work with individual clients, groups, and families—actually, it is very enlightening for families because members are often surprised by the answers other members give. It will also work with all ages—just make sure that the situations you adapt are appropriate for your participants' developmental level.

Before you introduce this technique to clients, it is helpful to generate a list of activities, experiences, or relationship that might evoke emotional reactions from your particular clients. You can use things like:

Giving a speech to your class.
Giving a speech to a group of 100 other teens.
Making a presentation to your boss.
Singing a solo at a choir concert.
Making a presentation to the president of your company.
Making a presentation to the president of the United States.
Singing a solo at church.

Taking a statistics/math/history/English pop quiz.
Attending a party where you don't know anyone.
Flying on an airplane.
Meeting your boyfriend's parents.
Jumping out of an airplane.
Taking a hot-air balloon trip.
Asking someone on a date.
The principal announcing that he or she would like to have you come
  to the office.
Your mom having a baby.
Your wife having a baby.
Having a baby.
Moving to a new town.
Changing schools.

Use situations that could actually happen in your clients' lives. If you run out of ideas, you can always ask clients to come up with their own ideas. Obviously, the list differs based on the kind, size, age, and experience level of your clients.

You will need an open space and something to mark your circles—we usually use masking tape or yarn, but you can also use rope or webbing. Choose whatever you are going to use as a "marker" to form two concentric (one inside the other) circles so that they look like a target. The middle circle needs to be big enough to fit in the whole group—so that they snuggle tightly. The outside circle needs to be at least several feet farther out. In a perfect world, the outside circle would be large enough that the whole group could stand shoulder to shoulder just outside of it. (If you have a single client, the circles can both be much smaller—we know—duh! But we thought we should mention it even if it was self-evident just in case it wasn't.)

To start, explain to your clients that the areas inside and outside of the circles represent different degrees of "comfort." The area inside the smaller circle in the middle is the "Comfort Zone." This is where people go when they are feeling relaxed and absolutely comfortable, feeling no stress or anxiety whatsoever. (Make sure you use developmentally appropriate language to describe "comfort.) Explain that the area between the smaller circle and the larger circle is the "Challenge Zone." When they are in this circle, people are feeling uncomfortable and emotionally challenged—stressed and anxious, but not in an overwhelming or necessarily unpleasant way. Finally, explain that the space outside the larger circle is the "Chaos" or "Crazy" Zone. In this area, people feel out of control, extremely stressed and anxious, and maybe even a little crazy. If you want, you can go back and review what each circle is—Comfort Zone, Challenge Zone, and Chaos or Crazy Zone. Next, ask the clients to move to a different area (i.e., Comfort, Challenge, or Chaos/Crazy) based on how they would react to the particular activity or experience as you announce them. As you name each possibility on your list, ask participants to move to the circle that represents how they would feel or react to each of them. Would that experience be "comfortable," "challenging," or "chaotic/crazy" for them? If you are doing this in a group or family format, after folks get settled into the circle that makes sense for them to be in, ask them to notice who is in the same circle as they are and who is not. If you are doing it with an individual client, you could ask him or her to imagine who among their friends and family would be in which circle.

Safety Cars

Safety Cars (Kottman et al., 2001) is a trust activity that can be done with individual clients or in a group to explore emotional and behavioral patterns, client character traits, emotional self-awareness, and capacity for self-regulation. It can be used with individual clients and in groups and families—though it is done in pairs; thus, if you have a group or family with uneven numbers, you will need to participate. We have done it with all ages of clients.

If you are playing Safety Cars with an individual client, decide who is going to "go first." (If you are doing it with a family or group, have them divide into pairs and decide the same thing.) Both people in each pair must stand facing the same direction, with the person who agreed to go first standing in front of the other person. Have the person in front hold his or her hands out in front at chest height, elbows bent, in a protective position. This person is the "car." The person in back (a.k.a., the "driver") puts his or her hands on the shoulders of the person in front. Explain that the driver's job is to keep the car safe and help the car feel safe and comfortable, and that the car's job is to let the driver know (through feedback and suggestions) what he or she needs to feel safe and comfortable. After the car and the driver have a brief conversation about what the car needs to feel safe and comfortable, explain that the car is going to close his or her eyes (or, if you want, you can distribute blindfolds—we just trust folks to keep their eyes closed—or open them if they need to do that; but we don't tell them that part) and the driver is going to keep his or her eyes open (important safety tip). Have them get into position and begin "driving" around the space. Give them about 2 or 3 minutes to "drive" around the room, and then tell them to stop. After they have "parked," tell them to switch, with the car becoming the driver and the driver becoming the car. Remind them of their respective positions and responsibilities, and give them a few minutes for the car to let the driver know what he or she needs to feel safe. Then tell the car to close his or her eyes, and put his or her hands up in the protective position. Remind the driver to keep his or her eyes open, and tell them to drive. After 2 or 3 minutes, let them know they can stop. If you have done this with an individual client, invite feedback about what he or she liked and disliked about each role—and other information he or she would like to share about feelings, self-regulation, and taking responsibility for someone else and/or not being in control of himself or herself. If you have played it with a group or family, watch for indicators of these elements while they do it (unless, of course, you have an odd number of members, and you were participating); afterward you can invite the members to have a conversation about all of these factors.

Shy Thighs

The main goal of Shy Thighs (Ann Randolph, personal communication, January 2015) is to explore clients' physical patterns, emotional self-awareness, and willingness to assess and take appropriate risks. You can do it with individual clients, families, and groups. While it can work with all ages, you will want to keep your feeling adjectives simple if you try it with younger children. We have done it mainly with older elementary students, and junior high and high school students, with a sprinkling of adult clients.

So, before you start the activity, it will help to develop a list of feeling words that can be used as adjectives, such as shy, bold, aggressive, angry, joyful, proud, peaceful, nervous, scared, lonely, curious, excited, curious, and powerful. Then tell the clients to walk around your space. As they walk, you will announce a pair of one of the feeling words with a body part (e.g., shy thighs, bold elbows, aggressive eyebrows, angry ankles, joyful shoulders). As they walk, watch them to see which combinations they like doing and which ones they dislike doing. Pay close attention to whether they chose not to do specific combinations because choosing not to do one of the combinations might tell you something about their ability to discern whether something presents too big of a psychological risk for them. To deepen the exploration of emotional self-awareness, you could follow this activity up with a conversation about what they liked about the combinations that felt comfortable to them and what they didn't like about the combinations that felt uncomfortable. You could also ask them to think about where in their bodies they usually hold those emotions you named. You could follow up this activity with a body outline activity in which your clients draw in feelings in the places on the body outline where they feel the physical sensations connected with specific emotions should be.

Welded Ankles

If you do Welded Ankles (Ashby et al., 2008) with an individual client, you can use it to examine emotional patterns, cognitive patterns, behavioral

patterns, and attitudinal patterns, along with client self-image, character traits, emotional self-awareness, and the ability to self-regulate. When
doing it with groups or families, you can use the activity to explore group
(friendship and/or classroom) dynamics and family dynamics. The activity will work with any age client, although for very small children, you
might want to tie their ankles together loosely with a soft piece of cloth
or bandana.

If you are doing the technique with a single client, the task is for the
two of you to walk across a space (20 to 40 feet across) with your movements coordinated, keeping your ankles attached as if they are welded
together. You can make a rule (and if you want to look at client self-
regulation, this is a good idea) that if your ankles come "unwelded," you
have to go back to the beginning and start over again. You can just keep
your ankles together with an imaginary tie, or, at least for the first couple
of passes, you can tie your ankles together with a soft cloth or bandana
to give you the experience of walking as a team. It is often helpful to have
a conversation about the best way to make the "welding" work, but that
discussion doesn't have to take place before you start. Sometimes it works
better if you try it for a while before you suggest that maybe it would be
helpful to brainstorm what is working for you both and what is not working.

If you are doing the activity with a group or family, tell the members
to stand in a straight line facing you, with the sides of their feet (or shoes)
touching the sides of the feet (or shoes) of the members to either side
of them, so that the whole group is "attached" to one another by having
their ankles "welded." Both of the members at the end of the line will
only have one ankle touching the one person next to them. Explain to
the members that their assignment is to cross the space without becoming "unwelded," and if their ankles do come apart, they need to start
over again. Depending on your sense of the group or family, you can
use the soft cloth method of welding for the first couple of tries if you
want. Again, you are probably going to want to use scaffolding to get the
members to have a conversation about what is working and what isn't and
what needs to change in their method of traversing the space to make
this work.

Storytelling and Creating Therapeutic Metaphors

Make Up a Story About . . .

This technique can be used to explore just about anything—self-image,
character traits, personal strengths and weaknesses, awareness of emotions, capacity for self-regulation, decision making and goal setting,
discernment about risks, and self-actualizing tendencies. It can also be

a way to explore relationships (family, classmates, co-workers, friends) and problem-solving skills. It can be used with individuals, families, and groups; children, adolescents, and adults. We often do this activity with clients who prefer to communicate with metaphor rather than directly. "Making up" a story can give them much-needed distance, which relating a "real" story cannot do.

The directions for this activity are ridiculously simple: "Make up a story about . . ." whatever you want clients to tell a story about. You can have them tell a story about animals or people; about fictional characters from books, movies, television shows, or video games; about a fictional version of themselves, and so on. You can show them photographs cut from magazines and ask them to make up a story about what happened before, during, and after the photography. You can use storytelling cards with words (e.g., Storymatic, Storymatic Kids, Spark Your Imagination Story Starter Cards) or pictures (e.g., Imagination Story Cards); play storytelling games (e.g., Lugu, Dixit, Tell Tale Fairy Tales, Once Upon a Time card game, Tell-A-Story), or play with storytelling dice (e.g., Story Time Dice, Rory's Story Cubes, Magic and Fairy Tale Dice). Because children are often fascinated with animals, we sometimes use a deck of cards called the Children's Spirit Animal Cards to help spark stories. If you are working with adolescents or adults, you might want to use cards featuring artistic masterpieces, like those in 250 Masterpieces in Western Painting, Famous Painting cards, or Professor Noggin's History of Art. You can even download art history flashcards from the Internet (*www.flashcardmachine.com/art-history.html*). Another way to set up a "made-up" story would be to put some things in a sand tray and ask clients to make up a story about what has happened or is happening in the tray. Obviously, because you are asking clients to "make up" a story, the information available in the story will be in metaphor form, so you will have to listen to the story metaphorically to figure out what it tells you about clients and their lives.

Tell Me a Story About . . .

Your goals with this technique would be similar to your goals with the "Make up a story about . . ." activity. You would be likely to use this version with clients who favor relating information directly, and you would still like the distance of a "story" rather than just relating information in an unvarnished format.

So, for this technique, you say to clients, "Tell me a story about . . ." You can ask clients to "Tell me a story about your tenth birthday," "Tell me a story about how your parents met," "Tell me a family story about how you got your name," "Tell me a story about when you learned about the birds and the bees . . ." The possibilities for stories about real-life events are endless. You can give them paper and drawing materials and have them illustrate the story, ask them to do a sand tray to show you what happens in the story, suggest doing a puppet show for the delivery of the story, introduce the idea of doing the story with buttons as characters in the story, and so forth.

You can also ask clients to tell you stories they have heard—like family stories, myths, and so on. For instance, my (Terry's) son, Jacob, has heard the story of his adoption about a thousand times—so many, in fact, that if I start a story with, "Would you like to hear the story about when Dad and I . . ." he interrupts me even before I get finished with the topic sentence. However, lots of clients like to repeat stories they have heard about their childhoods or family members and things that happened to them. All stories have information you will be able to use in understanding clients.

One-Word Story

The goal of this technique would be to get a distilled sense of something; it could be something connected to intrapersonal dynamics or interpersonal dynamics. It's kind of a quick-and-dirty procedure, and I (Terry) love it—with individual clients (children, adolescents, adults), groups, and families. We often use it with clients who are reluctant to talk at all (like those pesky sullen adolescents) and with clients who will not stop talking (you know who they are).

The way it works is this: you ask the client to use a single word to tell you a story about _____. The story can be about a specific situation or relationship, a possible solution to a problem, something that happened in the past, the client's week, and so on (whatever you are interested in learning a little bit more about). You can even expand it to two or three words if you want or (go crazy) a single sentence. You can have the client tell you a one-word story and then tell you a one-word story about the one-word story if you want. Sometimes we ask clients to act out the one-word story—with some kind of body movement or gesture or to choose one sand tray figure to go with the one-word story. (You have our permission to go wild with this one.)

Fortunately/Unfortunately

Fortunately/unfortunately (Ashby et al., 2008; Beaudion & Walden, 1998) is an activity we mainly use to help make some guesses about clients' character traits and gauge how well they take responsibility for their own difficulties and coming up with solutions to their problems. Because the original version requires an odd number of people, we usually use it with families or groups. You can adapt it to individual clients though if you use a bit of creativity. Since many younger children won't really grasp the abstract concept of being fortunate or unfortunate, this activity works better with older elementary children, adolescents, and adults. If you have a larger group, divide participants into subgroups of three (or five or seven–really, whatever works with your numbers, but each subgroup needs to have an odd number of members). If you have an even number, that just means you need to participate, which is okay because you can also model how to do it.

Have your clients sit in a circle and ask who would be willing to start a story. (If you have no volunteers, just start the story yourself.) To start off, ask the person who is going to start to begin the story with one or two sentences starting the first one with "unfortunately." (For example, "Unfortunately, when Tommy started walking his dog, the rain began to pour down on them.") Next, ask the person to the right of the story starter to continue the story by finding something constructive or fortunate that could also be a part of the story and add one or two sentences to the story, starting with "fortunately." ("Fortunately, Virgil, Tommy's dog, brought a very big umbrella that could cover both of them.") Then guide the next person in the circle to continue the story by finding something unfortunate about the circumstances, beginning the next part of the story with "unfortunately." ("Unfortunately, the wind was so strong that Virgil's umbrella snapped off.") Tell the participants to continue around the circle, alternating fortunate and unfortunate circumstances until the story comes to a natural conclusion (or you tell them that time is up), ending on a positive note with the last sentence beginning with "Fortunately. . . . "

It is essential to listen to what clients say when it is their turn because what they add to the story will tell you something about character traits and whether they take responsibility for problems and what kinds of solutions they tend to generate for handling problems This activity can be followed by a conversation about who liked being a "fortunately" person and who liked being an "unfortunately" person. You can also just observe the storytellers to gain a sense of their personality traits. If you want to use this activity with an individual client, you can alternate with each of you doing a "fortunately" sentence or two and then an "unfortunately" sentence or two.

Early Recollections

Early recollections (ERs) are moments–usually from the first four to six years–that a person chooses to remember from all the possible life experiences. Soliciting and interpreting early recollections helps the play therapist understand clients' intrapersonal and interpersonal dynamics (Kottman & Meany-Walen, 2016; Watts, 2013). Through early recollections, clients reveal their attitudes toward themselves, their relationships with others, and their view of life. When using this Adlerian technique (which can be helpful even if you are not Adlerian if you believe that clients' past informs and influences them in the present), if your goal is simply to use the technique to gather information, you do not have to share your interpretation with clients. If your goal is to use a pattern across early recollections to help clients gain insight, you will want to share your guesses about the meaning of the early recollections with your clients. This technique works best with children who are 8 years old or older, adolescents, and adults because it is often difficult to get younger children to describe a single incident contained in a memory. We tend to use it with individual clients, and we know therapists who use it in groups and families as a means of helping members understand one another.

Since you want to find patterns in clients' beliefs about self, others, and the world, you will want to gather six to eight memories. You don't have to do this in a single session, however; you can do it across several sessions. You can ask clients to verbally describe the memory; you can ask them to write the memory down for you; or you can ask them to draw a picture, make a sand tray, or do a puppet show of the memory. Ask for the memory by saying something like, "Tell me something that happened to you when you were little," or "What is one of the first things you can remember happening?" So that you have all the information you need, write down the ER exactly as clients tell them to you. When they have finished describing the memory, ask them how they remember feeling at the time, how they feel as they tell you about it now and how old they were at the time of the experience.

To figure out the significance of the early recollections, look for the central theme of each recollection, and then look for the overall pattern across the recollections. Look for patterns of interactions between the people in the memories, between the situations in the memories, between the communication that takes place in the memories, in the way problems are solved in the memories, and so on. As a way of coming up with the meaning of the pattern across the early recollections, ask yourself the following questions (Dewey, 1979; Kottman & Meany-Walen, 2016):

1. What is the "feeling tone" of the ER? Is there a pattern running through the ERs?
2. What is the focus of each memory? What stands out as being the most significant factor? Is there a pattern running through the ERs?
3. Who is in the memories? (The client, other children, family members, etc.?) If the client is in the memories, is it usually as an observer or as a participant? If the client is in the memories as a participant, is he or she active or passive?
4. What is the client's relationship to others in the memory? (Think in terms of both emotional relationship and familial relationship.)

5. How do the people in the memory (including the client if the client is part of the memory) interact with one another? Are there patterns of certain ways of interacting with others?
6. What is the attitude of the people in the memory? Is there a pattern running through the ERs?
7. If the client is in the memory, what role does he or she play? Is there a pattern running through the ERs?
8. If the client is in the memory, what is happening with him or her in terms of conformity or rebellion? Being taken care of or taking care of others? Controlling others or the situation or being controlled by others? Again, is there a pattern running through the ERs?
9. What emotions does the client remember? How strong are they? What are the emotions about? What emotions does the client feel as he or she is telling you the memory? Again, is there a pattern of emotions in the ERs or the present?

Movement/Dance/Music Experiences

Body Story

This is a combination storytelling and movement technique that I (Terry) developed for women's retreats—as a vehicle to explore how women (both teens and adults) feel about their bodies and how their body patterns developed over the course of their lives. You could also do it with men. I am not sure it would translate to children, just because it is a fairly abstract concept. You could certainly try it, though, if you thought it would work with a particular child.

The way you set it up is you ask clients to tell the story of their bodies from birth (or even from conception if you think it might be relevant) until the present. You could actually just leave it at that. However, I have found that asking them to act it out deepens the experience. Clients get a better sense of the impact of certain events on their bodies when they use movement to act the story out, and you get more information for helping you understand their physical patterns. So, after you ask them to tell the story of their body, the next part of the directive is to ask them to act it out—with their whole body. The "with their whole body" seems important—when I have not included that phase in my description of what I want them to do, they often just use their face, arms, and hands to tell the story, which does not have the same effect as using their entire physical self.

Storytelling Dances

It is often fun (and sometimes profound) to ask clients to use movement and dance to tell stories—stories about their childhood, stories about something that happened recently, stories about their vision for the future, stories about how they see themselves, stories about relationships with important people in their lives, and so forth. This technique can be a way to have them embody the feelings they have about the events featured in the story, help them remember specific features of a memory, or help them flesh out (pun probably not really intended) the details of an idea or dream. Depending on how you set up the topic for the story, you can use this technique for exploring self-image and recognizing personal strengths and weaknesses, and emotional self-awareness. In the interpersonal arena, you can set up the story so that you and the client can explore family dynamics, relationships at school or work, friendship skills, communication patterns, and problems and struggles. It is important to tailor your description of the topic of the story to whatever you want to explore, making sure to have the client look at the specific intrapersonal and/or interpersonal dynamic about which you wanted more information. This strategy can work with clients at every level of development. While we usually use it with individual clients (partly because we have found clients are much more likely to be inhibited about moving in front of other people), you could also do it with groups and families.

Because they will be acting out the story, sometimes the story will be longer than if they were just telling the story (so you would use this with clients who tend to give sparse details). For clients who are uncomfortable with embodiment, sometimes the story is significantly shorter than it would have been if they were just telling you the story. (We find that this is often a useful technique with clients who are so long-winded with stories that you constantly need to interrupt them to get them to get to the "meat" of the story.)

This is probably the easiest dance to set up. Depending on what you already know about clients, you might ask them to tell the story solely with their bodies without words or sounds; with regard to others, you might ask them to tell the story with words accompanied by movements and sounds; or you might ask them to tell the story with just movements and sounds, but no words.

For example, if you wanted to discover how your 5-year-old client, Amelia, thinks (or feels) about herself as a person and what she thinks about her assets and liabilities, you would say something like, "Use your words and your body to show me what you like about yourself," followed by "Now use your words and your body to show me what you don't like about yourself." Working with Chung, a 15-year-old struggling with self-confidence, you might say, "Show me how you move when you are feeling sure of yourself," then, "Show me how you move when you are feeling unsure." If you were working with Makayla, a 26-year-old struggling at work, you might want to say something like, "Show me how you move through work—how you feel about yourself as an employee. What does that movement sound like?" In the interpersonal arena, if you were concerned about family dynamics with 7-year-old Benjamin, you could say something like, "Please move like you move when you are with your mother . . . with your father . . . with your sister . . . with your brother." If this part goes well, then, in order to deepen your understanding, you could say, "Now do a dance and make some sounds that show me how you feel about your relationship with your mom . . . your dad . . . your sister . . . your brother." You could obviously do the same thing with friendships, communication patterns, and problems—with the "languaging" of the directive adjusted for the client's developmental level.

Music

We often ask clients (especially older elementary children, teens, and adults) to bring in music so we can listen to it together. Without asking any questions, you can tell a lot about people and how they think about self, others, and the world; how they solve problems; how they communicate with others; how they deal with and express their feelings, and many other things. (Really, whatever you want to explore, once you start thinking about music as a vehicle for finding more about clients, you can explore by listening to the music clients like.) With folks who like to dance or sing, having them dance to the music or sing the lyrics with the music can also be revealing. You might decide to ask some questions too, remembering to limit your questions to the ones you really need to answer to help you understand the client. Here are a few questions you could ask (and, as usual, don't rely on the questions we would ask—add your own and don't ask those on the list that don't appeal to you):

"What do you like/dislike about this song? Music? What do you like/ dislike about this type of music? What do you like/dislike about this musical group/singer?"

"What makes this song/music special to you?"

"What was going on when you first heard this song/music?"

"What does this song/music remind you of?"

"What does this song/music tell (us) about what is important to you?"

"What is the impact this song/music has on you and/or your life?"

"What is going on with you when you listen to this song/music?"

"What are you are thinking as you listen to this song/music? What is going on in your head as you listen to this song/music?"

"How do you feel when you listen to this song/music?"

"What feelings does this song/music evoke in you? (How do you feel as you hear it? How do you feel after you listen to it? How do you feel as you think about it later?)"

"What can we tell about you if we know you like/dislike this song/
music? What does this music/song tell (us) about you?"

"What does this song/music tell (us) about your life in general? What
does this song/music tell (us) about specific situations in your
life?"

"What does this song/music tell (us) about your relationships?
Friendships?"

"What does this song/music tell (us) about a particular relationship
in your life?"

"What does this song/music tell (us) about issues in your life?"

"What does this song/music tell (us) about how you solve problems?"

"How do you move to this song/music?"

"What do you want to do when you listen to this music? What do you
want to do after you listen to this music?"

"When do you want to listen to this song/music?"

"Are you more attracted to the lyrics or music?"

"Do you sing to it or just listen? If you sing, do you sing out loud, or
do you just sing to yourself?"

"What's the difference between singing or not?"

"How does the singer influence your enjoyment or dislike of the
song/music?"

"How would you feel if there was a different version?"

"Does the song remind you of regrets or other paths you could have
taken?"

You can also ask clients to bring in music or songs that represent the
important people in their lives or represent their relationships with certain people. If clients bring in songs/music to represent other people or
the relationships in their lives:

"Who does that song/music remind you of? What about that song/
music reminds you of that person?"

"Would that person also choose that song/music to represent himself
or herself? If yes, what would that person think about you picking
that song/music to represent him or her?"

"What song/music do you think that person would pick to represent
him or her?"

"What do you like about the music you chose to represent that person?"

"What do you dislike about the music you chose to represent that
person?"

"What song/music would you choose to represent your relationship
with that person (or some other person in their lives)?"

"What does that song/music tell us about your relationship with that person?"

"What song/music would you choose to represent how you would like your relationship with that person to be?"

Sand Tray Activities

The basic procedure for doing sand trays is described in Chapter 3. Here is a list of some specific sand trays you could do with clients, divided into specific areas you can use to explore:

Trays about emotions

1. Feelings they have had during their lives (or during the week, the day, at the present time)
2. A specific emotion and how that emotion affects the various aspects of their lives
3. Personification of a specific emotion

Trays about emotional patterns

1. What clients are afraid of or what worries them
2. What happens when they are afraid or worried
3. How they deal with being afraid or worried
4. Situations and/or relationships that stress them out
5. How they feel when things are stressful
6. Situations and/or relationships in which they feel uncomfortable
7. How they handle stressful or uncomfortable situations and/or relationships
8. How they feel/react when things don't go the way they are "supposed" to go
9. How they feel about making mistakes
10. Methods they use to avoid feeling out of control
11. Things that might be embarrassing to them
12. What it means to them to be embarrassed or humiliated
13. How it feels to be "out of control"
14. Situations in which they feel "out of control"
15. What it means to them to feel "out of control"
16. Feeling that they are not good enough
17. How they would have to live their life if they felt they were good enough
18. Times when they have felt inferior to others
19. How it feels to them to be rejected
20. A situation or relationship in which they were rejected

21. Things they do to try to avoid being rejected
22. Situations and/or relationships in which they have felt/feel angry
23. What anger feels/looks like to them
24. Situations or relationships in which someone got angry at them

Trays about behavioral patterns

1. The kinds of things that get them into trouble
2. What happens when they get into trouble
3. How significant others react when they do things that get them into trouble
4. How they get attention (both positive attention and negative attention)
5. How they get what they want (positive ways and not-so-positive ways)
6. Contrasting situations when they feel in control/out of control
7. How it feels to be in control/out of control
8. Times when they have felt picked on (or abused or bullied)
9. How they reacted when they have felt picked on (or abused or bullied)
10. Times when they have picked on, bullied, or abused someone else
11. How they felt before, during, and after they picked on, bullied, or abused someone else
12. What they do to get "back at" people who hurt them in some way
13. All the stuff they can't do/do badly/wish they did better
14. How they feel when there are things they can't do/do badly/wish they did better
15. What they do to express their dissatisfaction with themselves or others
16. What they do to prove they are good enough
17. Situations in which they compare themselves to others
18. Time when they have bragged about something or put someone else down
19. Situations or relationships in which they feel they need to put the needs of others before their own
20. How they take care of the needs of others
21. How they take care of their own needs

Trays about attitudinal patterns

1. Situations and/or relationships in which they feel they have a positive or optimistic attitude
2. Situations and/or relationships in which they feel they have a negative or pessimistic attitude

3. Situations and/or relationships in which they have been told they have a negative attitude
4. Situations and/or relationships in which their attitude was helpful to them or to others
5. Situations and/or relationships in which their attitude was harmful to them or to others
6. Situations and/or relationships in which they have given up easily
7. Situations and/or relationships in which they would never give up
8. Situations and/or relationships in which they tend to get into power struggles with others
9. Situations and/or relationships in which they tend to avoid getting into power struggles with others
10. Situations and/or relationships in which they tend to think or say "it's not my fault"
11. Situations and/or relationships in which they tend to take responsibility or ownership for their feelings, behaviors, attitudes, reactions, and so on

Trays about clients' self-image

1. How they see themselves
2. The things they like about themselves
3. The things they dislike about themselves
4. How they would advertise their positive qualities
5. What a "wanted" poster would include if it was highlighting their not-so-positive qualities
6. Something in their life they feel good about
7. Something in their life they feel badly about
8. Positive things others say about them (teachers, friends, grandparents, parents)
9. Not-so-positive things others say about them
10. Situations in which they feel self-confident
11. Situations in which they doubt themselves
12. The kind of daughter (son, sister, brother, granddaughter, mother, father, boss, employee, student, teacher, etc.) they are
13. Situations and/or relationships in which they believe they are competent
14. Situations and/or relationships in which they feel incompetent
15. Situations and/or relationships in which they feel that they take responsibility for their actions and reactions
16. Situations and/or relationships in which they feel that they do not take responsibility for their actions and reactions

Trays for exploring clients' strengths or assets and/or times when they "own" them

1. Things they are good at or proud of that they have done
2. Personality traits they have that they like
3. Things they like doing
4. Something(s) for which their friends would nominate them for an award
5. What they contribute to home/school/work
6. Ways they are helpful on home/school/work
7. How they make a positive impact on home/school/work

Trays for exploring family dynamics (can either be done directly or metaphorically about "a family")

1. The members of their family (one to three figures representing each member; one to three figures representing what each person brings to the family; one to three figures representing how each member sees himself/herself, etc.)
2. Ways the family gets along
3. Ways clients get along with the rest of the family
4. Conflicts they have with other members of the family (currently or in the past)
5. Conflicts other members of the family have with them (currently or in the past)
6. Conflicts other members of the family have with one another (currently or in the past)
7. How they deal with conflicts with other members of the family
8. How the members of the family deals with conflict
9. How they deal with conflicts between other family members
10. How the family members would solve a problem (either a specific problem experienced by their family or a more generic problem)
11. What it is like to be the oldest, second, and so on, among all the children in the family
12. What it is like to be in a particular birth-order position
13. How space aliens or total strangers would see their family
14. How other people in their town or neighborhood perceive their family
15. Family values ("What is important to the members of this family?")
16. What they think their parents' attitudes toward parenting are
17. How they think the members of their family show love
18. Family rules (about behavior, attitudes, feelings, conflict, solving problems, communication, etc.)
19. Family assets or strengths
20. Family struggles or problems

21. Family hierarchy ("Who is in charge in this family?")
22. Communication styles in the family ("How do people talk to/communicate with one another?")
23. Alliances in the family ("If there were family teams, who would be on which team?" "What would each of the teams stand for/be willing to fight for?" "Who would be in charge of each team?")
24. Their perception of their parents' marriage
25. Their parents' conflict resolution patterns ("What do your parents fight about?" "How do your parents solve disagreements with one another?" "What happens when your parents disagree about something?" "Who wins?" "How does that person go about winning?")

Trays for exploring clients' friendships
1. Their friends
2. What friendship means to them
3. How to make (and/or keep) friends
4. How they make (and/or keep) friends
5. What they look for in a friend
6. What kind of a friend they are
7. How friends see them
8. Personal strengths as a friend
9. How they get along with friends
10. How they get along with/feel about their friends having other friends

Trays for exploring attitudes and experiences at school/work
1. Their teacher/boss
2. Their favorite/least favorite experiences at school/work
3. Kinds of problems they have at school/work
4. Kinds of problems others have at their school/work
5. How the members of their class/work would solve a problem (can be specific or in general)
6. How people at school/work solve problems
7. School/work rules (which ones they like/which ones they dislike/which ones they follow/which ones they ignore/violate)
8. How they get along at school (in the classroom/on the playground) or at work

Trays exploring clients' experiencing and attitudes toward life
1. Wonderful, Fantastic Day or a Horrible, No Good Day
2. Three wishes they would make

3. Their favorite book, fairytale, movie, TV show, video game
4. A dream they have had
5. Things that bug them
6. A time/times when they felt successful
7. A time/times when they felt successful solving a problem
8. A time/times when they felt discouraged trying to solve a problem
9. "My life," "my week," "my year," etc.
10. Meeting a character who breathes fire (or other traits that symbolically represent something that they must deal with in another person or situation in their lives). A part of the setup will be the question "What will you need to take to be able to deal with this character?"
11. Going to a new world (a place they have never been before, like a dinosaur world; a new planet; outer space; some location connected to a movie, book, or video game they like; etc.). They pick a character that represents them and a character who knows something about this world and is going with them and can give advice. The tray is planning the trip and what they need to take with them.

Art Techniques

Safe Place Drawing/Painting

One of the first art techniques we use with many of our clients is a safe place drawing or painting (or even a sticker picture). It is a lovely vehicle for helping you understand what is important for clients' sense of safety, which is often important before you dive into in-depth exploration of client dynamics.

The setup (we acknowledge that this is a bit obvious, and we can't think of another way to describe it—it really is just this simple) is that you tell clients to draw or paint "a safe place." You can even (if you want to swing out and do something radical) ask them to create a sand tray showing a place where they would feel safe. After they are finished, you can make the choice whether you want to just let the experience stand on its own or you want to guide them in verbally processing how that place establishes or contributes to a sense of safety for them. We usually do this with individual clients, and you could definitely use it with a family or members of a group.

Sometimes at the end of this activity, we ask clients if we can keep the drawing or painting or take a photograph of the sand tray to bring it out whenever we start a session or whenever they feel anxious. Other times, clients want to take their creation home. (Okay, we don't let them actually take the sand tray and the sand tray figures home—we are generous, but not that generous—and you can send a photograph of it with them.) With clients whom you want to help learn to take responsibility for keeping themselves safe (because they are old enough to have that be part of what they are working on or because the adults in their life don't particularly do an amazing job of keeping them safe), you can also have them add in or do a separate drawing/painting/sticker picture/sand tray on what they can do to help keep themselves safe.

Kinetic Family, School, Work Drawings

Strangely enough, the goal of the Kinetic Family Drawing is to explore family dynamics; the goal of the Kinetic School Drawing is to explore attitudes toward, experience of, and relationships at school; and the goal of the Kinetic Work Drawing is to explore attitudes toward, experience of, and relationships at work. One of the best ways to discover interpersonal dynamics is to ask clients to use the basic format for the Kinetic Family Drawing (KFD) ("Draw a picture of the people in your family, all of them doing something)"or the Kinetic School Drawing (KSD) ("Draw a picture of yourself, your teacher, and several classmates, with everyone doing something" (Brooke, 2004; Knoff & Prout, 1985; Kottman & Meany-Walen, 2016; Nurse & Sperry, 2012). We adapted the basic procedure used in the traditional projective techniques of the KFD and KSD into a more casual exploration strategy and changed the standard questions into questions we might want to ask in Adlerian play therapy (Kottman & Meany-Walen, 2016). The following is a list of questions we could use to gather information with the KFD about family dynamics important for Adlerian play therapists. You can use these lists of questions if they work for you, or you can generate your own list of questions that would work better for what you want to learn about client dynamics.

1. Who is this person? (pointing to each of the people the client has drawn)
2. What is his or her relationship to you?
3. How old is this person?
4. Tell me a little bit about this person.
5. What is this person doing?
6. How does this person feel?
7. What does this person need the most?
8. How do you feel about this person?
9. How does this person get along with other people?

Choose several of these questions to ask about individual figures:

1. What does this person wish for?
2. What is this person thinking?
3. What do you like about this person?

4. What don't you like about this person?
5. What happened to this person right before the picture?
6. What will happen to this person right after the picture?
7. What will happen to this person in the future?
8. What does this person do well?
9. What does this person get in trouble for?
10. What is this person afraid of?
11. Which of the other children are you most like? How?
12. Which of them is most different from you? How?
13. With which of them do you spend the most time? Doing what?
14. Which of the children is Mom's favorite?
15. Which of the children is Dad's favorite?
16. Which of the children is most like Mom? How?
17. Which of the children is most like Dad? How?
18. Which of your parents are you most like? How?

Choose some of the following questions to ask about the family:

1. What is the family doing?
2. What will happen to this family right after this picture?
3. What happened to this family right before this picture?
4. What will happen to this family in the future?
5. If you could change anything about this family, what would you change?

Here is a list of questions we could use to gather information with the KSD about school and classroom dynamics important for Adlerian play therapists:

1. Who is this person? (pointing to each of the people in the drawing)
2. Tell me a little bit about this person.
3. What is this person doing?
4. How does this person feel?
5. How do you feel about this person?
6. How does this person get along with other people?

Choose several of these questions to ask about individual figures:

1. What does this person wish for?
2. What is this person thinking?
3. What do you like about this person?
4. What don't you like about this person?
5. What happened to this person right before the picture?
6. What will happen to this person right after the picture?

7. What will happen to this person in the future?
8. What does this person do well?
9. What does this person get in trouble for?
10. What happens when this person gets in trouble?
11. What is this person afraid of?
12. What does this person do for fun?
13. What does this person think about school?
14. Which of these friends do you most like? How?
15. Which of these friends is most different from you? How?
16. With which of these friends do you spend the most time?
17. Which of these friends is the teacher's favorite? Why?
18. Which of these friends doesn't the teacher like? Why?
19. How do things go for you in school?

Choose several of these questions to ask about school interactions:

1. What is the class doing?
2. What will happen to this class right after this picture?
3. What happened to this class right before this picture?
4. What will happen to this class in the future?
5. If you could change anything about this class, what would you change? What would you change about the school?

Because I (Terry) do a lot of play therapy with adults and teens, I modified the kinetic drawing procedure to create the Kinetic Work Drawing (KWD). You can modify the instructions for any situation you want to investigate—neighborhood, church, friends, groups, and so on. To set up the KWD, you would say something like: "I'd like you to draw a picture of your work. Put yourself, your boss if you have one, and a co-worker or two in the picture. Draw everybody *doing* something." When the client has finished drawing, ask the client the following questions about each of the figures:

1. Who is this person?
2. Can you tell me a little bit about this person?
3. What is this person doing?
4. How does this person feel?
5. How do you feel about this person?
6. How does this person get along with the other people?

Choose several of these questions to ask about individual figures:

1. What does this person wish for?
2. What is this person thinking?

3. What do you like about this person?
4. What don't you like about this person?
5. What happened to this person right before the picture?
6. What will happen to this person right after the picture?
7. What causes this person difficulties at work?
8. What does this person do well?
9. What does this person get in trouble for?
10. What happens when this person gets in trouble?
11. What is this person afraid of?
12. What does this person do for fun?
13. Which of these people is supportive of you? What do they do that is supportive?
14. Which of these people is most like you? How?
15. Which of these people is most different from you? How?
16. With which of these do you have the most conflict? What are the conflicts about? How are the conflicts resolved?
17. Which of these people is the boss's favorite? Why?
18. Which of these people doesn't the boss like? Why?
19. How do things go for you at work?
20. What do you like about your job?
21. What is difficult for you about your job?
22. If you could change anything about your job, what would you change?
23. If you could change anything about your workplace, what would you change?
24. Describe the "perfect" boss for you.
25. Describe the "perfect" co-worker.
26. If you could create your "dream job," what would it be? Describe what your workplace would be like and what you would do there.
27. What keeps you from creating your "dream job"?
28. What are you willing to do to move toward attaining your "dream job"?

Also (and this is really important to us), don't limit yourself to just drawing—be creative. You can do this in any modality you think will appeal to particular clients. We do things like kinetic family dance party (in which we ask clients to show us how the various people in their family dance); kinetic work fake song (in which we ask them to compose a "fake" song, with fake lyrics for their boss, several co-workers, and themselves at work); kinetic work PlayDoh sculpture (in which we ask them to make a sculpture of their teacher, several classmates, and themselves at school). If you have clients who like to express themselves in a certain way, having given yourself permission, you can just make up a kinetic family _____ when you are trying to explore family dynamics, a kinetic neighborhood _____, a kinetic friendship group _____, or a kinetic anything else you want to explore.

Buttons-As-Family

Another activity you can use to explore family dynamics would be the buttons-as-family technique. There are many variations of this assessment tool. I (Terry) learned it in a class at the annual summer school of the Adlerian Network of Ireland. (Embarrassingly enough, I don't remember the name of the teacher—as my grandmother used to say, "Getting old is hell!") You could do this with individual clients, groups, or families.

You start with a collection of buttons—big ones, little ones, old ones, new ones, metal ones, plastic ones, broken ones, and so on. Spread the buttons out on a table and tell clients to choose a button (be generous: you could let them pick two or three) for each person in their family. Then give them a piece of paper (again, you can be generous and give them a couple of sheets just to see if some of the buttons get placed in a separate piece of paper than the rest of the family), and tell them to arrange the buttons on the paper. Afterward, you can basically use the same procedure you would with a sand tray, starting with the experiencing, rearranging, touring, processing, noticing, rearranging, and so on. If you are feeling supergenerous (and you have a lot of buttons), you can let them glue the buttons to the paper once they decide whether they want them for good and take their family with them at the end of the session. We also like to use our buttons for "Button Stories," using buttons for characters in a story, because it gives clients who prefer to communicate via metaphor one more way to keep a safe distance between themselves and the events of the story.

Pokemon Character Creation

This is an activity that I (Terry) developed in response to the recent rise of interest in the video game Pokemon (and, with some clients, the game played with Pokemon cards). It can be used to explore both intrapersonal dynamics (especially self-image, recognition of personal strengths and weaknesses, and willingness to assess and take appropriate risks) and interpersonal dynamics (especially friendship). Because the focus is on characters from a video game usually played by elementary school children, it seems to work best with them (especially with that elusive population group—9- to 12-year-old boys). We have also used this activity successfully with adolescent and adult gamers.

The activity is pretty simple: you give clients some pieces of paper, some crayons or markers, and ask them to create a Pokemon character of their own. Folks who are familiar with the various Pokemon characters will jump at a chance to create their own; folks who are interested in this process but not familiar with Pokemon characters might need a little help to begin to imagine what a character would look like. With those clients, you can prime the pump by providing them with some examples—we have used stickers from a book of Pokemon characters or Pokemon cards. After the character is created, you can suggest that the clients make a list of three attacks (which is consistent with Pokemon cards) and three defenses (my own invention that is not part of the Pokemon cards) the character can use to keep himself, herself, or itself safe. Just like in the cards and the video game, the characters can also have health points (HPs)—the reservoir of strength that gets depleted during a battle with another character—the average Pokemon character will have about 100 (+ or –20) HP. With some clients, this initial art segment of the activity is enough. Lots of clients will want to describe their character, make up a backstory for the character, and explain how their weapons and defenses work. For clients who really get into this activity (and many do), you can have them create an army of these characters—or even two armies—and have them battle among themselves or battle the other army just like they would with the cards or in the video game. You can also use this in groups, with each member creating his or her own army of Pokemon characters and doing battle against the other members, forging alliances and collaboration teams for the battles.

Beware of those rigid clients who are offended at the idea that new Pokemon characters can be created outside the "real" game or at the suggestion that Pokemon characters can have defenses as well as attacks. These clients can sometimes get incensed by your audacity in suggesting a variation of how the game works. While it might indicate that this is an activity you would only bring up once with that particular client, this reaction can give you insight into how that particular client acts when others violate his or her own personal rules about how things should work. It would also give you something to revisit in future conversations as an "in our sessions" example of this reaction, which surely causes difficulty in other relationship outside of therapy. You can also keep it in your back pocket as a possibility for working on practicing flexibility and tolerance in future sessions during the "making changes" phase of play therapy.

Self-Portraits

Self-portraits can give you information about clients' self-image and self-perceived character traits. They can be useful with all ages and in all forms of play therapy. There are a number of different ways to do a self-portrait. Self-portraits can be representational or nonrepresentational. Clients who like to draw "realistic" drawings can actually do a representational drawing or painting of themselves—either their whole body or just their face. You can also ask them to draw shapes and patterns that show you how they feel about themselves, or you can ask them to tear construction paper and make a "portrait" of themselves. They can take stickers and make a "portrait" that way. They can draw a picture of themselves as an animal, plant, building, vehicle—the list is endless. They can make a picture of their energy in a variety of different situations or relationships. You can also suggest they draw two self-portraits—one of their "real" self and one of their "ideal" self. Folks who don't like to produce artwork can also make a collage—with animal photos, facial features, other pictures, or words cut from magazines—that represents who they are.

The Garden

This activity was inspired by Violet Oaklander's Rosebush technique, in which you ask clients to imagine themselves as a rosebush (Oaklander, 1978/1992). I (Terry) wanted something that would apply more to group and family dynamics, so I adapted the meditation and the questions to focus more on issues related to family, friend groups, and school/work. There are multiple potential goals for this activity. You could use it to explore self-image with clients of all ages. With children or teens who are struggling with family issues, with friends, or in school, or with adults who are struggling with work issues (or with family or friends), you could use it to examine interpersonal issues—exploring family dynamics, school/work relationships, and friendships. During the phase of play therapy in which you are helping clients make changes, you can also use this as a vehicle for clients learning to recognize and interpret social information and/or accept responsibility in interpersonal interactions. It may also be used as a tool for helping clients to ask for their personal needs to be met and set limits and boundaries.

Here's what you do: first of all, gather whichever art supplies work well with your client. Tell the client to get comfortable sitting or lying down (depending on your setting). Explain that you are going to lead the client through an imaginary journey, and ask him or her to listen and visualize whatever you ask him or her to see. Read the following guided visualization. *(Pause about 10 seconds whenever we have an ellipsis [. . .]. You can vary this depending on the client and your sense of how long he or she might need to actually visualize that aspect of the garden.)*

"I would like you to close your eyes. Just be aware of your body. Forget about what's been going on around you . . . just think about what's going on inside of you. Think about your breathing . . . feel the air move in through your nose and mouth, down into your chest—imagine that your breathing is like gentle waves lapping on the shore . . . As each wave rolls in, the more relaxed you feel.

"Think about your right arm. Feel it getting heavier and heavier . . . Feel the heaviness go all the way down the arm, down to your fingertips . . . Think about your left arm . . . Feel it getting heavier and heavier . . . Feel the heaviness go down, down, into your fingertips . . . Think about your left leg . . . Feel it getting heavier and heavier . . . Feel the heaviness go down, down, into your foot . . . Think about your right leg . . . Feel it getting heavier and heavier . . . Feel the heaviness go down, down, into your foot . . . Feel your body relaxing and feeling heavy . . .

"Now, I'd like you to imagine that you are a plant in a garden. Become one of the plants in the garden and find out what it's like to be a plant . . . What kind of plant are you? Are you very small? Are you large? Are you wide? Are you tall? . . . Do you have flowers? If so, what kind? They can be any kind you want . . . Do you have leaves? . . . What kind? . . . What are your stems and branches like? . . . Do you have any thorns? . . . What are your roots like? Or maybe you don't have any . . . If you do, are they long and straight? Are they twisted? Are they deep? . . . Look around you and see if there are any other plants in the garden. *(pause 15 seconds)* If there are other plants, imagine what they look like. *(pause 15 seconds)* Are there only a few of them or are there lots of them? Are the other plants the same as you or are they different? Do the other plants have leaves . . . flowers . . . stems . . . roots . . . thorns? *(pause 20 seconds)* How close are the other plants to where you are? Are they the same size as you or bigger or smaller? Is the garden in a pot or is it growing in the ground? Or through cement? Or even inside somewhere? *(pause 20 seconds)* Look around you. *(pause 20 seconds)* What do you see? *(pause 20 seconds)* Are there statues in the garden? . . . Animals? . . . People? . . . Birds? . . . Is there anything around you like a fence? If there is, what does it look like? . . . Does someone take care of you? If there is someone who takes care of you, what does he or she look like? . . . What does he or she do to take care of you? *(pause 20 seconds)* Does that person also take care of the other plants? What's the weather like for you right now? . . . What is your life like? . . . How do you feel? . . . What do you experience, and what happens to you as the seasons change? *(pause 20 seconds)* Be aware of yourself as a plant in a garden . . . look round carefully. Find out how you feel about your life in the garden. *(Pause a minute or two—relying on your clinical intuition to decide how long.)*

"In a little while, I'll ask you to come back to the present and reconnect with your body. Now come back . . . open your eyes and settle in. It is time take a piece of paper and drawing supplies and draw a picture of yourself as the plant and the rest of the garden.

When the client is finished drawing, ask the following questions you think will give you information you might find useful (and any others that might occur to you). (We want to acknowledge that this is a *lot* of questions, so tailor the number and which ones to the client.)

1. What kind of plant are you, and what do you look like?
2. Tell me about your flowers.
3. Tell me about your leaves.
4. Tell me about your stems and branches.
5. Do you have thorns? If so, tell me about them. If not, tell me how you protect yourself. Are you an unfriendly plant or a friendly plant?
6. Tell me about your roots.
7. Tell me about the other plants in the garden. Are they the same as you or different (bigger or smaller, the same kind of plant, etc.)?
8. Tell me about where you are in the garden. Are you close to the other plants or far away? Where are you located inside the garden (i.e., middle, outside, edge)?
9. Tell me about where you live. What kind of things do you see around you? How do you like living where you are? What else is in the garden with you?
10. Who takes care of you? How do you feel about that? How do they look after you?
11. Who takes care of the other plants? How do you feel about that? How do they look after the other plants?
12. What's the weather like for you right now? What happens to you as the seasons change?
13. How does it feel to be a plant? What is your life like as a plant?
14. How do you feel about living in this garden? If you could change the garden, what would you change?
15. If you could move to a different garden, would you? What kind of a garden would be the perfect garden for you?

You could use the "I notice" technique described in the sand tray play therapy section in Chapter 3 to explore things in the drawing you think might be important. Notice that this entire activity is done through metaphors. With most clients, you will want to just leave all the processing in metaphor without bringing it into the "real world." With clients who like to move back and forth from metaphor to the real world and back again, you can follow their lead and make some guesses about what various elements of the drawing mean in the real world or what they tell you about the client's "real" life.

Structured Play Experiences

Friendship Recipe

This activity is fun to do with children (either in a group or individually) with whom you want to explore friendship dynamics. It is pretty elementary for adolescents and adults. You ask clients to give you a list of "ingredients" that go into making friendships. Then you help them figure out how many "cups" of each ingredient they believe are important in making and keeping friends.

Friendship Dos and Don'ts

The goal of this activity is the same as that of the friendship recipe—to explore friendship dynamics. (You can also use it in groups for group member "dos and don'ts" and in families for family member "dos and don'ts.") In addition to having this be part of your exploration of dynamics process, you can have it be part of the stage of play therapy in which you work with clients to gain insight into their patterns.

This one is also pretty rudimentary, and we have had some good times with younger elementary students (and even preschool kids) with it. We use a body outline of a "friend" and have clients give us a list of the things they believe friends should do in order to be friends and things they believe friends should not do. (This is pretty simple . . . can't make it more complex than that we're afraid.) You can let this activity rest on its laurels (just having done it might be enough for some clients), or you can have a conversation after they finish the lists, talking about which of their friends follow these rules, whether they follow their own rules, whether they want to keep all of their rules, or whether they would like to change some of them.

Circles of Intimacy

The goal of this technique is to explore interpersonal dynamics—depending on which dynamics you want to explore, you make the activity about that. For instance, if you want to explore closeness, you design the circles around intimacy or friendship; if you want to explore safety, you do the circles around that; if you want to explore fun, do that. This technique works better with older elementary children, teens, and adults because younger children don't really understand the abstract concept symbolized by the circles. We find it can be a little tense if you do it in a group or family, so we tend to do it with individual clients.

This activity starts with a drawing of about six concentric circles—you can make the drawing for the client or explain how to do it to your client.

(I [Terry] even have a diagram of this on my computer that I just print out—you can make one for yourself—it takes about 5 minutes and then you have it available.) If you are doing the intimacy or closeness version, tell clients to put their name in the middle circle and then put the names of the people in their life to whom they feel the closest in the next circle out from the middle circle, followed by the names of the next tier of people to whom they are close in the next circle, and so on. I then ask them to describe each of these people they have included and (if this is developmentally appropriate) what qualities, characteristics, and/or behaviors they exhibit that earn them a place in that particular circle. If you want to gather information about intrapersonal dynamics (e.g., clients' character traits), you can also ask them what it is about their personality or behaviors that might be attractive to those people.

If you are satisfied with the information you have been given up until that point, you can stop there. However, if you want to deepen your understanding of the client's interpersonal dynamics, you can also ask clients if they are pleased with the number of people they have included or if they would like more or fewer people in their circles. You can also ask them who they would like to move closer to the inner circle (themselves) and who they would like to move further away from the inner circle. If you really want to get wild (and you want to violate one of our rules), you could ask them to elaborate on why. Depending on the variation of this activity you are using, you would adjust the client instructions to fit whatever you are exploring.

Role-Playing Dynamics

Another structured play technique you can use to explore interpersonal dynamics involves role-playing (i.e., asking clients to play a role). (We know this seems obvious, but we want them to actually show us how people act, and eventually show us how they react to those people.) It works well with all ages and with individuals, groups, and families.

There are several different ways to use this technique. One method is to ask clients to act out important people in their lives (their best friend, their least favorite person, the bully in their neighborhood, the other clients on the cheerleading squad, their grandmother, etc.). You can do this in a free-standing way (and kind of intuit how they react to those people), or you can make a follow-up request, which is to ask them to show you their reactions when the people they are imitating act that way. Another way to ask clients to role-play involves costumes. We usually use hats (which involves choosing a hat and then "channeling" the other person or choosing a hat and showing how they feel and react to that person), and you can use other costumes or a mirror with face paints if you want.

You can also use props, like weapons (if you have them in your playroom), sand tray play therapy figures, or some other toy, and ask them to choose a prop to help them show you how that person acts or how they react to that person.

THEORETICAL CONSIDERATIONS IN EXPLORING INTRAPERSONAL AND INTERPERSONAL DYNAMICS WITH CLIENTS IN PLAY THERAPY

In addition to the dynamics described in this chapter, many of the theoretical approaches have information and methods of exploration specific to that style of play therapy. We have already described what else Adlerian play therapists would want to know—information about the Crucial Cs, goals of behavior and misbehavior, personality priorities, and functioning at life tasks.

Most child-centered play therapists would not spend a great deal of time gathering information, though they might use observation to help them understand the gap between a client's "real self" and "ideal self." They might also use observation to notice what a client's conditions of worth are as a guide to places where the client could use extra unconditional positive regard.

Cognitive-behavioral play therapists combine the skill of observation and standardized testing to gather information about clients' affective/emotional, cognitive, behavioral, and language factors (Cavett, 2015; Carmichael, 2006; Knell, 2016). The standardized instruments often used by cognitive-behavioral play therapists include the *Child Behavior Checklist,* the *Minnesota Child Development Inventory,* and the *Puppet Sentence Completion Task.* These are supplemented by behavioral observation and play assessment like a feeling thermometer. The primary focus for exploration in cognitive-behavioral play therapy is always on the client's behavior and the factors in the client's environment that reinforce the behavior and the client's thinking patterns.

Ecosystemic play therapists engage in a much more formal evaluation process than that described in this chapter. They have a formal interview with caregivers, an interview with the child–client, and a family interview, all designed to assess current functioning and evaluate the ecosystems in which the client lives. Ecosystemic play therapists work with parents on completing the *Developmental Therapy Objective Rating Form-Revised* (DTORF) (Developmental Therapy Institute, 1992; O'Connor, 1993, 2016), which measures behavior, communication, socialization, and academics, and the *Marschak Interaction Method* (Marschak, 1960), an assessment tool that measures the parent–child interactional pattern (O'Connor, 2016). They may also use other standardized assessment instruments (e.g., *Wechsler Intelligence Scales for Children,* the *Personality Inventory for Children,* the *Developmental Teaching Objectives Rating Form,* and the *Connors Rating Scale*) and projective instruments (e.g., the *Children's Projective Drawing Battery,* the *Roberts Apperception Test for Children*) (Carmichael, 2006).

Gestalt play therapists seldom use formal assessment instruments in their exploration, relying on observation, questions, art techniques, metaphors and storytelling, and structured play techniques to explore dynamics (Carmichael, 2006; Oaklander, 1994). In Gestalt play therapy, in addition to the general dynamic factors described earlier in the chapter, practitioners are also interested in exploring client awareness of his or her process and contact boundary disturbances.

Jungian play therapists do little formal assessment in the process of play therapy. Because they are nondirective, their primary exploration tool is observation—of the client's actions and reactions in sessions (Carmichael, 2006; Green, 2009; Lilly, 2015). Jungian play therapists are always on the alert for picking up on the symbols present in their client's play, especially archetypes of the unconscious (Lilly, 2015). They might also ask the client to do a sand tray, though most of the time they would do a nondirective sand tray (asking the client to choose figures and put them in the tray without any more structure than that) (Punnett, 2016).

Practitioners of the narrative approach to play therapy would want to know more about the client's stories about himself or herself, the world and other people, the client's connection to the natural world, the client's culture and its wisdom and healing philosophies, and the client's willingness and ability to embrace his or her creativity (Cattanach, 2006; Mills, 2015). While narrative play therapists may occasionally ask questions, they would almost exclusively use observation (of the client's nonverbal expression during the client's stories and of the client's reactions as the therapist tells stories) and the techniques in the section on metaphor and storytelling in this chapter to gather information.

A psychodynamic play therapist would explore whether the client might be stuck in a particular psychosexual phase, whether the client could be struggling with an Oedipal or Electra complex, and how the client is getting his or her needs (for affection and approval, power, social recognition, personal admiration, personal achievement, self-sufficiency, independence, and perfection) met (Cangelosi, 1993; Mordock, 2015).

The primary focus of exploration in Theraplay is on the level of the client's attachment and the parent/child elements of structure, engagement, nurture, and challenge (Booth & Winstead, 2015, 2016; Jernberg & Jernberg, 1995). The tool used for exploration in Theraplay is the *Marschak Interaction Method,* which provides information about the family and how the parents interact with the children. Some Theraplay practitioners also use formal, standardized assessment instruments like the *Child*

Behavior Checklist, the *Beck Depression Inventory,* the *Connors Rating Scale,* and the *School-Aged Assessment of Attachment* to assess the patterns in the client's behavior and attachment.

In integrative/prescriptive play therapy, exploration of interpersonal and intrapersonal dynamics is extremely important because the course of therapy is determined by the play therapist's understanding of the dynamics. Of course, you know what we will say about which assessment tools each individual integrative/prescriptive play therapist will use—it depends. It is determined by his or her initial appraisal of clients' presenting problems and issues, the therapist's own training and expertise in both assessment and interventions, the cooperation of other family members, and many other factors.

MOVING ON . . .

Once you have figured out whatever you deem important in understanding clients' dynamics, you still might be stuck in the refrain, "What now?" You are probably going to want to make a treatment plan and proceed into the next phase of the process of play therapy, guided by your theoretical framework and beliefs about people and how to move forward. The next chapter is all about how to help clients gain insight in the process of play therapy (if you think that helping clients gain insight is important in play therapy).

Interlude 5

Developing a Conceptualization of Your Clients

$\mathcal{A}$ s you use the skills of asking questions and observing and the techniques designed to explore intrapersonal and interpersonal dynamics, you will be working to make sense of the information you are gathering. You want to apply your theory to help figure out what clients' patterns of intrapersonal and interpersonal dynamics tell you about where their issues are, what your therapeutic goals should be, and what is the best way to move forward. You have gathered a mass of information. The details on which you focus should reflect what you believe about people and how they grow and change and what you believe about the process of counseling and play therapy.

As a way of organizing the information you are gathering, you need to ask yourself, "What do my observations tell me about . . ."

- The emotional patterns of the client? As part of your assessment, you might ask yourself about whether the client is depressed, anxious, angry, despairing, discouraged, tense, insecure, ashamed, confused, disgusted, afraid, distrustful, guilty, hopeless, vulnerable, and/or hurting? (Notice that none of these feelings are pleasant or positive—remember that most of the clients we see in play therapy are not going to be happy campers.) Do the client's emotional patterns change in different situations or different relationships? How intense are the emotions the client is experiencing? Do the client's emotional patterns interfere with his or her functioning in any way?

What are the triggers that evoke the various emotions the client is feeling?

- The cognitive patterns of the client? For example, are there faulty convictions or irrational beliefs about self, others, and the world? Does the client think in a linear or a tangential way? Are the client's thoughts abstract or concrete? The client's cognitive patterns are the usual thoughts he or she has about self, others, and the world, and the way thoughts interact with emotions and behaviors.

- The behavioral patterns of the client? For example, is the client avoiding, isolating, uncooperative, impulsive, aggressive? Does the client argue, get into power struggles, or draw attention through inappropriate behavior?

- The body/physical patterns of the client? How does the client manifest his or her thoughts and emotions in his or her body (e.g., hunched shoulders, butterflies in stomach, dizziness, and so forth)? Has the client experienced traumatic events that have left physical symptoms?

- The attitudinal patterns of the client? What are the client's attitudes toward other people? Toward work or school? Toward his or her family? For example, does the client give up easily, get into power struggles, or have a pattern of believing "it's not my fault"?

- The client's self-image? What are the client's beliefs about himself or herself as a person? What is the client's sense of self in the various roles he or she plays in his or her life? What have you noticed about the client's self-confidence, sense of self-efficacy, and self-responsibility?

- The client's recognition of personal strengths and weaknesses? Does the client recognize personal strengths, and is he or she able to "own" strengths? Is the client being realistic about his or her assets? Does the client recognize his or her personal weaknesses? Is the client realistic about his or her limitations? Is the client willing to take responsibility for times when he or she is struggling?

- The client's emotional self-awareness? Can the client recognize his or her own feelings, as well as the triggers? Does the client know about the places in his or her body where emotions are experienced or stored? Is the client aware of the patterns of emotions he or she experiences on a regular basis? Is the client aware of the patterns in the intensity of his or her emotions? Can the client regulate the intensity of his or her emotions?

- The client's ability to self-regulate? Can the client monitor and control his or her emotions, thoughts, and behaviors? Where would the client fall on a continuum from "too loose" or "too tight"?

- The client's capacity for making decisions and setting and monitoring progress toward goals? How does the client make decisions and set and monitor progress toward goals? Does the client have the capacity for making and taking responsibility for his or her choices? What is the client's facility with and willingness to set short-term and long-term goals? How competent is the client in assessing movement toward goals?

- The client's willingness to assess and take appropriate risks? What is the client's willingness to take physical, intellectual, emotional, interpersonal risk? What is the client's aptitude for assessing which risks are "real" and which are psychological? What is the client's ability to assess which risks make sense for him or her to take?

- The client's movement toward self-actualization? What is the client's attitude toward self-actualization? Does the client manifest a desire to grow, to become, to change in positive ways and actual positive momentum toward becoming his or her best self? Is the client moving in the direction of self-actualization?

Each of the theoretical approaches to play therapy will have a unique pattern of focusing on these questions. Some will emphasize feelings, whereas others will emphasize thinking or interacting. Some will put more weight on emotional self-awareness, whereas others will pay more attention to the ability to self-regulate. You will have to decide how you want to apply your own theoretical approach and your personal way of thinking about people and how they change as you develop your conceptualization of each client. We have attempted to cover the elements most approaches to play therapy include in their conceptualization. There may be other factors you think are important, and they should be included in your conceptualization. You might want to consult Chapter 2 and even go to some original sources to begin to integrate your choice of a theoretical approach with your own ideas about people and how they change.

You will want to start conceptualizing your clients from your first meeting with them. However, the crux of conceptualizing your clients happens after you've gathered much of the information about clients' interpersonal and intrapersonal dynamics. Because, from our theoretical perspective, we can intervene on an emotional, cognitive, or behavioral level, we use the information we've gathered to decide how we believe clients will best be able to gain insight. Then, lo and behold, we use skills and tailor interventions to clients' unique styles of learning to move toward counseling goals. You will need to have a consistent way of taking the information you have compiled and organized to develop your treatment plan for clients.

We find it helpful to write out the areas that are important to us and our guiding theory and then decide (surprise, surprise . . . guided by our theory) how to proceed. By gathering information and tracking what we know about our clients, we can decide if we have enough information to move forward and in what ways we should move forward. Conceptualizing our clients according to our theory's constructs is like creating a road map of where we are, where we're going, and how we are going to get there. Developing a course of action helps to make the therapeutic process efficient and directed.

CHAPTER 6

Helping Clients Gain Insight

As you might have already guessed, when we talk about helping clients gain insight, we are referring to helping clients become more aware of their own patterns of behavior, emotion, cognition, attitude, and motivation. It may also involve helping them begin to understand the underlying meaning of their play and verbalizations. This chapter contains information about play therapy skills and techniques designed to help clients gain insight into patterns, underlying meaning, and anything else your theoretical approach or you yourself deem significant to bring to a greater awareness with your clients. Before detailing skills and techniques you can use to help clients gain insight, it would probably be valuable for you to consider several questions. Do you believe that gaining insight is necessary for change to occur in play therapy with clients? If so, do you believe that gaining insight is necessary for change to occur in play therapy for all clients or only for clients in a certain age range or in certain stages of development? Do you believe helping clients gain insight is an important component of your role as a play therapist?

As you consider these questions, it might influence your thinking to know that there are approaches to play therapy, such as Theraplay and cognitive-behavioral play therapy, based on the premise that insight is not necessary for change to occur—that change can occur without increased awareness. In child-centered play therapy, although therapists do sometimes use the skill of interpretation, they do not use techniques or activities to help clients gain insight because they believe that clients will come into a greater awareness without directive intervention by the play therapist. Other approaches to play therapy (Adlerian, ecosystemic, Gestalt,

Jungian, psychodynamic, and integral) hold that, with most clients, an increased awareness of their patterns is a key component of supporting positive change in play therapy; play therapists who subscribe to these approaches use both skills and techniques to forward this agenda. So, proceeding from the idea that you might have decided you believe increased awareness is important and are interested in helping clients gain insight, we move forward . . .

This chapter is based on the foundational premise that, for many clients, gaining insight is necessary for change to occur in play therapy, that the level of insight is dependent on clients' developmental level, and that helping clients to gain insight is an important component of the role of the play therapist. It is essential to remember that the answer to the question of whether to help bring certain material to clients' awareness is (get ready for it . . .) "it depends." To name a few of the factors on which it depends: (1) clients' developmental level, (2) their readiness to hear and accept a greater awareness, (3) the type of pattern to be brought to awareness, and (4) the potential impact of the increased awareness. You will need to use your best clinical judgment with regard to the timing, depth, and delivery of interventions designed to help clients gain insight.

In thinking about the impact of clients' developmental level on whether to help bring a greater awareness to certain patterns, it is helpful to keep in mind that most younger children and clients with intellectual disabilities need language and concepts to be simple and concrete, even when they are conveyed through metaphor. If you think an insight is too sophisticated for younger clients or for clients with intellectual disabilities, you may want to share your thoughts about specific patterns with parents and/or teachers rather than trying to communicate them directly to your clients.

No matter what the developmental level of your clients, it is essential to evaluate clients' readiness for insight before sharing what you have noticed with them or setting up activities designed to help them become more conscious of specific patterns that might be contributing to difficulties. When clients are ready, they tend to appear more open and curious about their own patterns. This can be manifested through comments they make during play sessions, through their narration as they play, or through the actual content of the play. With clients whose readiness is not obvious, sometimes it is necessary to attempt to help them gain insight through an interpretation or a metaphoric story. You will want to pay close attention to their reactions to help you determine whether they are open to greater awareness. If they have a negative or confused reaction, you know they are probably not ready, and you can go back to building the relationship or exploring dynamics. (It does not do any damage to have given it a shot though, so don't worry that clients are too fragile for you to make a mistake in timing.)

Some patterns are easier than others for clients to accept an increased level of awareness. Many times, clients who have experienced traumatic events are more resistant to insight than are clients who have not experienced traumatic events. There are other patterns that are easier for younger children to comprehend than others. For instance, most younger children would find it easier to understand your guess about an emotional pattern (e.g., "You usually seem worried when it is time to visit with your dad.") than a cognitive pattern (e.g., "You seem to think that you can't count on your dad to keep you safe.") Other times, what contributes to clients having difficulty hearing and accepting that certain patterns have an impact on them and their lives might be related to family or societal rules and values. For instance, in some families certain feelings are deemed acceptable (perhaps sadness and joy) and others are considered unacceptable (perhaps anger). You will need to consider the possibility that clients might not want to gain insight into specific patterns and be willing to accept insight into other patterns. Again, by observing clients' reactions to your working to help them gain insight, you can adjust what you are doing.

The potential impact of increased awareness on specific clients may also affect whether you use the skills and techniques from this chapter to help them gain insight into particular patterns. If the impact of gaining insight into a certain pattern would somehow create an overwhelming amount of cognitive dissonance or emotional upheaval, it might be better to wait until later in the therapeutic process or even at a later period in their lives. This would also be true for times in their lives when things are unstable or highly stressful, such as moving, the death of a family member, or changing schools or jobs.

It is critical that any messages designed to help clients gain awareness be delivered in a style consistent with their usual way of processing and expressing themselves, whether it be through direct communication or metaphor and symbols. As a reflection of a basic respect for clients, it is essential that they be given the distance created by communicating with symbols and metaphor if that is what they need. According to Yasenik and Gardner (2012), at times clients may be open to direct awareness, and at other times they may need something else: "The child's play could be very direct and literal, accompanied by verbalizations, indicating that the child is working with a certain level of conscious awareness. At other times, the child needs distance and protection from troublesome thoughts or feelings, and utilizes play scenarios and objects in a less conscious and more symbolic manner" (p. 46). We have also found that some clients almost always prefer to express themselves directly related to presenting problems, relationships, and situations in their lives; and there are others who almost always need the distance that is created by metaphors from consciously expressing themselves directly. There are also some clients who can switch back and forth between the two—with some topics and in some situations, communicating directly, and with other topics and in other situations, communicating through metaphors.

When dealing with clients who communicate directly, it is appropriate to have conversations with them in the playroom about their patterns of thinking, feeling, behaving, and so forth, and with clients who communicate through metaphor and symbols, you will need to do that. For instance, if you are working on impulsivity with 6-year-old Jeramiah, a client who always talks directly about his experiences, you can tell him you are going to play a game of pitch and catch designed to help him slow down and think before he does things. If, however, Jeramiah is a client who communicates in metaphor, as you are playing you could ask him how he thinks playing pitch and catch could help someone who has trouble slowing down and thinking before he does things. If Sally is a 16-year-old who communicates directly, when talking about a sand tray she has created about her dating much older men, you could make a guess about the connection between her abandonment by her father at an early age and her choices in men. If she is a client who communicates through metaphor, you could make a guess about the motivation of one of the figures in the tray instead of talking directly about what is going on with her.

When working with clients who communicate primarily through symbols and metaphors, you must work hard to match that style, avoiding "breaking" their metaphors by asking questions or making suggestions that bring them into reality (e.g., "I am guessing that guy who is hitting the woman in the doll house is like your dad," or "That 'friend' who is having trouble with his girlfriend is really you, right?" (ACK! That is what we would call "bad technique." Please try to avoid doing it.) In our experience, it is essential to avoid "breaking" clients' metaphors even when clients sometimes communicate directly and sometimes through symbols and metaphors. With these clients, it is important to match whatever method of communication they are currently using.

PLAY THERAPY SKILLS

Several skills can be used in play therapy to help clients gain insight into their patterns. Some of these are skills used in other forms of therapy that you can apply to play therapy (interpreting, using the client's metaphors, and confronting discrepancies) and one of them is specific to play therapy (designing therapeutic metaphors). Not all approaches to play therapy use all of these skills, and even the approaches that do use them vary in application. Following is a description of each of the skills and their use in play therapy.

Interpreting

Often clients are not aware that they are acting or reacting in a certain way; they frequently have no idea about how the patterns in their own intrapersonal and interpersonal dynamics are affecting them and their lives. Even those who are cognizant of their patterns may lack the abstract verbal reasoning ability to conceptualize what these patterns mean about them and their interactions or what to do in order to change them. Interpretation is a skill designed to help clients begin to notice and understand their own patterns. When play therapists use interpretation, they observe clients' play and verbalizations and make comments intended to help clients make meaning of what they are doing in the playroom and gain insight into their patterns, both inside and outside the playroom. By commenting about what is going on (and frequently, what it means), the play therapist can help clients think more clearly about their behavior, emotions, cognitions, reactions, attitudes, motivations, relationships, communication, problems, and so forth.

VanFleet et al. (2010) focused on interpreting play themes. They suggested that play might have special meaning for clients if the play is repeated, if they do similar activities with different toys, if they are playing with unusual intensity and focus, if specific play sequences happen in several different play sessions, if the play continues across sessions, and/ or if there is a shift in the emotional tone. By paying attention to play that has any of these qualities, you can begin to determine which play themes might be important to clients and consider interpreting them as a way of helping clients gain an awareness of what their play might mean. Van-Fleet et al. (2010) listed some common play themes for children: power and control, aggression, emotions, good against bad or evil, winning and losing, mastery of developmental tasks, mastery of anxiety or fears, reenactment of trauma, identity exploration and formation, boundaries and limits, grief and loss, nurturance and love, regression, attachment and connection, safety or protection paired with threat and danger, resilience, persistence, problem identification and solutions, wishes, and cultural symbolism. In our work with adolescent and adult play therapy clients, we have observed them to have the same themes in their play. (We add, however, that many times, no matter what the age of the client, even after all our years of experience in play therapy, we don't always know what play means, so don't get yourself in a tizzy if you have no idea what it means. You can still share the idea that you noticed it seemed important to clients even if you don't have a clue about why it is important to them.)

O'Connor (2002) suggested that if interpretations were going to help clients gain insight in ways that would help them solve problems, they needed to be delivered in developmentally appropriate language and in small enough increments that clients would not be overwhelmed. He suggested several different levels of interpretation of play themes and patterns. The play therapist can comment on the first level (content, which is about clients' overt behaviors and activities); the second level (feeling, which is about clients' emotional expression, including nonverbal cues, facial expressions, and voice intonation); the third level (intention, which is about the purpose of clients' play), the fourth level (psychological meaning, which is about deeper motivations and explanations of play filtered through psychological theory); the fifth level (relationship of the play to prior sessions, which is about the session-to-session pattern and what it might mean); and the sixth level (relationship of the play to daily life or events, which is about the connection between clients' behavior in sessions to actual events, situations, or relationships in the rest of their lives) (O'Connor, 2000). Obviously, the first and second levels require less interpretation about meaning than the subsequent levels.

According to Kottman (2011; Kottman & Meany-Walen, 2016), your interpretations can focus on:

1. Clients' nonverbal communication (e.g., "You looked over here like you were checking whether it was ok with me if you buried the stuffed animals in the sand.").
2. Clients' reactions to the therapist's statements and questions (e.g., "You looked nervous when I said we were going to do a puppet show. I am thinking that you aren't sure 20-year-olds are allowed to do puppet shows.").
3. Clients' subtle reactions to or feelings about interactions between the therapist and the client (e.g., "I am guessing you think I am crazy telling you we are going to blow bubbles together. It seems like a weird thing for grownups to do together.").
4. Clients' subtle reactions to the relationship between themselves and the therapist or to the play therapy process (e.g., "It seems like maybe you are wondering how playing with me is helping you.")
5. Nuances in the ways clients communicate (e.g., "I have noticed that it seems like when you are nervous, you talk more quietly, almost like you are hoping I don't hear what you are saying.").
6. The underlying meaning of clients' behavior (e.g., "Mrs. Hedgehog hides every time I reflect that she seems to be feeling irritated or annoyed. It seems like Mrs. Hedgehog thinks she is not allowed to get mad, so she hides when I notice that is how she is feeling.")
7. The underlying meaning of clients' verbalizations (e.g., "When you asked me whether I was going to Texas this year, I am thinking you were trying to tell me you wish I wouldn't go away for a long time this year.")

You can interpret patterns within a session (e.g., "I have noticed you appear to be kind of agitated today whenever your job is mentioned," or across several sessions (e.g., "The little bunny often has trouble finding someone to play with him, and he always seems sad when that happens."). You can also make interpretations of patterns that typify clients' personalities, coping strategies, communication style, approach to problem solving and conflict resolution, and any other aspect of their overall intrapersonal or interpersonal dynamics. Some theoretical approaches also use interpretations of patterns in clients' patterns that extend into relationships or situations outside of the playroom (e.g., "I have noticed that you are determined to be in control in the playroom. I am guessing that you also like to be in control at home and at school too.").

The various approaches to play therapy have several different labels for interpretations. While most approaches call interpretations "interpretations" (something like "a rose by any other name"), Adlerian play therapists call them "metacommunications" (Kottman & Meany-Walen, 2016), whereas some child-centered play therapists call them "enlarging the meaning" (Ray, 2011) or just "interpretations" (VanFleet et al., 2010). Regardless of what you choose to call them, here are some guidelines that will help you structure interpretations so that they can be optimally helpful to clients.

- Match clients' style of processing and expressing themselves. (We know we already said this in other contexts, but it bears repeating here.) You can make your interpretations directly, or you can embed them in clients' metaphors. This is really important because if you leave a metaphor to make an interpretation, you will most likely lose your clients' willingness to "hear" the interpretation. You will have more of the impact you intended if you make your interpretations using the characters and settings of the client's metaphors. If 4-year-old Leonard always uses a lion to represent himself, make your interpretations about what the lion feels and means. When 34-year-old Josie describes her life as a rat race, suggest that the rats must be awfully tired, always having to keep moving and competing with one another.

- Make sure your language is consistent with clients' developmental level. Gauge clients' verbal sophistication, and use vocabulary and concepts that they will be most likely to understand. Even when you make the world's most insightful and brilliant interpretation (and we have confidence that you will be doing just that), if clients don't understand what you are talking about, they will not gain insight into anything (other than maybe the disconnection between yourself and them).

- Always be tentative when delivering interpretations. You need to be careful to avoid jamming your ideas down clients' throats. By sharing your ideas in a tentative way (e.g., "I am guessing . . ." "Could it be that . . ." "Might it be true that . . ." "I am thinking that . . ." "It seems as though . . ."), you can make guesses about patterns, the meaning of the patterns, and the underlying meaning of the play without imposing your opinions or interpretation on clients.

  • Be intentional with your choices of what to interpret. (We know we are harping a bit on this intentionality, and we thought we hadn't mentioned it in a while, so we could just slip it in.) Pay attention to clients' readiness and openness to certain ideas and themes and make sure you share interpretations about the patterns and situations they are likely to be ready to examine, rather than places where they are stuck in denial or resistance.

  • Share your interpretations in small enough portions that clients are able to digest them. It is helpful to avoid making global interpretations that would be overwhelming to clients and result in stomachaches for them (either literal or metaphorical).

  • Watch clients' reactions to your interpretations. Notice whether clients seem open to hearing what you have to say or are uncomfortable with or resistant to your comments. Usually when clients find your interpretations to be helpful, they will do something that indicates they hear you and agree with what you said. This is often called a recognition reflex (Kottman & Meany-Walen, 2016) and can be anything from a smile or nod to verbal agreement. When clients either disagree with your interpretation or the interpretation was too much or too soon, they will almost always have a visible reaction. You need to look for some kind of a reaction. It might be a nonverbal reaction, which could be a play disruption (where clients interrupt what they are doing and abruptly switch to doing something else; Kottman, 2011), a frown, a shrug, a head shake, or some other subtle way of rejecting what you said. They could also make a verbal rejoinder, refuting what you said or the way you said it. When this happens, pay attention to the vehemence of their response. If they overreact, many times you were correct in your observation, but you were either too early or not gentle enough with your interpretation. This is your chance to say, "Well, it's something to think about" (the most valuable phrase I [Terry] learned in my entire doctoral program—again from my mentor Dr. Byron Medler). Don't get into a power struggle with them about whether or not you were right; just let it go, store it away in the back of your mind, and try it again later or in a different form. If they simple disagree, it could be that you were wrong. . . . if you think that it is possible you were mistaken, you can always apologize and suggest a reset.

  • Don't get attached to clients agreeing with your interpretation. Sometimes you will just be wrong. And sometimes you and a client will have a different idea of what something means. It is okay to make a mistake, and it is okay for clients to construe the meaning of something differently than you do. Many times, even if you are right, they may still need to disagree with you. That's okay too. Other times, you might be right, and clients will just ignore you. (Actually, this is the most prevalent situation with us and with many of our students.) Again, let it go. It isn't clients' job to affirm or confirm you . . . it is vitally important for you to let go of needing someone else to tell you that you are right, which is not what therapy (play or otherwise) is about (though many of us who are drawn to therapy really do want someone else to tell us we are right).

Using the Client's Metaphors

With clients who speak in metaphor, use their metaphors. (We know it might feel like we are beating a dead horse here, and we want to make sure you get how important this is . . . do you see what we just did there?) If Ronan uses the shark puppet to represent himself, you can ask the shark questions, make interpretations about the meaning of the shark's behavior, reflect the shark's feelings, and so forth. You can also tell stories about the shark and his relationships, problems, adventures, solutions, and so on. When Sissy uses a tornado figure to represent her boyfriend, you can talk about the tornado, you can ask the tornado questions, and you can talk to her about her and other people's reactions to having a tornado in their lives. When your adult play therapy clients use figurative language (like "rolling stones gather no moss," "barking up the wrong tree," "catching a hot potato," "crying over spilt milk," "being caught between a rock and a hard place"), jump right in and use this language with them. They will feel more understood and more open to hearing your "wisdom."

Confronting Discrepancies

Often clients are not consistent. Many times, those inconsistencies (e.g., between what they say this week and what they said last week, between what they are doing and what they are saying, between what David's teacher tells you about what happened on the playground and what David tells you, between how they say they feel and what their body tells you they are feeling) need to be confronted. Remember that, in therapy, confrontation means something different than it means in regular life. It doesn't mean you have to get in Imelda's face and yell at her; it just means you get to point out inconsistencies, gently bringing about clients' awareness of something they may have overlooked or avoided. Here are some guidelines that can help you use confrontation effectively in play therapy:

• Be gentle. This is important whenever you do a therapeutic confrontation, whether it is in play therapy or some other modality. When you are pointing out discrepancies, quite often clients' initial reaction will be defensiveness. One way to keep them from going into full-blown counterattack is to make sure you are not attacking them—you are just sharing a noticing of an inconsistency.

• Use humor. One way to make sure clients don't think you are attacking them is to use humor to point out inconsistencies rather than being in clients' faces with your confrontations. You can say things with a small smile or a kind laugh, starting with "And last week, you said. . . ." "Even though you say you are not mad, you are pounding on the floor with your fist." "It seems like maybe you and your mom don't exactly see what happened in the same light." Be careful, especially when you are working with children and teens, that you don't present your humor in ways that can be construed as teasing or sarcasm, which is actually counterproductive, invoking the very defensive reaction you are trying to avoid.

• Use confusion. We often use what we call the "Columbo" technique, named after the lead character from a television show from the 1970s, in which Columbo, a police detective from Los Angeles, solved crimes, at least partly, with his signature "confusion." (No, we don't tell our clients we are imitating a TV detective, even though some of our adult clients recognize this ploy.) When we are using this technique, we start sentences with something like "I'm kind of confused, Mr. Tiger. Last week, you said you didn't care if you have any friends, and this week you tell me that you are angry and sad because the other animals don't want to play with you." Or, "This is really confusing to me. You say you want a girlfriend who cherishes you, and you still stay with Katrina even when she is really mean to you." (Notice how we also watched our language choices and avoided using "but" because it also evokes a defensive reaction.)

• Pay attention to timing and readiness. Notice whether your clients are ready to hear what you have to say with your confrontation. Sometimes clients' denial is essential to their ability to cope, so recognize that there are times when confrontation is more effective than at other times. You need to have a solid relationship with clients before you can use confrontation. You also need to be sure that clients are ready to deal with the specific material being confronted.

Designing Therapeutic Metaphors

One of the skills essential in the process of helping clients gain insight and in helping clients make changes (just so you know, this is a skill for Chapter 7 too, and we are not typing all this again in forty pages or so) is designing therapeutic metaphors—made-up stories designed to communicate indirectly about a pattern that is not working or to teach something without being obvious about it. While we recognize that a whole category of strategies is dedicated to storytelling and therapeutic metaphors, we believe the creation of basic metaphors is a skill rather than a technique. Here are the steps for designing therapeutic metaphors (Gil, 2014; Kottman & Meany-Walen, 2016; Mills & Crowley, 2014):

1. Decide your goal in telling the story. This is the most important step in the whole process. Your goal should be concrete, uncomplicated, and achievable because if you try to use a story to accomplish something nebulous or all-encompassing (e.g., "pointing out that Tate has low self-esteem," "helping Sophia recognize her relationship with her mother is dysfunctional," "teaching Anthony anger management skills," or "ensuring Brianna's happiness"), the story is sure to fail in its purpose. So, keep it simple with goals like "Teaching Dakota deep breathing can serve as an anger management tool," "Highlighting Sophia calling her mother names is contributing to the difficulties in their relationship," or "Helping Mateo recognize when his negative self-talk is affecting his school performance." We recommend actually writing the goal of the story down in one concrete sentence like "The goal of this story is to help Akako recognize it is normal to experience two contradictory feelings about a person or situation." That way, if you get lost in the middle of telling the story, you can reorient yourself by revisiting your goal and making a story course correction.

2. Based on your previous interactions with the client, decide (a) whether you want to use toys or props in the telling of the story; (b) whether you believe that the client will be more responsive to a story that is reality-based or fantasy-based; (c) how close you can get in the telling of the story to the actual situation in the client's life; and (d) how you want to deliver the metaphor (just telling the story, drawing a picture to illustrate the story, making a book with or for the client, doing a puppet show, asking the client to act out the story as you tell it, etc.).

3. Decide when and where you want the story to take place. It is best to dislocate the story in time and space so that the client can maintain the desired emotional distance between the story and his or her experience. By dislocating the story in time, telling the story as if it happened in the past or will happen in the future, the client can deny that the story is about him or her. Dislocating the story in space, using some other town or country as the setting for the story, will also allow this. Even if the story takes place just a short time ago in the past or the future (i.e., "last week" or "next month") or in a location a short distance from where the client lives (i.e., "in the town next door" or "a country close by"), by dislocating it in time and space, you create an emotional distance that allows the

client to listen to the story without automatically having to entertain the possibility that it might be about him or her.

4. Make the description of the physical setting of the story very clear and concrete. It is important that it not be completely the same as the child's situation, and it can have several parallels. The scene can be a natural setting ("in the jungle . . ."), a mythical setting ("in a place where all the animals could talk . . ."), or a realistic setting ("in my old neighborhood when I was a kid . . .").

5. Be very specific when describing the characters in the story. Each character should have a name and a description of both physical and emotional characteristics. At the least, characters should include a protagonist (this is usually an animal or a person who represents the child) and an antagonist (an animal, person, or situation creating difficulty for the protagonist). Sometimes it is also useful to include a character who is a resource person (someone who can provide advice or help for the protagonist—this character might represent the play therapist or some other important person in the client's life) and an ally or two (an animal or person who can provide support or encouragement for the protagonist).

6. Describe the difficulty or dilemma experienced by the protagonist in concrete terms. The problem can be related to a person and a relationship or to a situation that is causing the protagonist's struggles. This problem can be similar to the situation facing the client; however, the similarity should not be too obvious. It is important for you to avoid pointing out any similarities between the story and the client's life because the power to consciously recognize or acknowledge the parallels must belong to the client.

7. As you tell the story, especially if your client is an older elementary student, teen, or adult, it will make it more real (and helpful) to the client if you can elaborate on the sensory information, including visual, auditory, olfactory, kinesthetic, and tactile data, to enhance the experience. For example, you might emphasize the visual aspects (i.e., "the sea was blue green, with waves taller than a redwood tree"), auditory properties (i.e., "Gabriella, the pirate, heard the screeching of the seagulls and the crashing of the waves"), olfactory experiences (i.e., "she smelled the stink of rotting seaweed and dead fish"), kinesthetic information (i.e., "walking in the surf, Gabriella was hit over and over by the huge waves, staggering and almost falling on her face"), and tactile experiences (i.e., "she felt the salt air and sand on her skin, uncomfortable and scratchy").

8. As you tell the story, while the protagonist should make progress toward overcoming the problem, there should also be obstacles to overcome. The story needs to feature a certain level of struggle so that the client feels that the protagonist has earned the final solution, rather than

simply having it magically happen. If you have a resource person and allies, they can help the protagonist when needed. And, ultimately, the protagonist needs to make the decisions and be responsible for the biggest part of the effort involved in overcoming any obstacles and resolving the struggle.

9. Be sure you describe the resolution of the problem in concrete and clearly defined terms so that the client recognizes things are better than they were at the beginning of the story. The resolution does not have to completely eliminate the original difficulty, and it should show that the protagonist has made progress in learning to cope with the situation.

10. Keep referring to the goal you wanted to accomplish with the story as you tell it because everything in the story (initial setup, obstacles, progress, resolution, and moral) should be related to the lesson you wanted to communicate to the client through the story.

11. After the resolution, you can have the characters have some sort of celebration and affirmation of the changes in the protagonist. In our experience, it is useful to have the end of the story feature a statement that makes clear exactly what the protagonist has learned (i.e., "Gabriella learned to understand that sometimes her choices get her into trouble," "The pirate learned that she could take care of herself even when she was in a scary situation," or "Gabriella learned that, when she was angry, she could count to ten slowly to calm herself"). (Yikes! Not all three of them—that would be overwhelming *and* it would contradict our dictum that you should just have one concrete goal for your story.) With older children, teens, and adults who are more able to grasp abstract lessons, the moral or learning does not have to be obviously stated; it still needs to be clearly illustrated in the story.

12. You will want to watch the client's nonverbal reactions to the story as you tell it. Depending on the client's responses to the story (body language, eye movement and eye contact, activity and energy levels, verbal comments, level of participation), you may want to make shifts in the story—either in content, action, or length. For instance, with a client who seems bored, you might need to be more dramatic in the telling, add more engaging information, or cut the story short, and with a client who seems engaged in the story, you might expand the story, adding more detail or having a sequel in some future session.

13. Decide if and how you want to process the story with the client. With some clients, just telling the story is enough, and they don't want to talk about the story after you are finished. With other clients, they want to talk about the story, and at the same time it is important to them to retain the plausible deniability regarding the fact that the story is really about them or their lives; so for these clients you need to keep the processing

about the characters and content of the story without ever drawing a parallel to what is happening with them. Other clients actually introduce the idea that the story has elements similar to the things that are happening to them or even that they recognize the story is about them and want to talk about that. They may even want to brainstorm ways they could use the possible solutions described in the story in their lives. (This is when you want to stop yourself from doing a little happy dance to celebrate the fact that progress is, indeed, happening.)

TECHNIQUES FOR HELPING CLIENTS GAIN INSIGHT

By now, you know the drill—for each of the techniques we give you the goals you can hope to achieve, the age range that they work best with, and whether we see them working with individual clients, groups, families, or all of the above. Most of the techniques we use for helping clients gain insight are metaphoric, so we have more activities in the section on storytelling and creating therapeutic metaphors than in the other sections. To do justice to metaphors, you really need to let yourself go and get creative. Go wild.

Adventure Therapy Techniques

Balloon Bop

Several years ago, I (Terry) was in Ireland presenting on Adlerian play therapy at a conference. I wanted to do something interactive and didn't have my usual suitcase full of toys and materials. The only things I had in my suitcase were some balloons and tongue depressors (don't ask why), and I invented this game to play with the audience. It is useful with clients who are rule-bound or rigid; clients who are "too tight"; clients who habitually get angry at others; clients who have difficulty taking the emotional or cognitive perspective of others; and clients who have difficulty cooperating or communicating with others. The goal would be to help clients understand that they have lots of different rules governing their behaviors, emotions, and thoughts (in many cases, out of their awareness)—the idea behind this technique is to bring those rules into clients' awareness. You could also use it to help clients examine the things they think "make" them angry and help clients consider that others may have different cognitive or emotional perspectives. During the "making changes phase," this activity can help loosen "too tight" clients and give clients a chance to practice communicating and cooperating with others. Because the processing requires some degree of abstract thinking, it works best with clients who have reached formal operational thinking because there are some nonconcrete concepts in discovering their rules, so it is more appropriate with preteens, teens, and adults than for younger children. Because you can do it with individual clients, groups, and families, we are going to give you two separate sets of directions (one for individuals and one for groups and families).

When using this technique with individual clients, small groups, or families with fewer than eight members, you will need one tongue depressor and one balloon; when using it with large groups or really big families, you will need enough tongue depressors and balloons so that there is one tongue depressor and one balloon for every six to eight participants. (You can play this with very large groups if you are introducing play therapy to lots of people and want an activity that will be guaranteed to make them think.)

If you are doing this activity with an individual client, here is the procedure:

1. Give the client the tongue depressor and the balloon. Ask him or her to blow up the balloon and tie it off.
2. Explain that these are the rules for the activity:
   a. Don't hurt yourself.
   b. Once you start the activity, you can only touch the balloon with the tongue depressor, not with your hands.
   c. Every time you touch the balloon with the tongue depressor, you must say one positive thing about yourself.
3. There is a very good chance the client is going to ask you about other rules—just repeat the rules you have already recited.
4. Give the client about 5 minutes to do this. When you stop the client, ask him or her to tell you what the rules of the activity were.
5. After the client recites the rules, ask him or her if there were any rules he or she made up. If the client denies making up rules, feel free to point out the rules you noticed, like making up that the balloon could not touch the floor, making up that they could not touch the balloon with elbows or heads, staying in a specific place, and so on. (Even if the client doesn't deny making up rules, you can list the ones you noticed they made up—their list won't contain all of them.)
6. Point out that in our everyday lives, we all have many rules that either we made up or someone else made up rules that we have to follow. Give a couple of examples to get clients thinking (e.g., on the highway, I have made up that I can't go more than 10 miles over the speed limit, which some legislators made up; my son made up that he cannot go an entire day without checking his Facebook account; my niece made up that she can't go out of the house without straightening her hair; our family made up that you can't lose hugs, even if someone is mad at you—if you ask for a hug, you get it).

7. Invite clients to talk about what rules they are living by that are made up; then invite them to consider which of those rules are serving them and which are getting in their way. This is a jumping off place for considering whether to make changes in our rules.

8. Often, it is also helpful to discuss the fact that we frequently get angry when other people do not follow our rules—even if they do not have the same rules, and (in many cases) we have not had a conversation with them about our own rules. It is also important to note that when we get angry with ourselves, it is usually because we are not following our own rules; when we get anxious, we are either violating our own rules or the rules someone else has set that we think we need to follow.

With a family or a group with fewer than eight members, give one member the tongue depressor and the balloon. With a family or group with more than eight members, subdivide the group into smaller groups, and give one member the tongue depressor and the balloon. Ask that member to blow up the balloon and tie it off.

1. Explain that these are the rules for the activity:
   a. Don't hurt yourself.
   b. Once you start the activity, you can touch the balloon with the tongue depressor, not with your hands.
   c. After every time someone touches the balloon with the tongue depressor, that person must give the tongue depressor to someone else. A single person cannot touch the balloon two times in a row.
   d. Everyone in the family (group) must participate.

2. There is a very good chance one of the members will ask you about other rules; just repeat the rules you have already recited.

3. Give the family/group about 8–10 minutes to do this. When you stop them, ask the members to recite the rules of the activity.

4. After they list the rules, ask them if there were any rules they made up. If the members deny making up rules or just list a few rules they made up, feel free to point out the rules you noticed (e.g., like making up that the balloon could not touch the floor, making up how they were going to handle making sure one of the members did not touch the balloon twice in a row, making up that "everyone needs to participate" means that everyone needed to wield the tongue depressor, etc.).

5. See number 6, 7, and 8 from the discussion with individual clients—you can talk about those points with families and groups as well.

This is one of those activities in which it is important to verbally process so that your clients will gain an awareness of what the rules are. (It isn't one of those games in which clients have a lightning bolt of insight hit them without talking about it.) Here are some sample questions you could ask in the processing:

"What were your reactions when you first heard the rules for the activity?"

"How did you feel when I asked you if anyone had made up any rules?"

"What rules did you make up for doing the activity?"

"How did you feel when you realized you had made up rules for doing the activity?"

"For family or group play, how did you communicate the rules you made up to the other members? How did you react when someone didn't follow one of your rules?"

"For family or group play, when someone else made up a rule, what was your reaction?"

"For family or group play, what was your reaction when someone else didn't follow one of your rules?"

"How do you usually react to rules laid out by your family? At school or work? By your friends? By society?"

"How do you decide which rules you are going to follow?"

"What are some of the rules you made up that you are following in your life?"

"Which of those rules is still working for you? How can you make sure you keep following those rules?"

"Which of those rules is no longer working for you (or never did work for you)? What would you be willing to do to let go of those rules?"

"Choose one or two of the rules that are no longer working for you. Imagine you have made the necessary changes to let go of those rules. How would your life be different?"

If you have a client who cannot use a balloon because of an allergy to latex, you can use beach balls and rulers or you can use the activity called "Guidelines" in Ashby et al. (2008, pp. 82–85).

Storytelling and Creating Therapeutic Metaphors

Goals of Misbehavior Show

While this is really an Adlerian technique (Kottman & Meany-Walen, 2016; Manly, 1986), the goals of Misbehavior Show can be used by play therapists from other approaches to play therapy. We would mostly use this technique with individual children rather than in groups or families.

It is designed for children rather than adolescents and adults, though you could probably use it to help individuals with intellectual disabilities, no matter what their age. The primary goal of this activity would be helping clients gain insight into their goals of misbehavior. It is a little different from most of the other activities because it is a technique the play therapist does for the client rather than something the therapist asks the client to do.

According to Dreikurs and Soltz (1964), children demonstrate four goals of misbehavior: attention, power, revenge, and proving inadequacy. In this technique, using puppets, dolls, or sand tray figures, you would do a short show featuring a character who demonstrates a selected goal of misbehavior. The "misbehaving" character would have "lines" typical of individuals who manifest the particular patterns of thinking, feeling, and behaving emblematic of children who have specific goals of misbehavior. This character could also narrate what he or she is feeling and thinking while saying those "lines" and acting out the negative behaviors. As part of using this activity to help the child gain insight, after the initial show, you could ask what he or she thinks about that character, you could invite the child to give the character feedback about the impact of his or her behavior on other people, you could suggest that the child might want to play another character who would react to the target character, and/or you could ask the child to play out a character who did similar things. It could also be enlightening to add characters to the show who would represent the reaction of other people (adults and other children) to a character who manifests that particular goal of misbehavior and observe the child's reaction to this or engage the child in a conversation about the interaction between the characters.

Attention-seeking characters would do things to draw attention to themselves. They might bother others, brag, show off, act silly, be really loud, make messes, and the like. They could be mildly inappropriate, and then when one of the other characters corrected them, they would stop for a little while, but later resume the inappropriate behavior. Other characters would express frustration and annoyance at this pattern. Attention-seeking characters would say things like: "I want others to notice me," "I want others to do more for me," "I want to be special," "I should get all the attention," "Why aren't others playing attention to me?" "I don't get enough attention," and "I feel sad/mad/disappointed when no one is noticing me."

Power-seeking characters would do things like having temper tantrums, arguing, lying, getting into power struggles with others, refusing to cooperate, and/or being disobedient or defiant. When one of the other characters corrected them, they would escalate their acting out, which would result in the other characters getting angry with them. Power-seeking characters would say things like: "I want to be in charge," "I want others to do what I want them to do," "I want/need to show others they cannot control me," "I want others to stop telling me what to do," "I want/need power," and "I must have power/control to be safe/protect myself."

Revenge-seeking characters would do things like deliberately hurting others (either physically or emotionally), saying malicious or cruel things to others, being violent toward others, and/or threatening others. If one of the other characters asked them to stop or set some kind of consequence or punishment, these characters would become even more violent, aggressive, or vindictive. Revenge-seeking characters would say things like: "I have been treated unfairly," "I want to get even with others," "I need to pay others back for hurting me/jerking me around," "I am going to make others feel what it is like to be hurt," "They are going to pay for what they have done to me," "I need to keep others at a distance so they can't hurt me," and "I am going hurt them."

Characters who are displaying or *proving inadequacy* would do things like . . . well, they wouldn't do much, actually. They would give up easily or would not even make an attempt to do things. They might say they can't do things, they might be mute and refuse to answer others, they would be reluctant to try new things, they would express extreme self-doubt, they would basically be the manifestation of discouragement. They might seek isolation from others. In extreme cases, they might be suicidal or self-destructive, but with younger children this would probably be an inappropriate subject for a show. When other characters gave them feedback or tried to be encouraging, these characters would sink lower into their own self-doubts and discouragement. Characters who are set on proving their own inadequacy would say things like: "I wish others would stop asking me to do things," "Stop asking me to try harder," "People should feel sorry for me," "Leave me alone," "I might as well not try because I won't be successful anyway," "I can't do anything right," "I can't do it," "I'm a loser," and "I am not important."

Mutual Storytelling

Mutual storytelling was originally developed as a therapeutic technique by Richard Gardner (1993), who used psychodynamic theory as the filter to understanding the story and designing the retelling. I (Terry) adapted his approach to work with Adlerian methods of conceptualizing and reorienting (Kottman & Meany-Walen, 2016). You will want to listen to the client's story through the filter of your own theoretical approach to play therapy and use your understanding of how the client's story represents his or her issues, assets, and struggles and use your retelling to help the client move toward resolving those issues, capitalizing on his or her strengths, and learning to cope with struggles. This is an activity you can use to help clients gain insight or to teach them new ways to handle situations or relationships, so you could use it in this phase of play therapy or the final phase of play therapy. You just need to be clear about the goal of your retelling and target the message toward what you want to accomplish with the story. You can do it with individuals, groups, or families, though it is easier to do with individuals because you don't have to consider the impact of your retelling on multiple people. If you do it with groups or families, you would need to decide how you are going to choose the person who is going to tell the story that you will retell or if you are going to have all of the members collaborate on a story that you would then retell. We have used it with all ages of clients, though most teens and adults will be pretty canny about your purpose in retelling the story. (This doesn't have to be a problem unless you let it be one, so don't.)

Here are the basic (cross-theoretical) steps for mutual storytelling:

1. Ask the client to tell you a story with a beginning, a middle, and an end. Depending on the age and sophistication of the client, you can ask the client to choose several animal figures, puppets, or dolls, pretend they can talk, and tell a story using them as characters. Or you can just ask the client to tell a story without props. If the client is resistant to coming up with a brand-new story and he or she has already told you a story, you can use that story as the base story for your retelling. We let clients tell us the plot to a favorite television show, movie, video game, or book if they say they can't think of an original story. (We know this isn't "pure," and it still works because they filter what they remember and how they tell the story through their own world view.)

2. Listen to the story for the underlying meaning—it may present aspects of the client's personality; a current situation in the client's life; the client's relationships with significant others; the client's usual ways of thinking about self, others, and the world; the client's usual method of solving problems; and other aspects of the client's life important to understanding the client and his or her journey.

3. As you listen to the story, think about what the following elements tell you about the client and his or her life:

   What is the overall affective tone of the story? What does the affective tone of the story tell you about the client's life?

   How do the actions of the characters in the story fit with what you already know about the client and the people in his or her life?

   How do the situations or problems in the story resemble situations or problems encountered by the client in his or her life?

   Which character (or characters), if any, represents the client?

   What are the difficulties encountered by the character that represents the client? How do they relate to the difficulties in the client's life?

   How does the character who represents the client feel in the story?

How do the other characters in the story feel/respond to the behavior of the character who represents the client?

What does the story tell you about the client's view of self?

What does the story tell you about the client's views about and attitudes toward other people?

What does the story tell you about the client's usual approach to relationships?

What does the story tell you about the client's attitude toward life?

What does the story tell you about the client's usual approach to problem solving?

4. Explain to the client that you would like to tell another story with those same characters. (Be sure you don't imply that the client's story was deficient, which could be why you need to retell it—that would be bad. Retell the story, using the same characters, setting, and beginning as the client's story. You will want to change the middle and the ending of the story. If you are using the story to help clients gain insight, the retelling could include: (a) an internal monologue with one or more of the characters talking about how they are thinking, feeling, and/ or behaving; (b) one of the characters gaining insight into something parallel to something that the client needs to become more aware of; (c) one of the characters noticing a pattern that is causing him or her difficulty; (d) one or more of the characters giving constructive feed- back to the character that represents the client; (e) one or more of the characters confronting a discrepancy expressed by or present in the character representing the client; or (f) one of the characters talking about a play theme that has been present in the client's play. If you are using the story to help clients change their behaviors, the retelling could include (a) a more appropriate resolution of the story conflict; (b) alternative ways of viewing self, the world, and others; (c) different ways of building relationships and getting along with others; (d) varied interpretations of personal issues that may be interfering with clients' ability to function; (e) more socially appropriate methods of resolving conflicts; or (f) more appropriate strategies for coping with problems. As you design your retelling, think about the following questions:

What is your goal in telling the story? What do you want to teach the client with your narrative?

Which character(s) would you leave in? What will you try to accom- plish with these characters? Would you add any character(s)? What traits would you incorporate in any added character(s)? Why would those character(s) be important with this client?

How can you emphasize the client's strengths?

How can you illustrate strategies for connecting with others, becoming and feeling capable, gaining confidence in being sig- nificant, and having courage?

Do you want to incorporate some kind of consequences for any negative behaviors in the story? What kind of consequence would be realistic, related, and respectful?

Do you want to incorporate some kind of positive consequences for positive behaviors in the story? What kind of consequence would illustrate the importance of positive behaviors?

What method of conflict resolution or problem-solving strategy would you like to illustrate in the retelling? How could you resolve the conflict in an appropriate and realistic way in the retelling?

How can you use the characters to model more positive attitudes toward solving problems?

How can you have the characters resolve the conflict in an appropriate and realistic way?

How can you incorporate more positive ways for the characters in the story to view themselves, the world, and others? How can you incorporate more positive attitudes in the characters?

How can you illustrate more appropriate ways of building relationships and getting along with others?

How can you illustrate a variety of interpretations of personal issues that may be interfering with the client's ability to function?

What social skills or other skills do you want to illustrate with the retelling?

5. Watch the client's nonverbal reactions as you retell the story to help you decide whether to end the story early, extend and expand the story, or pause the story to talk about the client's reaction to the story you are telling.

6. When you are done with the retelling, consider whether and how you want to process the story and the impact of your retelling with the client.

Creative Characters

Creative Characters is a metaphor/storytelling technique devised by Robert Brooks (1981) and Crenshaw, Brooks, and Goldstein (2015) that uses several different characters to co-tell a story with the client. It is a lovely way to help clients gain insight into underlying thoughts or feelings and into patterns of thinking, feeling, behaving, and relating. You can use the reporter character to make interpretations or ask questions designed to help clients look "underneath" their behavior to the underlying dynamics and recognize their own patterns. In our experience, although you can use it with a variety of developmental levels in play therapy, this technique seems to work best with individual preteens and young teens. We have also successfully used it with groups and families—you just have to alternate the teller of the story so that all of the members get a chance to co-create the story. Make sure everyone gets to be the reporter; often the questions individual members ask can be as revealing as people's answers to the reporter's questions. We frequently record (either audio or video) the presentation of the story so that clients can watch it later—either in session or at home. Here is our adaptation of the technique:

1. Describe the setting, the characters, and the beginning of the story.

   a. The setting can be either real or imaginary; however, it should have some elements that relate to the client's life. The more detailed description of the setting and the beginning of the story, the better chance that most clients (especially children) will get into the story.

   b. In casting the story, include a character who represents (a) the client; (b) the play therapist (yes, once again, you get to be the wise person) or another wise person with whom the client can consult about problem situations; (c) the difficult situation or an antagonist in the client's life; (d) at least one ally for the protagonist; and (e) a reporter who asks the other characters for information, reactions, feelings, attitudes, plans, and so forth at various intervals throughout the story.

   c. With a child client, invite him or her to help you choose a puppet, doll, stuffed animal, sand tray figure, or some other toy to represent each of these characters. You can also engage the client in drawing the characters, rather than using toys. As you develop the description of the character, include details from the physical appearance of the representative toy. If you are working with an older person (like a teen or adult), you can still do this part if you think the client would be willing. Otherwise, you can just tell the story without any props or art work.

   d. Explain that each of the characters can talk and that you and the client will take turns telling the story. You and the client can either rotate who speaks for which character or switch off, with one person taking responsibility for speaking for all the characters in the story for a while and then handing off the telling of the story to the other person.

   e. Describe the beginning of the story with some kind of dilemma facing the protagonist (yes, that's the character representing the client). The dilemma can resemble the client's presenting problem or some other challenge facing the client. Be sure to make the connection relatively subtle and oblique—not emphasizing the parallels to the client's life.

2. Begin telling the story. Usually, at least the first time you use this technique with a client, you will probably want to speak for all the

characters at the beginning of the story to model how the process works. As the client seems to get the "hang" of telling the story, you can pass the telling to him or her. It is especially important to start out with you speaking for the reporter and the wise consultant, as the client may not understand how to speak for either of these characters or may not have any questions or advice to insert into the story.

3. As the story unfolds, whether you are telling the story or the client is, you the reporter interviews the other characters to find out how they are feeling and what they are thinking, and the wise consultant provides advice, different perspectives, and information to the other characters as the story progresses.

4. Eventually, as clients more clearly understand the process, they will express a desire to take over speaking for either the reporter or the wise consultant. (We think it is super cool for clients to recognize that they are curious about how others are thinking and feeling and that they might have some sage thoughts to share with others, so let them have at it!)

5. The end of the story should resemble the end of a therapeutic metaphor—with some socially appropriate resolution of the dilemma or challenge facing the protagonist and a celebration of the lessons learned along the way or the skills demonstrated by the protagonist and his or her allies.

Bibliotherapy

In bibliotherapy, you use books to provide a therapeutic story designed to convey a message or teaching to clients (Karges-Bone, 2015; Kottman & Meany-Walen, 2016; Malchiodi & Ginns-Gruenberg, 2008). Bibliotherapy can help clients gain insight into situations and relationships in their lives, help them understand themselves better, learn to take someone else's cognitive or emotional perspective, or consider new and different ways of relating to other people. By reading a book to a client or suggesting a client read a book, you can use the book to create awareness, provide information, promote conversations, suggest solutions to difficulties, enhance empathy, and/or help clients recognize that other people might have similar struggles. Bibliotherapy is appropriate for all ages and any configuration of play therapy—individual, group, and family. It can also be used as homework with young children (have caretakers read to them) or school-aged and older clients, who can read to themselves. (If you work with special needs clients, make sure any book you ask them to read is within their reading level.)

If you are working with children, it is important that you choose a book that has appealing illustrations, interesting story content, useful information that the child can understand and use, and recurring refrains that keep the child interested (Kottman & Meany-Walen, 2016). With many children, it also helps if the book has broad (and obvious) humor and surprise elements. With teens and adults, you want to recommend stories that are well written with characters and situations that will be appealing and engaging to them. (Again, we know—duh . . . No matter what the age of your client, it is important that the story depicted in the book have some parallels to the client's situation. It is also helpful to make sure that the book is developmentally appropriate.)

Whether the book is read in a session or for homework, you will need to decide whether and what kind of follow-up activities you want to provide. With clients who like to verbally process experiences afterward, having a discussion about either (1) what happened in the book and/or (2) how the situation or relationships in the book are similar to the client's life can be helpful. Other clients might prefer some kind of activity designed to help them process. For example, this could be a drawing or painting depicting people, places, animals, and other objects mentioned in the book or showing the feelings of the characters in the book or the client's feelings in response to the book; constructing collages out of pictures or photographs depicting key events, characters, feelings, or activities in the story; or making puppets or using commercial puppets to depict key events, characters, feelings, or activities in the story. Clients can dictate or write about how they feel about the characters, their situation, or any other part of the story or dictate or write a letter to one of the characters in the story or create an alternative ending to the story. It is also fun to work with clients to role-play various characters and situations from the book. (Remember, the possibilities are endless—let your imagination and creativity go wild.)

Appendix B presents a list of some of our favorite books for working with child clients on specific goals. Because books for teens and adults are so dependent on their individual interests and tastes, we hesitated to make suggestions for them. Your local public librarian or a local school librarian is a great source of information, as are folks who work in bookstores (as long as you don't mention the person for whom you are seeking a book is one of your clients—remember confidentiality applies even in your favorite stores).

Movement/Dance/Music Experiences

"Here's How I Feel" Dance

This activity is designed to help clients become more aware of their feelings. It can be used with any age, any configuration. You can provide the music for the dancing, or you can ask clients to bring in music. With our younger clients, we usually bring music on our iPads or phones and ask them to dance. You can also dance without music.

The basic activity is pretty simple—ask clients to move/dance how they feel in different situations. Initially, you can provide the list of situations or experiences based on what you know about them or what they need to explore (e.g., when I get in trouble from my mom, teacher, boss, spouse; when I have to do my chores/I have to go to work; when I have a fight with my brother, boss, dad, wife, partner; when I have a problem I can't figure out how to solve; when I feel sad, lonely, mad, happy, irritated, frustrated; when I feel like no one understands me; when I can't get my emotions under control; when I feel out of control; when I feel like no one loves me; when I am afraid I can't do my homework, meet my deadlines, find a partner). Later, if you want, you can ask them to create their own list of situations or experiences that engender specific feelings or reactions. After or during the dancing, of course, with clients who like to verbally process, you can lead them in a conversation. With clients who do not like to verbally process, many times this activity is enough, all by itself, to increase awareness of the feelings associated with different situations or experiences.

Role Dancing

All of us fill a variety of roles—student, boss, employee, mother, sister, son, girlfriend, and so on. We also have other, less structured roles—the one who is always responsible, the one who takes care of everyone else, the one who rebels, the one who rights wrongs, the one who can't do anything right, the perfect one, the grouchy one, and the like. In this activity (Dan Leven, personal communication, February 2015), you can give clients an opportunity to gain insight into how each of their roles affects them at the bodily (and probably emotional) level. While we have done this activity with younger children (keeping the list of roles pretty simple), we usually use it with preteens to adults just because they are able to understand the roles they play on a more abstract level than younger clients. It can work with groups and families, but we usually use it with individual clients because sometimes they tend to be more willing to move when they are in a session by themselves than they would be in front of others.

Again, as in the "Here's How I Feel" dance, the directions are pretty simple.

You invite clients to move/dance about one of their roles. There are lots of ways you can structure the dance and what clients do in it. They can dance the way they move in that role, they can dance how they feel in that role, they can dance how they feel about that role, they can dance how they perceive they got the role, they can dance how they perceive others box them into that role, and so forth. After they get the hang of it, you can also invite them to use movement/dance to break themselves out of any role in which they feel stuck or uncomfortable. You can invite them to move just a little—to gently shift out of the role; you can invite them to totally break out and move in ways that feel like they are the complete opposite of that role. You can stop with just one role, or you can ask them to move in several different roles. You can also invite them to suggest roles they would like to dance. Again, you can verbally process or not—both work.

Composing Music

For musical clients, it can be very helpful for them to write songs about the various things going on for them. Using an app like Music Maker or Loopacks, you can give them a vehicle for expressing themselves and gaining insight into specific issues in their lives. In our experience, this works best with preteens and teens. You can use it with individual clients, groups, and families. Once your clients have composed their music or written their songs, you can invite them to move to the music if they are inspired to do so, which adds another layer of insight for some clients.

Sand Tray Activities

Many of the sand trays designed to help clients gain insight are trays the play therapist does for the client or trays the play therapist and clients co-create. Here are some possible directed sand trays that help clients to gain insight:

Trays you would do for the client
1. Tray showing clients your perception of how they see themselves
2. Tray showing clients your perception of how they see others
3. Tray showing clients your perception of how they see the world
4. Tray showing clients your perception of how they gain significance
5. Tray showing clients your perception of their emotional patterns
6. Tray showing clients your perception of how they solve problems
7. Tray showing clients your perception of how they build relationships
8. Tray showing clients your perception of the ways their thinking patterns are getting in their way
9. Tray showing clients your perception about a specific problem they are trying to solve and what is keeping it from being solved
10. Tray showing clients your perception about a specific relationship in which they are struggling and the factors that are causing difficulties
11. Tray showing how you think clients' lives would be different if their presenting problem were solved

With clients who need possible insights presented in a metaphoric way, you can do a tray about a character without revealing that the tray is about them and their struggles. You can also design a metaphor played out in your sand tray following the procedure detailed in the skills section of this chapter.

With co-created trays, you and your clients make the tray together, either taking turns putting in objects or having a conversation together about objects you both think you want to put in the tray, then putting them into the tray.

Interactive sand trays you can co-create with clients

1. Tray reframing a problem situation for clients
2. Tray depicting a problem and then adding things to the tray or taking things out of the tray to explore possible solutions
3. Tray telling a story together—first the client puts an object into the tray and tells a sentence or two using the object as an element of the story. Next the therapist chooses an object that will help move the story along and tells a sentence or two using that object. Alternately, the therapist and the client choose objects and tell a sentence or two that moves the story forward.
4. The client puts figures into the tray depicting a situation in which someone has a problem similar to the problem the child is experiencing; then the therapist puts some figures into the tray that might be important things to think about regarding the problem.
5. Mutual storytelling—the client tells a story in the tray/creates a world in the tray. The therapist retells the story or redoes the world in a more constructive manner.
6. Creative characters—the therapist (or the therapist and the client) picks figures to represent characters (including one for the client, one for the problem encountered by the client, one for a resource person or ally, and one for a reporter who is going to interview other characters) and they take turns telling the story with the client. The therapist occasionally interrupts the action so that the reporter can ask questions, make comments, or interpret what is going on in the story
7. The therapist picks therapeutically relevant figures and asks the client to use them to tell a story

Trays the client does

1. Tray depicting a maze (or obstacle course), using objects in the tray as obstacles. The client names the destination and chooses a figure to represent a character traversing the maze, finding solutions for dealing with the obstacles along the way.

2. Tray to show what his or her life (job, family, world, school, inter-actions with other people, etc.) would be like if the presenting problem was solved

3. "Solutions" tray to consider alternative ways to solve/alleviate his or her problem

4. Tray to show his or her ideal world, self, job, spouse, family, class, and so on

5. Tray depicting a world in which the client knows how to do every-thing (or a specific thing he or she struggles with)

6. "Perspectives" tray (or series of trays) depicting a bunch of differ-ent ways of viewing a situation or problem, and the client chooses one he or she would be willing to take on for the following week

7. Tray using the metaphor of seeing the world through different lenses (sunglasses? rose-colored glasses?) to reframe or get a dif-ferent perspective on a problem situation or relationship

Art Techniques

Body Outlines

The goal for this activity will vary, depending on where you want to help clients gain insight. Depending on your goal, you would use this tech-nique with many different populations. For instance, it is hugely helpful in working with clients who are unaware of where in their bodies they store feelings; it is useful for folks who have distorted or negative body images; it is informative to clients who are insecure or do not own their assets. We have used it with groups, families, and individual clients of all ages.

All you need for materials are some markers or crayons and a piece of paper (roll of white paper or newsprint) that is as big as the clients you want to outline. If you have clients who are reluctant to draw on the out-line, you can have them use stickers or stamps and stamping pads. Have your clients lie down on the paper and trace around their bodies with the marker or crayons. (When you get to their knees, stop so that you do not violate their private space close to their genitals. After you are done with the outline, have them get up and draw an inverted V connecting their legs together.) Then you can either brainstorm what they would like to fill in on the body outline, or you can give them a directive. Here are some directives we have used with clients:

1. What I like about me
2. Where I keep my feelings
3. Secrets I keep inside myself
4. Things I tell myself about my body

5. Things I love about my body
6. Things I am ashamed of about my body
7. Things I got from my birth family (on the inside of the outline) and things I got from my adoptive family (on the surface of the outline)
8. Things I think (in the head), things I feel (in the heart region), things I do (in the rest of the body), things I say (in thought bubbles connected to the head)

You know the drill by now—use your imagination to come up with directives to help specific clients gain insight. One modification of this technique that you can use with folks who are too self-conscious to actually use an outline of their own bodies is to have them draw a gingerbread person on a big sheet of paper and have them fill it in as if it were an outline of their body.

Secret Feelings

The goal of Secret Feelings is to help clients recognize that they can have more than one feeling at a time, particularly feelings that might seem to contradict one another. It can also be used to help clients gain insight into the layers of feelings they have in response to specific situations and feelings they might be denying, especially feelings they believe are "negative" and unacceptable. It works best with children from 8 years of age to adulthood. (In our experience, even with the visual aid of the picture, younger children are still confused by the idea that several emotions that feel incongruent with one another can coexist.) You can use it with individuals, groups, and families.

You will need white card stock paper (this paper works better than just copy paper, which is a bit flimsy for multiple layers of crayon), one white crayon, one orange or yellow crayon, and one dark (black or blue works best) marker. Tell clients to use the white crayon to draw a shape, scribble, or word that represents a feeling they have about a particular relationship, person, or situation. This technique seems to work best when clients use the white to draw an emotion they do not like feeling or with which they are uncomfortable but that isn't necessary. You may have to suggest a specific relationship, person, or situation that you believe has evoked contradictory or layered emotions. It can be helpful to ask the client to draw about a relationship, person, or situation you feel they have strong feelings about that they are denying or sublimating. Ask them to look at the drawing and talk about how it feels that it is almost impossible to actually see what they have drawn. (Some clients might be relieved that the drawing is indiscernible, or they might be frustrated by the invisibility of the drawing, etc.)

Next, tell clients you would like them to use the yellow or orange crayon to draw a shape, scribble, or word that represents a different feeling they have about that same relationship, person, or situation. This can be a feeling with which they are more comfortable, a feeling that is closer to the surface, or of which they are more aware. This drawing can be anywhere on the page, even on top of the first drawing. After the drawing is finished, ask clients to talk about what it feels like to add a drawing that is more easily observed about the same relationship, person, or situation as the first drawing.

Now ask clients to take the marker (we find that darker markers seem to work better) and completely color the whole page with marker, even covering up the drawings they have made. As they color, ask them what they are noticing about the drawings. They should be able to see both of the drawings emerging from the marker cover-up. Hopefully, they will notice that both of the feelings are still there, even though the one they drew with the lighter color was difficult to see initially. Help them process how two feelings/reactions to the same situation can occur at the same time, in many cases with one of them being hidden, denied, or suppressed. (Obviously, use developmentally appropriate language designed to help them explore this concept.)

Aquariums

This is a variation on a technique we learned from Eliana Gil in a workshop at an APT conference. Our version is more metaphoric than the one we learned from Eliana. We have used it with individual clients, families, and groups. (There are directions for how to do it with families and groups at the end of this section.) You can use it to gather information about clients' relationships if you are in the exploring dynamics phase, or to help clients learn to better understand their relationships if you are in the gaining insight phase. Depending on how you describe the activity, it can be focused on the client's family relationships or on relationships in the other places in clients' lives—classroom, neighborhood, work, friend groups, and so on. It can work with any age, with the caveat that cutting paper with scissors or tearing it are part of the activity.

You will need a large piece of poster board, assorted colors of construction paper, scissors, and glue (glue sticks or rubber cement works best). Set the poster board on a table and tell clients that the poster board is an aquarium and that their job is to stock it with fish. Give them the scissors and construction paper and ask them to make fish for some of the following: the meanest fish, the fish that hides the most, the fish that the other fish don't like, the fish the other fish pick on, the bravest fish, the fish who is scared all the time, the fish who takes care of all the other fish, the fish the other fish wish would move to a different aquarium, the fish nobody ever notices, the fish everyone in the aquarium thinks is cute, the fish who doesn't get taken seriously, the fish that everyone else blames for things that go wrong, and so on. (You choose which ones you want to do based on what you know about the client and his or her circumstances. And remember, use your own imagination; you don't have to limit yourself to the ones we have generated.) Watch them as they work and make interpretive comments about how they do the activity when you think your comments will help them gain insight into their process. After they have finished making all the fish, tell them to use the glue to attach each of the fish somewhere on the poster board. After they have finished gluing, if they are willing, ask them to identify each fish—they can name the fish and describe the attributes of each one.

Remember, with clients who are willing to verbally process, you can process the product and the process of art techniques. You can ask them how they decided where to put each fish, how they decided which colors to make each fish, how they decided which ones were going to be big or little, and so forth. You can also guide them in a discussion about the relationships between the various fish—either using the "I notice . . ." method of inviting processing or asking questions about how the various fish get along, which ones are friendly, which ones are enemies, and so on. You can also ask about how the fish in the aquarium solve problems, how they negotiate getting their needs met, how they resolve conflict—you can even use the metaphor of the fish to make suggestions of other ways to handle things when situations in the aquarium do not seem to have an equitable solution.

If the fish who represents clients (like the client is the fish who is the most scared or the least likely to be heard or seen), you can help them brainstorm how to make changes that would optimize the life of that fish. For example, you can suggest to clients that they can move things around, add structures, make another fish to protect a vulnerable fish, and so on. With clients who can/are willing to come in and out of the metaphor, you can also talk about (drum roll) who in their lives each fish represents and which fish represents them as a vehicle to talking more directly about situations that are problematic for them.

If you want to do a different version of the activity, you can give the following instructions: "Stock the aquarium with fish that represent the people in your family." (Or classroom, neighborhood, workplace, or friends group—whichever group you want to explore with the client.) With clients who are more guarded, instead of asking them to take ownership (by saying "your" family . . .), you can say "a family," "children and teacher in a classroom," "people who live close together in a neighborhood," "some people who work together," or "a group of friends" as a way to let the client keep a safe distance from the material.

If you are working with perfectionistic clients, have them tear the construction paper rather than using the scissors. Since they won't be able to tear paper perfectly, this can be used to help clients gain insight into the issues connected to any maladaptive perfectionism, or it can be used to help clients practice being okay even when things are not perfect or don't go the way they want them to go.

For working with a group or family, you can do this activity at least two different ways—you can give each person his or her own piece of poster board and let the person create an individual aquarium with fish representing every person in the group or family and when they are done have them describe what they have done and compare notes. You can also have each person in the group add "one fish" to the poster board without specifying that the fish represents him or her. After everyone has contributed a fish, have the group members/family members process the product they have made and the process of doing the activity.

Animal Phototherapy

This is an adaptation of an activity I (Terry) learned from Robert Segel in 1991 at a workshop he did at the Texas Association for Marriage and Family Therapy Annual Conference in Dallas, Texas. (I have changed it a million times since then, so I am not even sure he would recognize the technique, and I like to give credit when I remember where I learned things—that is becoming more difficult as I get older and my brain gets feebler.) It is a technique that works best with teens and adults—sometimes I use it with individuals and sometimes with groups. I almost always use it to help clients raise their awareness of what personality traits are important to them, what they would need to change to cultivate those traits, and what would prevent them from making the changes they would need to make to cultivate them.

The only preliminary step before you can do this activity with clients is to gather some magazines that have photographs of animals in them and cut the photographs out so that you have a selection of different "types" of animals—wild, domestic, aggressive, sweet, farm, jungle, forest, desert, sea, mammals, birds, insects, lizards, amphibians, and so on. (I have several hundred photographs in my collection because I always think the more, the better—but that might just be me.) Have your clients go through the collection, looking for a photograph to which they feel a strong connection. After they choose the animal with which they resonate, lead them through a conversation that includes the answers to the following:

1. Describe this animal.
2. What drew you to pick this animal?

3. What positive qualities do you share with this animal?
4. What positive qualities does this animal have that you wish you shared but don't?
5. How would your life be different if you did have those positive qualities?
6. What keeps you from having those positive qualities?
7. What changes are you willing to make in your life to cultivate those positive qualities?

One variation of this technique is designed to help clients (usually preteens, teens, or adults) gain a greater awareness of the patterns in the relationships in their family of origin and an understanding of how they fit in their family. You could also use this activity in the exploration section of therapy if you would rather—or use it in the exploration phase and then in the insight phase as well. This version is predicated on clients' ability to go back and forth between using a metaphor and being literal. If you have clients who can't go back and forth, you can just have them pick animals to make up "a family" instead of their own family and then skip the descriptions at the beginning of the directions and just ask the questions in the metaphor. With your animal photographs, ask the clients to choose an animal to represent themselves and one to represent each member of their family of origin. Ask them to describe each animal with an emphasis on the strengths and weaknesses of the animal, explain how the personality of the family member is similar to the animal, and describe the relationship between each of the animals and the animal that represents you. Then ask the following questions:

1. "Which of the children in this family of animals is the mother's favorite?"
2. "Which of the children in this family of animals is the father's favorite?"
3. "Which of the children in this family of animals is most like the mother animal?"
4. "Which of the children in this family of animals is most like the father animal?"
5. "Which of these animals is most like you or your animal? How?"
6. "Which of these animals is most different than you or your animal? How?"
7. "Which of these animals fight with one another? What do they fight about?"
8. "Which of these animals play together? What kinds of things do they play?"
9. "What is the relationship of the parents with each other?"

10. "What is the relationship between each of the parents and the children?"
11. "What are this family's strengths?"
12. "What are this family's struggles?"
13. "How could an observer tell if the family was struggling?"
14. "If you could change anything in this family, what would you change?"

Here is another variation, also designed to help clients consider the relationships in their family of origin. To do this one, you will need a different set of photographs—pictures selected from magazines that have groups of animals—I like to have some photographs of a group of animals from the same species and some photographs of a group of animals with animals from several different species. It is especially revealing to clients when you have some predators and some prey animals in the same group. Have clients choose a family from the selection (you can specify that the family is their family, or you can just call it "a family," depending on clients' need for distance). And (of course) there is a set of questions for this one too:

1. "Describe this family."
2. "What are the strengths and weaknesses of this family?"
3. "What does this family do well? What does this family do poorly?"
4. "What would the members of this family like to change about the family?"
5. "What is the main difficulty encountering this family?"
6. "How would the lives of the family members be different if this difficulty was eliminated?"
7. "How do you think the family could go about eliminating this difficulty?"

With clients who do not need to communicate with a metaphor, you can also ask the following (less metaphorical) questions:

1. "How does this family resemble your own family?"
2. "What strengths does your family share with this family?"
3. "What weaknesses does your family share with this family?"
4. "What would you like to change about your family?"
5. "What is the main difficulty in your family? How does it resemble the difficulty of the family in the picture?"
6. "How would the lives of the members of your family be different if this difficulty was eliminated?"
7. "How would the lives of the members of your family be the same if this difficulty was eliminated?"

Quick Draw

The Quick Draw technique is a way to get clients over their feelings of insecurity about how well they draw and give them permission to use drawing to gain insight into specific topics, relationship, feelings, or situations. You can do this activity with children, teens, and adults (and we have specific directives for children and others for adolescents and adults). You can do it in groups and families, as well as with individuals.

The setup for Quick Draw is pretty easy. First, we give clients several sheets of paper and ask them to fold them in half or quarters. Then we tell them we are going to ask them to draw something for each of the situations we name—they can use shapes, textures, and colors to depict those situations; they can draw in a representational way or a nonrepresentational way. The only thing they can't do is to draw a traditional feeling face, like a smiley face or a frowny face; they have to do something more than that. Finally, before you give them the situation they are to draw, tell them they have only one minute to do each of the drawings you ask them to do. Choose at least two (but it can be as many as eight, though we seldom do that many because we want to leave time for processing) of the following to ask them to draw:

For kids

1. The last time you were mad at someone
2. The last time you were sad
3. The last time you were incredibly happy
4. The last time you were disappointed in yourself
5. The last time you were proud of yourself
6. The last time someone was mad at you
7. The last time you felt badly about something you did
8. The time you felt the most loved
9. The friend you like the best
10. The grownup you like the best/the least
11. The relative you like the best/the least
12. The last time you were scared
13. The thing you worry about the most
14. Something you did that you feel bad about
15. The person you spend your happiest times with
16. The work/school experience that you feel really good about
17. The time you were madder than you have ever been
18. Your most exciting experience
19. The most fun you have ever had
20. Your best time at church (for kids who go to church)
21. Your worst time at church

22. Your worst time at school
23. Your proudest moment
24. Your biggest disappointment
25. Your best moment
26. Your worst fear
27. The thing that is hardest for you in your life
28. The thing in your life you would most like to change
29. The thing in your life you would most want to stay the same

For adults/teens

1. The last time you were mad at someone
2. The last time you were sad
3. The last time you were incredibly happy
4. The last time you were disappointed in yourself
5. The last time you were proud of yourself
6. The last time someone disapproved of you
7. The last time you were disapproving of someone else
8. The last time you felt guilty
9. The last time you had a spiritual experience
10. The last time you felt totally loving toward yourself or someone else
11. The last time you were terrified
12. The last time you were scared
13. The thing you worry about the most
14. The thing you did you feel the most guilt about
15. The relationship in which you feel the happiest
16. The work/school experience in which you felt the most successful
17. The time you were madder than you have ever been
18. Your most exciting experience
19. The most fun you have ever had
20. Your first spiritual or religious experience
21. Your most significant accomplishment
22. Your biggest disappointment
23. Your best moment
24. Your worst fear
25. Your greatest challenge
26. The impact you would like to have on the people you love
27. The impact you would like to have on the world
28. Your best self
29. Your evil twin
30. The thing you are most ashamed of
31. The relationship that is most important to you
32. The thing you are afraid others will find out about

33. If you let yourself shine, it would look like . . .
34. If you reached your highest potential, you would look like . . .

These are just some of our ideas, so don't limit yourself to this list. (You knew we were going to say this, but we couldn't resist.) After they finish drawing, use the drawing as a basis for a conversation, processing how it was to do the drawing and what it was they learned about themselves from what they chose to draw and how they drew it. You can use this activity as a springboard for lots of other things—such as conversations, puppet shows, other drawings, movement and dance.

Mandalas

The more traditional definition of a mandala is a Hindu or Buddhist graphic depiction of the universe, with the circle outline creating a boundary that signifies wholeness or unity. Practically, when used in therapy, a mandala is a circle in which clients draw pictures to represent various aspects of their lives. A therapist can give clients very specific directions on what to include in the drawing or go with a more free-form directive to "draw a picture of your life" or "draw what is important to you in your life." Your clients can gain insight into their own feeling, thinking, behaving patterns, attitudes, values, and all sorts of things from a mandala, depending on how you use your instructions to set up the goal you have for the client. While most play therapists use mandalas with preteens, teens, and adults, we have even used them with younger children; we just kept our directions simple and straightforward with the younger clients, using the more free-form version of the directive. With older clients, we are usually more specific—the directive in the following paragraph is an example of one we would give a teen or adult. Individuals, groups, and families can all get "enlightenment" from mandalas.

You can draw a circle outline on a large piece of paper (which is what we do with elementary school-age clients) or have clients draw their own circle. Explain to them that you want them to color a mandala. For a more directive version of a mandala (Edna Nash, personal communication, 2006), you would say something like this in your directions:

"The mandala is a picture of your life. Before you draw, you will choose a different color to represent each of the areas of your life (physical environment, health, money/finances, career, intimate relationship/romance, family of origin, children, personal growth, spiritual/emotional, fun and recreation, friends). Be sure that the color you choose represents your feelings about that particular area. Next, draw something (you can use symbols, realistic figures, shapes, textures, etc.)

that expresses how you feel about that particular area and how things are going with that aspect of your life. As you draw, think about how much energy and time you devote to each area in your life and fill the space in the circle accordingly. (In other words, if you spend the majority of time at work, you will want to color most of your circle the color that represents work, and so forth.) Do not just make a pie graph—that won't give you a sense of how your life is going."

With some clients, just doing the drawing is enough for them to get insight into the various parts of their lives; with other clients, it is often helpful to talk about the process and the product of the procedure. We ask clients some of the following questions:

"What did you notice as you drew your life?"
"What were the areas that are taking up the most energy and time?"
"Were you surprised at any colors or symbols you chose to represent a particular area?"
"What about that surprised you?"
"Which symbols/colors did you feel most comfortable with?"
"Which symbols/colors were you uncomfortable with?"
"How much space did you leave for doing nothing?"
"Are there specific areas that seem to dominate/have too much of your time and energy?"
"Are there areas that are important to you that are not getting much of your time and energy?"
"Anything you would like to change?"

You could also ask questions like:

"What do you think/how do you feel about each area? Do you see any area where you want to/need to spend more time or energy or less time or energy?"
"What is each symbol/thing in the drawing, and what does it mean to you?"
"What do the colors mean to you?"
"Turn the picture around in a different way. Now what do you see from this different perspective?"

Another version of the mandala activity would be to ask clients to do a mandala focusing on "the issue" or on what they feel could be their next step in dealing with the issue. Another would be to ask them to draw their ideal life, relationship, job, and so on, and another would be their wish for the future. The possibilities are endless.

Structured Play Experiences

Friendship Want Ads

We have both had success with asking older elementary children and teens to write want ads for what they would want in a friend. We have used this activity for a couple of different purposes. For example, you can use it to help clients look at whether the people they have been choosing as friends actually meet their criteria for a friend and do a bit of reality testing if they don't. This works much better for helping them gain insight into their relationship patterns than arguing with them about whether their friends are "true friends" or "real friends," which is often what adults do with children about their friends. It is also sometimes enlightening for clients to look at whether they meet their own criteria for what makes a desirable friend. You can also use it with teens to help them look at boyfriend/girlfriend relationships in the process of helping them become aware that they often choose to connect with people of the opposite sex who they don't really like. Sometimes it helps them recognize that there are certain people they have in the "friend zone" that they might want to reconsider in another, closer role. We tend to do it in individual sessions just because, if you do it in a group, teens are often less likely to admit in front of other teens that they have been choosing boyfriends or girlfriends who would not even come close to being someone they would want as a friend.

(This description is probably going to be visiting the obvious zone again, and here it goes.) You ask clients to write an advertisement they could put in the newspaper (or on a dating website). Sometimes you have to bring in some want ads so they know what they look like . . . or you might visit a dating website so that they can see what people write in advertisements. (Make sure the website is appropriate before you visit it with kids.) Then you can have a conversation with them about whether the people they are choosing to have in their lives would meet the criteria they have listed in their want ad. You can also ask them about whether they would hire themselves as a friend if they answered a want ad that listed the things they listed.

Importance Jars

Quite often people get stuck in paying more attention to what is urgent and less to what is important. This activity is designed to help clients gain insight about their priorities by having a physical procedure for examining what is important to them. It is an activity that works better with pre-teens, teens, and adults, probably because relative importance is a pretty abstract concept. However, we have also used it with third- and fourth-grade students. It works better with individual clients and with families because in a group it is difficult to get folks to agree on what is important to the entire group.

To do this activity, you will need three jars—they can even be recycled jars. Label them as Very Important, Important, and Not Important. Before you show clients the jars, give them twenty to thirty small strips (2″ × 5″) of paper and have them write one of the things they have to do in their lives—like a "To Do" list—on each of the paper strips. You can have them write the things they need to do this week, this month, every day, and so forth—use any time period that works for specific clients. After they have the list, show them the jars and ask them to sort the paper strips into the appropriate jar. When they have done this, you can have them empty each jar one at a time and have a conversation about what makes each of the tasks very important, important, and not important and whether they want to move some of the strips to other jars as they reevaluate.

One variation on this technique that you could use with clients who need help recognizing that trying to control everything and everyone doesn't actually work would be to use jars that say "Things I have control over" and "Things I have no control over" and have your clients make a list of things they want to control and to sort the paper strips into the jars. Another variation designed to help clients who worry excessively determine which of their worries is reasonable and which isn't would be to use jars and ask them to make a list of their worries and sort them into the jars—you can choose the labels you want to put on each jar.

Invent a Pet

This activity can be used to build a relationship with clients in the first phase or in the gaining insight phase. We tend to use it to help clients figure out what their emotional needs are and begin to determine how to get those needs met in appropriate ways. The activity is a safer way to explore this topic than just to make a list of needs (that might or might not get met by the people in their lives). It can be used with any age, for individual clients, groups, and families.

You will need some supplies for this technique—craft materials (pompoms, yarn, Styrofoam balls, toothpicks, ribbon, felt, googly eyes, pipe cleaners), recycling materials like egg cartons and medicine bottles, glitter, glue, and scissors. If you are feeling adventurous and your clients are older elementary kids, teens, or adults, you can even use hot glue. (But remember—and remind the clients—hot glue is HOT!) Have clients make a list of the things they need to feel loved. If you are doing this with a family or group, they will need to brainstorm and come up with a combined list of what the members need. Then invite them to figure out how to use the materials to create a pet who could meet those needs. After the pet is created, with clients who like to process activities, you can ask how they think their new pet can meet their needs—or you can even ask the pet to tell you how it thinks it will meet the clients' needs. If clients are inclined, you can even generalize to their real lives and how they can get their needs met—but be sure they are ready and able to go there before you take that leap.

Stains

We learned this activity from Rebecca Dickinson (personal communication, January 2017), who developed it to work with older elementary, adolescent, and adult clients who have had bad experiences in life (sometimes involving trauma), that have left "marks" on them physically, emotionally, cognitively, or relationally. This activity is designed to help clients gain insight into how experiences from the past affect them in the present and help them recognize that positive things (perhaps even beauty) can be created from negative experiences.

Because of the nature of the process, this activity will take place over several sessions, so it is helpful to let the client know that you will not be able to finish it in a single session before you begin. For this activity, you will need a plain light-colored cloth bag, a variety of materials that can stain cloth (like dirt, mustard, ketchup, tomato sauce, grass, etc.), Sharpies or fabric paints, and laundry detergent. To start the technique, invite the client to experiment with the "staining" materials, trying to see which ones leave a lasting mark on the cloth bag. As the client does this, depending on the age of the client, the client's verbal abilities, and/or the need to stay in the metaphor, you can have the client consider (and share if the client is so inclined) which of the individual stains represent specific negative past life experiences. With a client who has the capacity for this kind of processing, you can even invite him or her to speculate as to which of the materials will actually leave a lasting mark on the bag. Leave the potentially staining material on the bag until the following session, when you invite the client to hand wash the bag with the laundry detergent. With a client who enjoys verbally processing, you can have a conversation about which of the materials actually left a stain, which did not, and what the experience of trying to wash out the stains was like for them. Unless you have access to a dryer in your play space, you will need to leave the bag to dry before the following session. In that session, invite the client to use the Sharpie or fabric paints to draw on the bag, transforming the stains into beautiful creations that are more pleasing to the client. When the transformation is complete, you can ask the client some questions if he or she is inclined to verbally process:

"What was it like creating the stains?"
"Which of your experiences did each of the stains represent?"

"What was it like trying to wash out the stains?"

"Were some easier to get out than others?"

"Did you put more effort into getting out some stains than others?"

"What do you think about the stains that remain? Do they affect how the bag looks to you?"

"We never completely erase difficult things that have happened in our lives. What difference did it make for you to be able to transform the stains into something you could be satisfied with, especially knowing that the original stain didn't disappear completely?"

THEORETICAL CONSIDERATIONS IN HELPING PLAY THERAPY CLIENTS GAIN INSIGHT

Remember, not every approach to play therapy is predicated on the preposition that insight is necessary for change to occur in play therapy. Theraplay therapists focus on using the therapeutic relationship with clients to build a sense of attachment, and they work with parents to make a bridge so that the parents of their child and adolescent clients learn to foster attachment with them. They do not believe clients need to become more aware of the factors that have prevented attachment, nor do they believe clients need to understand the factors that will help create attachment through the therapeutic process.

While cognitive-behavioral play therapists may use some interpretation to help clients deepen their understanding of the meaning of their play, they do not believe that insight is a requirement for change to happen. They tend to work with clients on developing new, more adaptive patterns of thinking and behaving, without needing for clients to understand what made those patterns maladaptive in the first place.

As we have mentioned, child-centered play therapists do sometimes use the play therapy skills of interpretation and clients' metaphors but would seldom use confrontation because confrontation would be too close to blatantly leading clients. They would not use the techniques and activities described in this chapter for that same reason.

The other approaches to play therapy we are describing in this book would all use the skills of interpretation, using clients' metaphors, confrontation, and designing therapeutic metaphors. They would also use the techniques we have outlined in this chapter. Adlerian play therapists would be likely to use the Misbehavior Show and many of the sand tray techniques described in this chapter. Jungians especially like to work with clients using sand tray techniques (though they are more likely to use nondirective sand trays rather than any of the directives we have listed) and mandalas (again—with less structured instructions than the ones we have provided for you). Psychodynamic play therapists make use of "soft" interpretations, confrontations, and the client's metaphors; they would not usually use most of the more directive techniques. Gestalt play therapists would be especially interested in the dance and movement activities, along with the body outline technique listed in the art techniques section. Integrative/prescriptive play therapists would probably use most of the skills in this chapter with at least some of their clients and, depending on their interests and the interests of their clients, they might be willing to incorporate any and all of the techniques designed to help clients gain insight.

MOVING ON . . .

So, we now know where we are going, we have started down the path of how to get there, and there is still more to learn. If you believe that a major part of your job as a play therapist will be in helping clients to make changes in their thinking, feeling, and behaving, the next chapter will provide you with a foundation for that process.

Interlude 6

Language Choice

L anguage choice can be very important in play therapy. Some specific examples of ways to be intentional with your language choices are (1) avoiding the word "but" (replacing it with "yes and . . ."); (2) eliminating "try" from your play therapy vocabulary; (3) avoiding using "we" (unless it really is a "we" situation), and (4) (mostly) using the same words clients use to describe their experiences, with some exceptions.

• Avoid "buts" (instead use "yes, and . . ."). It is important to avoid using the word "but" in your interactions with clients (and with the other important people in your life). Instead, you can use the "yes, and" approach, which is a key component of the central philosophy of improv theater. When you use "but" in a sentence, other people, especially children, tend to feel that the "but" discounts or negates anything positive you might have said in the rest of the sentence. For instance, if Penelope says to clients, "You worked really hard on that, but you still didn't succeed." what clients hear is, "You failed." or "You are a loser." If Jorge says to clients, "You are really excited about building that tower, but it isn't very high." what clients hear is "You didn't do that as well as you should have done it."

There are two ways to use the "yes and . . ." approach. By substituting "and" for "but," you can avoid the disconnection of "but" and convey something much more positive to clients, which can foster connection and provide encouragement. So, with the examples from this paragraph, to Penelope you could have said, "You worked hard on that, and you still didn't succeed. I bet that was disappointing to you." To Jorge you could have said, "You are excited about building that tower, and you wish it could have been even higher." Using this version of "yes, and," instead of being discouraging to clients, the play therapist is simply acknowledging what happened and is recognizing the feeling that accompanied it.

Another way to use the "yes and" strategy (even in a situation in which you disagree with what clients are doing or saying) is finding something you can encourage or agree with in what clients say or do. You then let them know you agree by starting a sentence with a "yes" (either by using the actual word or just by having a part of the sentence that conveys agreement) and bridging into a correction if it is needed with your "and." For example, when the client is cheating during a game, you can say, "You are being very creative in your interpretation of the rules, and sometimes that might be upsetting to people you are playing with because it keeps everyone else from being able to win." Sometimes we start the "yes" part of our response with reflecting a feeling, like when you have a client who is ranting about her boss being unfair because he is docking her pay when she is late for work, and you say, "Yes, I can hear that you are mad because the boss is docking your pay, and you do acknowledge that you are getting in to work late."

- Avoid "try." We often quote Yoda from *Star Wars* in our supervision sessions and with clients: "Do. Or do not. There is no try." This actually echoes an idea that Alfred Adler posited a few years before the *Star Wars* movies. He suggested that, when people say they are going to "try," it means they have no expectation that they are going to succeed; they are acknowledging (and maybe even welcoming) failure. So, we avoid saying "try," and we often point out the inherent underlying meaning of "trying" to clients. (Clients seem to prefer having the confrontation about "try" that uses the Yoda quote to the Adler quote, just so you know.)

- Avoid using a "nursey we." (We know—we are a bit locked into the things you should avoid, and yet . . . we think these are important.) If you have ever been a patient in a hospital, you might recognize this reference—we have noticed nurses in hospitals seem to use a kind of royal we that announces "we" are going to get a shot, wonders if "we" slept well, and so on. (As I [Kristin] was delivering my second child—unexpectedly and rapidly, without an epidural—my nurse [attempting to be empathic and encouraging] said, "We're going to do this" I looked her in the eye and asked, "Exactly what is it that you're going to do?") So, when you are suggesting to clients that you would like them to paint a picture of their families, instead of saying, "We are going to paint or draw a picture of your family," you would say, "Please paint or draw a picture of your family."

- Match vocabulary words with clients, except . . . It helps build connection with clients if you know and understand vocabulary words that they use (unless, of course, you have clients who are fluent in profanity and you are super uncomfortable with profanity, or you think that it would be counterproductive to match those kinds of words). For instance, if you are working with clients who play video games, it behooves you to know and use vocabulary words that gamers use; similarly, if you have clients who are interested in trains, it helps to know terms related to trains. With young children, when you are tracking clients' behavior, it is helpful to use the same words they use to label objects. Even if you know the thing acting as a golf club is really a sword, not a golf club, you should call it a golf club rather than a sword. If a client is calling a puppet a puppy and it is actually a wolf puppet, you should call it a puppy.

We believe there is an exception to this guideline though. When clients use evaluative or judgmental words to describe characters in the play (like "good guys" and "bad guys" or "nice kitty" and "bad kitty"), we work to avoid using those words because we don't want to reinforce that all-or-nothing, moralistic thinking. It is important to help clients to shift the way they are thinking about the world, moving them away from categorical good versus bad thinking because it is helpful for them to recognize people are not all good or all bad. Because many clients referred for play therapy believe they are coming to play therapy because they are "bad," and tend to think of themselves as "naughty" or "evil," it is essential to help them change this pattern of thinking. One way you can do this is through your language choices. So, when a child is playing at being a bank robber and wants you to be a police officer, instead of labeling the robber "the bad guy," you could call him "the guy who is breaking the law," and instead of labeling the police officer the "good guy," you could label him or her "the person who is trying to make sure people follow the rules" or even "the police officer." Sometimes this involves more words than the "evil bad guy" and will require you to be creative in thinking of ways to shift the categorical words like "good," "bad," "evil," "mean," "nice." (And we believe it is worth the effort.)

CHAPTER 7

Helping Clients Make Changes in Play Therapy

Now, in some ways, we get to the heart of the matter—helping clients to make changes. While there are some theoretical approaches to play therapy (e.g., child-centered approaches) that do not emphasize the counselor using directed activities to help clients make changes in behavior, cognitions, emotions, and/or interactions, all approaches to therapy really have these types of changes as the end goal of the process. (Or why would people come to see us if they didn't want to make some kind of change? We don't know anyone who goes to therapy just to stay the same. Well, someone wants clients to make some kind of change—in the case of some child clients and lots of teens, someone else, like parents or teachers, wants them to change—but they don't necessarily want to change.) Of course, we want to invite you to consider whether you think deliberately guiding people to make changes and/or offering directed interventions is important in play therapy and what the role of the play therapist should be in helping clients to make changes. The other question is, if you do think it is appropriate for you to use skills and techniques to help people make changes, which skills and techniques do you think will work best for you and for clients?

In getting ready to write this book, we made a list of ineffective patterns of behaving, thinking, feeling, and interacting that people who come to play therapy (or the people who sent them to therapy) usually want changed. Then we used that original inventory as a jumping off point for making several lists of things we thought play therapy could change. We have noticed that desired change is usually directional, so we have lists of things we think would be good to increase and lists of things we think would be good to decrease. (And, in some cases, there are reciprocal things on the increase and decrease lists—like risk-taking.) Some of these goals make more sense for child clients or adolescents than for adults, so we have tried to be pretty generic in the things on the list so that you can apply them to whichever population you desire. And we know there are lots of things folks want to change that we have not thought to include in our lists. Remember—adopt and adapt—you can use the skills and techniques described in the chapters for any clients, with any presenting problems, and adopt any goals that will work for you and your clients. Just modify them in the ways you need to change them so that they will be helpful, or give yourself permission to invent your own activities. (We give you ours—permission, that is—not kids, husbands, or money.)

Okay, here's the list:

Related to behaving–decrease

1. Impulsivity, out-of-seat/off-task behavior, inattentiveness
2. Noncompliance with rules, requests, and/or commands
3. Defiant behavior
4. Physical aggressiveness
5. Power struggles with other people/arguing
6. Bossiness or demandingness
7. Blaming others, lack of willingness to take responsibility
8. Bragging
9. Inappropriate or dangerous risk-taking

Related to behaving–increase

1. Cooperation skills
2. Negotiation skills
3. Assertiveness skills
4. Willingness to act on/follow through with possible solutions to problems
5. Self-control
6. Attentiveness, ability to stay on task
7. Willingness to take responsibility
8. Willingness to take appropriate academic, physical, and interpersonal risks
9. Willingness and skills involved in "resetting" after a problem occurs
10. Willingness and skills involved in self-scaffolding new learning and behavior

Related to thinking–decrease

1. Negative self-talk
2. Negative self-talk
3. Negative self-talk
4. Negative, pessimistic thinking
5. Negative, pessimistic thinking (Sorry, almost everything we could think of connected to thinking patterns we wanted to decrease was related to negative self-talk or negative, pessimistic thinking.)
6. Denial of personal assets
7. Unwillingness to take the cognitive perspective of others
8. Denial or obliviousness to personal needs

Related to thinking–increase

1. Positive self-talk in place of negative self-talk
2. Positive, optimistic thoughts
3. "Owning" personal assets
4. Skills involved in considering others' cognitive perspectives
5. Skills involved in optimistically reframing situations and experiences
6. Skills related to recognizing their own needs
7. Skills related to accurately assessing risks and consequences
8. Problem-solving skills

Related to feelings–decrease

1. Denial of emotions
2. Getting "stuck" in anger, sadness, depression
3. Obliviousness to physical manifestations of emotions
4. Negative feelings about self
5. Difficulty managing frustration, anger, and/or stress
6. Unwillingness to take others' emotional perspective or recognize the feelings of others
7. Self-doubt

Related to feelings–increase

1. Feeling vocabulary
2. Recognition of multiple (sometimes contradictory) feelings
3. Awareness of the emotion–body connection
4. Awareness of specific feelings
5. Getting through and out of anger, sadness, depression
6. Skills for appropriately communicating about feelings
7. Skills related to recognizing the feelings of others
8. Skills related to considering the emotional perspective of others

9. Positive feelings toward self, self-confidence, sense of self-efficacy
10. Skills related to tolerating and managing frustration
11. Skills related to dealing appropriately with anger
12. Skills for dealing with stress

Related to interacting–decrease

1. Obliviousness to or denial of the impact of personal behavior on others
2. Difficulty with setting personal boundaries
3. Unwillingness to take personal responsibility
4. Difficulty with good sportsmanship
5. Unwillingness to ask for help

Related to interacting–increase

1. Skills related to recognizing and accurately interpreting social information
2. Skills related to accepting responsibility in interpersonal interactions
3. Skills related to recognizing and appropriately asking for personal needs to be met
4. Skills related to setting appropriate limits and boundaries
5. Willingness and ability to share power with others
6. Recognition of appropriate and positive roles in peer group and family
7. Skills involved in realistically assessing the characteristics of self and others
8. Willingness to take personal responsibility
9. Skills for winning and losing gracefully, taking turns, and otherwise being a good sport
10. Skills necessary for actively listening to others
11. Skills necessary for cooperating in group activity and with family members
12. Skills necessary for encouraging others
13. Social skills (beginning and ending conversations, maintaining developmentally appropriate conversations, apologizing gracefully, etc.)
14. Skills necessary for keeping out of fights/using self-control in social situations

We are pretty sure we have left lots of things out of these lists, and it is time to move on to the ways to actually help folks make changes. Without further ado (we have always wanted to write that in a book), on to the skills and techniques.

PLAY THERAPY SKILLS FOR HELPING CLIENTS MAKE CHANGES

You will, of course, want to use the skills you have worked with up to this point to help clients make changes. And there are skills that are particularly relevant to this phase of play therapy (that can, of course, be used in earlier phases—this is just where they seem to fit into the book). They are paying attention to timing, looking at secondary gain, being realistic and helping others to be realistic, and teaching.

Paying Attention to Timing

This one is pretty simple—pay attention to timing. It is important to make sure you introduce activities designed to help people make changes at a time when they are ready and able to undertake change. (You didn't think we could be so succinct, did you?)

Looking at Secondary Gain

Lots of times people don't change because some part of them is getting something from the behavior (or thinking, feeling, interacting) that is causing them difficulties. Secondary gain is the desired or positive (at least as perceived by the client) side effect of a thought, emotion, behavior, or interaction. A secondary gain to arriving late to work could be missing a boring morning meeting or an awkward interaction with a colleague. A secondary gain of choosing to continue to abuse alcohol or drugs could be avoiding addressing past pain or trauma. If your child is throwing a temper tantrum because you refuse to buy her a candy bar in the store and she keeps throwing tantrums every time you take her to the store, despite the fact that you are putting her in time out, yelling at her, and spanking her to get her to stop, her behavior probably continues because there is a secondary gain. The secondary gain for her might be that when she is being punished you are paying attention to her or that you do give in and buy her a candy bar every fifth time she has a meltdown. Secondary gains can be in or out of the client's awareness. Whatever the secondary gain, we believe it is essential to the change process that you help clients ferret out what it is because the only way change is going to occur is if they become aware of what it is that is sustaining the inappropriate/ineffective pattern.

In trying to understand what a person's secondary gain is, your theory can come in handy in exploring what his or her motivation might be. Secondary gain is not important in every theoretical orientation. The theories that would be most likely to use secondary gain as a vehicle for helping clients change would be Adlerian, cognitive-behavioral, and psychodynamic. Adlerians believe that all behavior is purposeful, and thus they intently consider "secondary gain" as part of what keeps a client "stuck" and, by gently bringing the secondary gain to the client's attention, hope to liberate them from being stuck. Cognitive-behavioral play therapists are always looking for the circumstances that reinforce maladaptive patterns, and so they would ask the client to examine and give up the secondary gain. Psychodynamic theory followers believe that people have a drive to get their needs met and that those needs are often unconscious. In this theory, secondary gain is probably buried in the unconscious motivation of the client, perhaps involving avoiding pain and maximizing pleasure—at least momentarily.

What does your theory teach about how people get stuck in maladaptive patterns of feeling, thinking, behaving, and/or interacting? What do you believe about this? That will help determine whether you think about exploring secondary gain and revealing your hypotheses about secondary gain to clients as a tool to help them make changes.

Being Realistic and Helping Others Be Realistic

This is another easy one—we are not miracle workers, and play therapy isn't magical—it's pretty cool, but it's not an enchantment. (In over 30 years of doing play therapy, I [Terry] have had three miracle cures that weren't really miracles because we had put lots of work into the play therapy, parent and teacher consultation, and family play therapy before the clients got "miraculously" better.) So, in order for you to avoid discouragement in the process, you need to know that all of your clients' problems are not going to disappear overnight (and some of them may never disappear). This doesn't mean you are not doing good work; it means people are human. There will be behavioral, emotional, cognitive, attitudinal, and interactional patterns that are resistant to change; and there will be patterns that only change a small amount. It is essential to help parents and teachers (and adolescent and adult clients) think about what would be a reasonable and acceptable degree of change for them to be satisfied with the outcome of the play therapy process. Do this at the very beginning of the play therapy process. By front-loading reasonable and realistic expectations for the process, you will help clients more than if you let clients (or parents or teachers) cling to hopes for miracle cures.

Teaching

There are many ways to teach clients new skills or help them acquire new ways of thinking, feeling, behaving, or interacting, and that is really a whole book of its own (which we are not writing and are never going to write). We are just going to provide you with some tools we use when we teach clients in play therapy: scaffolding, modeling, direct didactic teaching, indirect teaching, and reinforcing/encouraging.

Scaffolding

Developmental psychologist Lev Vygotsky posited that learning new behaviors and mastering new skills happened in what he called the "zone of proximal development" (ZPD). He defined the ZPD as "the distance between the actual developmental level as determined by independent problem solving and the level of potential development as determined through problem solving under adult guidance, or in collaboration with more capable peers" (Vygotsky, 1978, p. 86). (That's a fancy way of saying there is a period of time between when you start to learn things and when you have mastered them.) During the ZPD, you might struggle or you might have a steady improvement; you might even feel as though you are failing and give up.

Vygotsky was a developmental psychologist. He explained what might be happening, but he didn't particularly see a need to help folks figure out what to do to make things better. Wood, Bruner, and Ross (1976) came up with the idea of something they called "scaffolding"—a way to help folks get through the ZPD with as little pain as possible. Scaffolding can include modeling a skill, providing hints or cues, and adapting material or activity in order to help people master that skill. We especially like providing hints or cues for our clients—charts, lists, gestures, facial expressions, and the like. We have noticed that scaffolding can happen anywhere—at home with parents scaffolding their children; in newlywed couples scaffolding one another in the process of figuring out how to build the kind of family they both want; in school with teachers scaffolding their students' acquisition of skills; in play therapy sessions with play therapists scaffolding children, adults, adolescents, family members, parents, and teachers in making changes.

You should consider several things as you begin to scaffold a specific skill or particular pattern of thinking, feeling, behaving, or interacting: (1) Does this particular person need scaffolding at this particular time to be able to move toward mastery of this specific skill or pattern? (2) What kind of scaffolding works well for this specific skill or pattern? (3) What kind of scaffolding works best for this particular person? (4) How much scaffolding does this particular person need at this time in the ZPD to be able to move toward mastery of this specific skill or pattern? (This isn't from Vgotsky or Wood et al.; I [Terry] just made it up, but it works for us.)

Modeling

Modeling is showing clients how to do things (we think you probably already know this, but we want to reinforce that it is an important skill for teaching things in play therapy). Sometimes you show them yourself by modeling in a session; sometimes you get someone else in your clients' life to show them how to do it; sometimes you (with informed consent, of course) invite another person into your session to show how it is done; sometimes you ask your clients to watch a television show, movie, or instructional video so they can see someone else doing it; sometimes you videotape them doing it in a session and send the recording home with them to watch it. We model, or find models of, being imperfect, winning or losing with grace, recovering from a mistake, building relationships, taking directions or giving directions, being disappointed, being proud, being sad, being happy, touching appropriately, listening to others, and lots of other things that happen spontaneously during a session (or are preplanned before a session).

Direct Didactic Teaching

This tool consists of situations in which you tell clients how to do something, you structure a discussion about how to do something, or you set up an activity designed to give them an opportunity to acquire a new skill or pattern and/or practice it. If you use an activity, for it to be direct didactic teaching, you need to provide a chance to verbally process their experience.

Indirect Teaching

This tool consists of setting up an activity for having people acquire or practice a new skill or pattern and then not inviting them to verbally process. It could also be using storytelling, metaphor design, or bibliotherapy to help clients learn something new.

Reinforcing/Encouraging

Lots of time, growth is slower than clients would like (and slower than we would like too), so it is helpful to make sure you give lots of encouragement for changes, even small ones. So, build in reinforcement and encouragement into your sessions—it can be simple, like a nod, a smile, a pat on the back; or it can be more complex things like you pointing out progress and acknowledging effort—all of those elements that keep people from giving up and that help motivate clients to pay attention to your teaching. We teach other people in the client's life to do this, too. Parents, siblings, teachers, partners, or children can be fantastic reinforcers or encouragers for children, siblings, students, partners, or parents.

PLAY THERAPY TECHNIQUES FOR HELPING CLIENTS MAKE CHANGES

Clearly, you can use many of the skills and techniques we have described in earlier chapters to help clients make changes. The techniques in this chapter are specifically focused on helping clients make progress toward the goals we have listed earlier. *And* to make up your own or adapt these techniques to work better for you and your clients!

Adventure Therapy Techniques

Slow Motion Races

We both volunteer at elementary schools, working with children who would otherwise not get play therapy services. This is a technique we made up to get students back to their classroom without running through the halls and leaving us behind in their dust (a "no-no" in schools everywhere). It works best with preschool and elementary-age children who have some characteristics of ADHD—impulsivity, short attention span, and the like—to help them learn to manage those traits. Another goal for this activity is to help children who have a tendency to engage in power struggles to learn ways of interacting with others (even "authority figures") without getting into power struggles and to practice cooperation skills (even though there is still an element of competition).

It's pretty simple: you challenge the client to walk somewhere as slowly as possible; whoever gets to the destination last, wins the race. We even like to use the inclination toward melodrama seen in children in this population and reframe it into the more positive quality of theatricality by making acting out the effort and challenge of going slowly part of the activity, which translates to visibly straining muscles, grimacing faces, and the like.

Blindfolded Basketball

This trust activity encourages clients (of all ages) to practice staying attentive, taking responsibility, accessing risks and consequences, taking the emotional and cognitive perspective of others, sharing power with others, listening to others, cooperating with others, asking for others to meet their personal needs, and being a good sport. It is easier to do with individual clients, and with some adaptation, you can do it with families and in small groups.

For an individual client, it requires three props—a Nerf basketball, a blindfold, and a small- to medium-sized trashcan. Between the two of you, decide who is going to "go" first. Whichever person is going to "go" first is the guide, and the other person is the basketball player. Explain that it is the guide's responsibility to keep the other person both physically and emotionally safe and to steer the basketball player to the basket without touching him or her, and it is the basketball player's job to let the guide know what he or she needs to feel safe and to make baskets. The basketball player orients himself or herself to the trashcan (aka, the basket), puts on the blindfold, and takes the basketball. Before you actually start playing, clarify that the only way to get points in the game is to guide the basketball player to make the baskets because the only person who gets points is the person who is guiding at the time, not the person who has the basketball. After each goal, trade roles so that you take turns being the guide and the basketball player. (Because you are just taking turns, there is really no point to keeping score because no one is going to win, but it isn't necessary to tell clients that little detail.)

If you are playing the game with a small group or family, have the members take turns being the blindfolded basketball player and rotate the responsibility of guiding so that each member gives the player one set of instructions to get the player closer to making a goal and then passes the responsibility for guiding on to the next member. With folks who are willing to process, this is a great activity to process, with questions like the following: "How did it feel to have responsibility for someone else?" "What was it like to have to trust someone else to keep you safe and help you complete a task successfully?" "What was it like knowing that the only way to be successful was to work as a team?" "How was it possible to figure out how to steer someone without being able to touch them?"

Show Your Feelings

The possible goals with regard to this one are extensive. You can use it for enlarging feeling vocabulary, increasing awareness of the emotion–body connection, enhancing skills for appropriately communicating about feelings and recognizing the feelings of others, increasing skills related to recognizing and accurately interpreting social information, and realistically assessing the characteristics of self and others. Again, it is an activity that can be done with any age clients and any therapeutic grouping.

For preparation, you need to take a pile of 3″ by 5″ cards, cut them in half, take a list of feeling words, and write one feeling per card. (The Internet is a great place to get a list.) Take turns drawing a card from the pile and acting out the feeling word, with the other person/people making guesses about what feeling is being acted out. You can make a rule that the person acting out the feeling is to use his or her whole body with no sound, just his or her face, just his or her voice without words, his or her whole body with sound effects, and so on. If clients are interested in verbally processing, you can talk about which feelings were easy to express, which feelings were easy to guess, situations in which they have felt those feelings, times when they couldn't figure out how others were feeling, and so on.

Storytelling and Creating Therapeutic Metaphors

The first set of techniques we are going to describe in this section are all specific change metaphors. Specific change metaphors have a definite formula and format aimed at helping clients make particular changes in (1) self-image thinking, (2) affect, or (3) behavior (Lankton & Lankton, 1989). Although the core of this process was developed by Lankton and Lankton (1989), I (Terry) have modified the basic metaphor formulas to make them applicable to play therapy. All of the specific change metaphors seem to work better with individual clients because they are custom-designed to fit the needs of specific clients; you could use them with a small group if the clients shared similar issues or presenting problems. We have used them with all ages.

Self-Image Thinking Metaphor

The goal with self-image thinking metaphors is to shift negative self-talk into more positive self-talk; increase clients' positive feelings toward themselves, their self-confidence, and sense of self-efficacy; and increase clients' willingness to "own" their strengths. Here are the steps for creating a self-image thinking metaphor:

1. Construct a central character (the protagonist for you English majors out there) who represents a positive central self-image. With younger clients, use a puppet or figure to represent this character; with older clients, you can decide whether a puppet or figure would be appropriate—if not, you can just tell the story without props.

2. Describe the protagonist as having positive traits that strongly resemble the positive traits of the client, even those the client does not acknowledge. Include in the description of the protagonist several qualities or characteristics the client might like to have (or characteristics that you wish to enhance, even if the client doesn't actually want them yet).

3. In the first part of the story, include a section illustrating how the central character embodies each of the desired qualities. Include specific visual cues for each quality (e.g., "bright smile," "strong arms," "looks other people in the eyes").

4. As the story progresses, verbalize the protagonist's internal monologue, emphasizing his or her positive self-image and faith in himself

or herself and his or her ability to solve problems (e.g., "I know I can do this, even if it is a little scary" or "I couldn't jump that far last week, and I know I can do it now").

5. Invent a supportive ally/friend and show the protagonist interacting in a positive manner with this ally. It is often useful if the friend struggles a bit with self-image and still works to be helpful to the protagonist. (Again, with younger clients, you can use puppets or figures to act out the story.)

6. Develop several scenarios in which the protagonist of the story deals with different situations, demonstrating the positive characteristics and positive self-talk about self-image.

7. Describe a positive or routine situation and describe the main character coping successfully with it, demonstrating his or her positive qualities, with the internal monologue illustrating a sense of self-efficacy. Have the ally help operationalize the solution generated by the protagonist.

8. Describe a stressful, anxiety-provoking situation and portray the protagonist coping successfully with it, demonstrating his or her positive qualities. Have the protagonist muse about the feelings evoked by the problematic situation and his or her accompanying self-talk in an internal monologue and some dialogue with the ally. Make sure that there is a realistic struggle in the process of resolving the situation, with perhaps a smidgen of self-doubt, also recounted in the internal monologue and dialogue with the ally.

9. Have the protagonist and the ally have a celebratory conversation about what happened, featuring a summary of how the protagonist's positive qualities and affirming self-image helped get the main character and his or her friend to the resolution of both situations.

Affect Metaphor

In designing an affect metaphor, it is important to decide whether you are going to use the metaphor to help a client explore the layers of feeling that could occur in a situation (where the goal would be to learn to recognize multiple, sometimes contradictory, feelings), help a client change or shift a feeling state (where the goal would be helping clients to get through and out of anger, sadness, depression, or some other feeling where they were feeling stuck), or help a client learn to better manage a specific feeling (where the goal would be learning to handle anger or frustration in appropriate ways). If you are working with a client on layered emotions (like having two contradictory feelings about a person or situation or having a feeling on the surface as a reaction to a person or situation with emotions layered underneath that surface feeling), you would follow these steps:

1. Describe a protagonist and a resource person. If you are using puppets or figures to represent the characters, include both a physical description and a description of the character's emotional palette (for example, "He was a person who had a lot of different emotions and knew just what he was feeling about the people and situations in his life"). The resource person should be wise and understanding, providing encouragement and emotional support for the main character. When describing the actions of the resource person, make sure he or she does not solve the problems experienced by the protagonist. Rather, the resource person should reflect feelings and normalize the protagonist's emotional experience.

2. Develop several encounters or situations. In your description of the encounters or the circumstances of the situation, keep your focus on the character's emotional reactions.

   a. Have the character encounter a person or a situation that is positive or routine. In the description of this encounter or situation, include the various layers of the emotions felt by the character. For instance, "One happy day, David got a puppy. He was excited and a little nervous about how he was going to take care of the puppy. He was pretty confident about feeding the puppy, but he was anxious about taking the puppy for a walk during the very cold winter days. David told his dad that he was happy and nervous." (Notice that in this description there are only two feelings, which is often the case with positive or routine circumstances, and the emotions really are not particularly problematic.)

   b. In the description, have the main character acknowledge that he or she has several different feelings and articulate a recognition that it is not problematic to have two different feelings at the same time. Sometimes you will want to have the protagonist recognize this for himself or herself, and sometimes you will want to have a resource person help the protagonist understand this phenomenon. For example, "His dad pointed out that lots of kids, even though they were excited to be getting a pet, worried about being able to take care of the pet. His dad asked David to tell him about what he was worried about and listened carefully to his happiness and his fears."

   c. Next, have the character encounter a person or situation that is negative or stressful. In the description of this encounter or situation, include the layers of the emotions felt by the character, with an acknowledgment of the complex (and sometimes even contradictory) nature of the emotions. For instance, "Sheila's father had gone to jail for beating her up, and when her grandmother wanted Sheila to visit her father, she told her grandmother that she would not go because she hated her father. That night, she cried herself to sleep because she really missed her father. Sheila loved her father, and she hated him. That was confusing to her."

d. Although you can have the protagonist sort through the layers of emotions all alone, it usually helps to have a resource person listen to the protagonist's various feelings, help clarify them for the protagonist, and help him or her understand that having layered feelings is normal, even when it is a bit scary or confusing. "When Sheila talked to her grandmother about how she was feeling, her grandmother told her that she understood that sometimes Sheila felt like she loved her dad and hated him at the same time. Sheila's grandmother told her that of course she was angry at her dad for hitting her when he got drunk and she still missed doing fun things with her dad when he was sober. She said, 'It is confusing, sweetie. Sometimes I get confused feelings about your dad too—with me mad at him mixed up with my love for him.'"

If you are using a story to help a play therapy client modify a feeling state that is causing him or her difficulty or helping a client learn to cope with a specific feeling in a more functional way, you could use puppets or figures to facilitate the following process (or you can just tell the story without props if you think that would work better with a particular client):

1. Describe a protagonist who is struggling with a particular feeling, using the details of the characterization to "flesh out" the person, emphasizing the specific emotion you want to feature, how the character reacts to this feeling, and how the feeling is manifested in the body. It is often helpful to include a description of the facial expressions and other nonverbal evidence of how the character is experiencing the feeling. For example, "Fernanda hated school. Every time she thought about going to school, she got a stomach ache. When Fernanda's mother woke her up to go to school, she frowned and burrowed back under the covers because she just didn't want to go because she hated school that much."

2. Describe another character who has a relationship with the protagonist, or describe a place, object, or situation that evokes an emotional reaction in the protagonist. For instance, "Mrs. Young, Fernanda's teacher, was very strict and assigned lots of homework. Mrs. Young was very loud, and when she got very impatient with Fernanda, she always talked to her in a loud voice. Fernanda felt frustrated with Mrs. Young and by midyear, she kind of hated her."

3. Recount an interaction between the protagonist and the other character (or the place, object, or situation), with the focus on the protagonist's affective state (such as sadness, frustration, depression, fear) evoked by the interaction. Be sure to suggest that the protagonist is struggling with the emotion itself or with the way he or she is handling the emotion. For instance, "One day, Fernanda forgot to bring her homework to school, even though she did it. Mrs. Young talked in her loud voice at her for not having her homework, 'once again.' Fernanda was so very frustrated and angry with Mrs. Young because Mrs. Young would not believe she had done the homework. She felt that Mrs. Young always yelled at her for not doing her homework, and she gave her a 'hate look' whenever the teacher talked about her doing her homework. The next day, Fernanda brought her homework to school, tore it up, and threw it at her teacher. Mrs. Young looked very sad and disappointed, but she did not yell at Fernanda. She just shrugged and walked away. Fernanda was ashamed that she had destroyed her homework and felt sad that she could not figure out how to get along better with her teacher."

4. Introduce some sort of change or movement in the story that causes an alteration in the relationship or situation. This can involve the characters moving closer together, further apart, and so on, or the protagonist experiencing something that changes his or her reactions to the person, place, object, or situation. The protagonist can also learn some coping strategy that allows a better way to handle the problematic emotion. For example, "Fernanda went to talk to Mr. Lei, the counselor in her school, about her problem with her teacher. Mr. Lei listened to her feelings and told her that he understood that she was feeling frustrated and angry with her teacher. He suggested that she might also be a little embarrassed about forgetting her homework. He asked her whether she would like to figure out a way to start remembering to bring her homework to school, and they came up with a way for her mother to remind her to put it in her school folder. Fernanda said she was still mad at Mrs. Young for yelling at her. Mr. Lei asked her to pick some puppets to represent herself, Mrs. Young, and several other students to show him how Mrs. Young talked to her and how she talked to the other children in her class. When Fernanda showed Mr. Lei how Mrs. Young talked to the other children, she realized that Mrs. Young had a very loud voice and maybe she wasn't really yelling at her. She was still mad though that Mrs. Young had not believed she did her homework. Mr. Lei asked her if she would be comfortable having Mrs. Young come to the counselor's office so they could talk about what was happening between them. Fernanda said that she was willing to do it, and Mr. Lei asked Mrs. Young to come in. Mr. Lei asked Fernanda to be so brave as to tell Mrs. Young how she was feeling. This

was hard for Fernanda. She decided it would be worth it because she wanted things to be better for her at school, so she told Mrs. Young that it hurt her feelings when Mrs. Young did not believe she had done her homework and she got mad at her too. She also told her that she didn't like it when Mrs. Young yelled at her. Mrs. Young told Fernanda that she was sorry she hurt her feelings. She told Fernanda she was frustrated because she knew how smart Fernanda was and she believed Fernanda was hurting herself by not bringing her homework to school. Mr. Lei asked Fernanda to tell Mrs. Young about their plan for getting her homework to school. Mrs. Young smiled and told Fernanda she would try to talk in a quieter voice when she talked to her."

5. Complete the story with a description of the learning undergone by the client, along with any observable changes, including body sensations and expression and behavior resulting from the shift experienced by the protagonist. You can also focus on the character's enhanced ability to deal with the feelings that have caused difficulties in the past. For instance, "Fernanda was excited about the plan she and Mr. Lei had made up. She smiled and her stomach didn't hurt the next day when her mother woke her up. She had already put her homework in her folder the night before after she finished it. She hopped out of bed to get dressed and catch the bus. When she walked into her class, Mrs. Young smiled at her, and she smiled back. Mrs. Young told her she was proud of her for bringing her homework in a soft voice. She just knew she was going to have a good day at school. She would remember that if she and Mrs. Young were having a problem, they could go to Mr. Lei's office and talk it out."

Behavior Change Metaphor

Behavior change metaphors could work to increase any behavior you wanted to help clients cultivate. To develop a behavior change metaphor, you would follow the following steps (again, using puppets or figures to represent characters when you think it is appropriate):

1. Determine a clearly defined observable behavior you would like the client to learn to use.
2. Describe the protagonist, using as many details as possible emphasizing physical appearance, behavior, cognitions, and emotional reactions. Have the character be similar in age and situation to the client (but not so similar that it forces the client to acknowledge that the protagonist is a "stand in" for the client).
3. Set up a situation in which the protagonist displays the desired behavior. Include a description of the character's internal

monologue to support the introduction of this behavior in response to the situation.

4. Develop several different "chapters" for the story, changing the context in order to allow the protagonist to demonstrate the desired behavior several different times. As part of the character's internal monologue, include some self-affirmations for using the new behavior.

Nightmares

I (Terry) originally developed this activity for my godson, Kent, who used to have a lot of nightmares when he was in elementary school. Since he is now almost 30, I have been using this technique for a long time. This strategy can give child clients a tool they can use to stop nightmares or reduce the anxiety about bad dreams. It can also help them develop a sense of control over other fears. The primary vehicle for this technique is the creation of a metaphor that externalizes fears and helps to make them more manageable. It can also be helpful for teaching children to begin to recognize negative, self-defeating thinking, substitute positive thoughts for negative thoughts, and develop skills necessary to optimistically reframe situations. It can give children an opportunity to practice cooperation skills and follow through with possible solutions to problems, along with the skills involved in "resetting" after a problem occurs, and self-scaffolding.

The metaphoric story can be created by the therapist for children or can be co-created by the therapist with children. When the therapist and clients co-create the story together, this technique can be used to encourage clients' willingness to take risks, solve problems, and recognize their needs, self-confidence, and sense of self-efficacy. You could even teach parents and teachers to do this technique with children outside the play therapy session as a way to generalize the learning.

To do this technique, you will need four or five miniature horse figures; several other figures (of either people or animals, depending on what might be most interesting or appealing to the client); several pieces of string or yarn (10–12 inches long), and multiple small fences (they can be plastic, wooden, or metal). Set the horses, the other figures, the string or yarn, and the fences on a table or on the floor. Explain that the horses, which happen to be mares, usually run wild in the night, and when they run wild, they feel scared and they scare other animals (and maybe even people). You can ask the child to name the night mares and the other figures if he or she wants. If you are telling the story to the child, demonstrate how wild and crazy the mares can get (you can even verbalize how scared they feel being out of control this way). Have the night mares get very close to the other figures (animals or people)—maybe even acting like they are going to kick the other figures, jumping over the other figures, knocking the other figures down, or crashing into things and hurting themselves. Verbalize how the other figures are feeling (i.e., scared, unprotected, unsafe, etc.). If you are co-telling the story with the child, ask the child whether he or she wants to move the night mares around, move the other figures around, or do the verbalizing about the feelings of the night mares and/or the other figures. You do the parts of the storytelling that the child does not want to do.

Ask the child what he or she thinks might help to calm down the night mares, keep the night mares safe, and keep the other figures safe. Point out that sometimes, in order to create safety, structure (restraints, rules, boundaries) needs to be imposed, and ask the child to help figure out something that could happen with the string or yarn and/or the fences to make sure everyone is safe and feels safe. You can guide the child in exploring the idea of using the string or yarn to rope the night mares in order to help them calm down, suggesting if the night mares were put in a corral created by the fences, they might feel less wild/more safe and everyone else would be safe too. You will probably need to help the child follow through with this action, building a corral, gathering up the night mares with the string or yarn, and putting them into the corral. The child can use the other figures to help accomplish this or can do it on his or her own. As the night mares move into the corral, verbalize that they feel safer, calmer, more peaceful, and so on. At the same time, you would probably also want to verbalize the feelings experienced by the other figures (relief, lower anxiety, less stress, etc.). You can use encouragement to highlight the child's contribution to the resolution, especially related to the child's willingness to take risks, solve problems, recognize his or her needs, self-confidence, and sense of self-efficacy.

There are several variations on this technique you could try. You could have the child physically act out the part of one of the night mares, using pillows or chairs to create fences for helping create and maintain control and safety. You could ask the child to draw a safe place where the night mares could run wild but not risk hurting themselves or others or a place where the night mares would know what the rules were so that they didn't hurt themselves or others. You could ask the child to draw or paint or use stickers to re-create a nightmare he or she has experienced and then help generate ideas for keeping safe inside that nightmare or strategies for calming himself or herself down upon waking up after a nightmare. You could use construction paper labels that say "Nightmare Repellent" taped onto spray cans of air freshener, and send them home with the child so that the spray around his or her bedroom can keep the nightmares (or monsters) away from the room. You could have the child draw a time when he or she felt out of control, then recount what happened before, during, and after this experience, emphasizing factors that help him or her feel more in control.

With clients who are able to "come out of the metaphor" to have a conversation about the relationship between the story and events outside the playroom, you can have a discussion about ways they can actually introduce the idea of roping and corralling the night mares as part of their dreams . . . sometimes you can actually teach them to preload a dream, using self-talk to suggest that they are going to have a positive dream before it is time to go to sleep.

Here are some questions you could ask children who like to verbally process when you are done telling the story:

> "How do you think the night mares felt when they were running wild and sometimes hurting others and sometimes hurting themselves?"
>
> "What do you suppose they were thinking as they were running wild?"
>
> "How do you think the other characters felt when the night mares were running wild?"
>
> "What do you suppose the other characters were thinking about the night mares when the night mares were running wild and scaring them?"
>
> "What are some ways that the night mares could have calmed themselves down?"
>
> "What are some ways the other characters could have helped the night mares calm down?"

Inner Knowing

This technique invites clients (any age, any grouping) to trust their "inner knowing" using photographs of people cut from magazines. The primary goal of this activity would be to help clients practice recognizing and accurately interpreting social information and realistically assess the characteristics of others. You could also use it to help clients practice self-scaffolding, taking safe interpersonal risks, accepting responsibility in interpersonal interactions, sharing power with others, actively listening to others, cooperating with others, considering the emotional and cognitive perspective of others, and optimistically reframing situations and experiences.

In order to make this activity work, you will need to develop a collection of photographs cut from magazines. The photographs should feature people—together, alone, in groups, facing one another, with their backs turned to one another, talking, laughing, arguing, fighting, and so on. You need a variety of different pictures of feelings, relationships, and situations. Have the client choose one of the photographs (either at random or after perusing them) and develop a story (with a beginning, middle, and an end—you knew we were going to say that) about the photograph. It is often helpful to start them off by asking some questions (yes, we are scaffolding the storytelling) about who the people are and what their relationship is, what happened before the photograph was taken, what is happening at the moment the photograph was taken, what happened after the photograph was taken, what the people are saying to one another, and so forth. You can even invite clients to take several photographs and put them in some order and develop a story with several chapters. If you have a client who does not feel comfortable with people, you can even have them do the same activity with the photographs of animal groupings you used for the animal phototherapy.

Metaphor Shifting

All people, whether they are young or old, speak and think in metaphors. As Lakoff and Johnson (2003) suggested, metaphors actually structure our perceptions and understanding. For instance, when you are working with an underachieving student who thinks of himself as a sloth, this way of thinking about himself gives him an excuse for the choices he makes and the way he lives his life. He does not have to put out a lot of effort because, after all, sloths move slowly and avoid doing much of anything. If you are working with a family whose members describe the identified client as a tornado, you will know (basically) how the members of the family perceive that child and (even if you are the most amazingly objective person who is not easily influenced by the thoughts of others) you will probably begin to consider the possibility that the child has out-of-control behavior problems or has ADHD.

   Metaphor shifting is a way of reframing something for clients using symbolic language to shift how they think and feel about specific people, relationships, or circumstances. During the exploration phase, listening to clients' metaphors for themselves can help you understand their intrapersonal dynamics and listening to their metaphors for other people can help you discover their interpersonal dynamics. Pointing out the meaning of their metaphors can help them increase their awareness during the insight phase. During the making changes phase, if you can help clients shift their metaphors, many times you can assist them in modifying their thinking patterns from pessimistic, self-defeating patterns into more optimistic thoughts and attitudes; you can also help them move from negative self-talk to more positive self-talk; and you can help them alter many of their dysfunctional interactional patterns. This is a relatively sophisticated intervention, so you need to make sure you are paying attention to the client's developmental level. Because it takes abstract verbal reasoning skills that children don't usually develop until they are about 12 years old, it is a technique you would usually use with parents about their children, themselves as parents, or their family or with preteen, teen, and adult play therapy clients.

Part of what you do to help clients shift their metaphors is listen to the metaphoric ways they describe themselves, others, and their situations and relationships. As you listen, you consider which metaphors are helpful to clients (e.g., "My son is a gem." "My car flies like a jet plane." "My life is like a journey—sometimes smooth and sometimes rough.") and which are a hindrance (e.g., "My daughter is the devil's spawn." "Our family is like a zoo where all the animals escaped." "My teacher is a witch."). After you have figured out which metaphors might be undermining a positive attitude or the ability to make necessary changes, the next step is to help clients to explore other possible metaphors for the same person, situation, or relationship. So, instead of "My daughter is the devil's spawn," you could help the client consider other metaphors like "a roller coaster," "a carnival ride," or even "a fun challenge I can master." For "like a zoo where all the animals escaped" you could suggest "circus act with those cool performing dogs," "penguins playing on an ice flow," or "otters frolicking in a stream."

Dance/Movement/Music

Walk Like an Egyptian

This activity was the result of my (Terry) having several clients who had difficulty with social interactions—they just could not make and keep friends, which was very frustrating to me because they were (mostly) likeable kids. (Well, at least I liked them.) They were also kinesthetic-tactile learners, so just having conversations about how you make friends or doing puppet shows about how friends are made was not helping to change anything. You can use variations of this technique with any age and with individual clients, groups, and families. Depending on how you set it up, you can use it to work toward many different goals, including "owning" personal assets, making a connection between emotions and the body, being more willing to take responsibility, self-scaffolding, improving social skills, and gaining self-confidence and an increased sense of self-efficacy.

When I was working with some kids who were less confident and were starting to feel defeated, I decided I wanted them to consider how the "popular" kids in the sixth grade moved through the hallways at school, so I asked them if they would be willing to observe that rare breed in the wild (or at least in the elementary school). As I explained that I thought the popular kids moved through the hallways differently than the not-so-popular kids, it looked as though a light bulb lit up over the heads of my clients. The following week, they were incredibly eager to show me (with their entire bodies) how the popular kids move through the hallways. When I wondered (out loud—okay, sometimes I am a bit manipulative) whether someone who was not particularly popular would get a bump in popularity if he or she moved through the hallways like the popular kids did, I got several volunteers. And, lo and behold, the popularity polls of the kids who were willing to try moving differently through the halls went up—a lot, actually. The feedback from the students who tried it was that when they moved in a "popular kid way," other people responded more positively to them. So, I decided to expand this technique with a whole bunch of variations—I have my clients walk like successful bankers, like teens other people want to date, like students who are going to make an A on their spelling test, like women who are going to figure out ways to make their marriage work, like athletes who are going to win the MVP trophy for football, and so forth and so forth and so forth. If I have one technique that has made the biggest bang for my buck, it is this one, which has changed the lives of children, adolescents, and adults in many positive ways.

Being-With Dances

There are times when clients just need to allow themselves to "be with" certain feelings or memories. This happens when it is important for a client to actually experience certain feelings instead of pushing them away or ignoring them. By slowing down enough to let the feeling in and making room for the feeling to come into consciousness, the client can actually feel and explore the emotion. Sometimes this leads to letting go of the resistance and accepting the feeling when it arises, which can actually help clients eventually get through those feelings and out the other side. One of the best ways we have found to be helpful in this process of recognizing and accepting emotions is a being-with dance. This technique works better with older elementary, adolescent, and adult clients because the idea of "being with" is pretty abstract. If you have a family or group with members who are able to be uninhibited with one another, you can certainly do this in that setting; in our experience, this technique seems to work better with individual clients. The primary goal of this technique is to help clients get through specific feelings, like anger, sadness, depression, and grief. You can also use it to help clients become more aware of their feelings and of the emotion–body connection, learn to recognize multiple feelings about the same issue or relationship, and practice dealing with stress and frustration in healthier ways.

To introduce a being-with dance to clients, first you would ask them to just sit, paying attention to their bodies—maybe even inviting them to do a body scan. As they get more centered and grounded in their bodies, you would invite them to make room for the feeling they have been resisting or holding against. When they are ready, you can suggest that they get up and move with that emotion, however that feels in their body. You will want to stress that this is not a releasing dance; rather, it is a being-with dance. With younger children, you would use fewer words and be less formal in your instructions. You would just ask them if they are willing to let the uncomfortable feeling they are having come in, and if they are, just have them move with the feeling. For clients who are willing to verbally process, you could ask them to name the feelings they were choosing to "be with," where in their bodies they felt certain feelings, and how it felt to move with the feelings instead of against them. You could even use some kind of a scaling to ask them how comfortable they were with the particular feeling they were experiencing before and after the dance.

Releasing Dances

Releasing dances are designed for helping clients to release something. (Remember—we made up these names.) Releasing dances usually come after being-with dances, but they can just be stand-alone if that works better with particular clients. Again, these dances work best with older elementary, adolescent, and adult clients because the underlying concept is not really concrete enough for most younger elementary or preschool clients. However, you can also just do this technique with younger clients without explaining the premise. We actually have done this with families and groups—with folks who are very comfortable with one another, and we usually do it with individual clients in order to avoid having self-consciousness get in the way of them releasing the feelings they need to release. Clients can use release dances to let go of feelings that are difficult for them (anger, frustration, grief); to release painful memories; to release old patterns that are no longer serving them; to release relationships they no longer have; or to release attitudes that cause them interpersonal problems. (We know—all of these are not on our list of goals, and sometimes you just have to change things up and not follow the rules—especially if you are the ones who made the rules up. If you recognize something else clients need to release, don't limit yourself to this list of potential "releasings." Again, use your best clinical intuition and give yourself permission to be creative.)

Introducing a releasing dance is pretty easy. Have clients imagine the thing they want to release in expanded sensory detail—how big it is, what color it is, what texture it is, what sounds it makes, how it moves, and so on. Then ask them to figure out how they could let go of it with a movement or dance and then tell them to move in the way they imagined to let go of whatever it is they want to let go of. (Sometimes we just skip the figuring out step and ask them to move in ways that release whatever they want to release. With some clients who are doers and not thinkers, this works much better than asking them to figure anything out—just moving works better.) This technique is great with children who are habitually angry, it encourages them to develop a "releasing that anger" dance or movement that they can use at home, in their neighborhood, or in their classroom. (You usually need to pre-warn the parents and teachers [and maybe even other family members and classmates] before you invite clients to "unleash" their releasing in public.)

Celebrating Dances

One thing that often gets neglected in therapy sessions (both talk and play) is celebration. We believe it is important to pay attention to the positive aspects of clients' lives as well as the problematic aspects. Hence, we have celebrating dances. We want to celebrate victories in clients' lives, clients' strengths, positive memories, and fun times. Suggesting these dances is pretty easy. You ask clients to stand up and dance their happiness, joy, pride, and the like, connected to whatever they want to celebrate. Sometimes clients don't recognize occasions that deserve celebration, so you might have to suggest that certain things are worth celebrating—things like a whole week without getting sent to the principal's office, resisting the temptation to check on Facebook for the ex-boyfriend's status, being a helpful friend, and so forth. You can do these dances with any client in any setting—just make it fun. This is also a great homework assignment for families as a way to help them put positive energy in their positive energy bank as often as possible.

Invoking Dances

Invoking dances (we want to acknowledge that our naming of the types of dances we do is not particularly imaginative) are designed to invoke a feeling, a memory, or the energy of a particular person or relationship. They are meant to help clients connect either to a specific feeling or to a time or person outside the session to help inspire them. They can be useful in helping clients consider "owning" their assets; shifting into more positive, optimistic thinking patterns; recognizing the feelings of others; taking the emotional and cognitive perspective of others, recognizing their own needs, and getting through and out of "negative" emotions. This particular type of movement is usually more appropriate for teens or adults in play therapy rather than for young children because the idea of "invoking" may be a little abstract for younger elementary students. If, however, you ask a young child to dance the way a person who believed in them would want them to dance, they might be able to understand what you mean. (Go ahead—take a chance. What's the worst thing that could happen if it doesn't work?)

To set up an invoking dance, you would ask clients to think of a particular emotion they want to feel, a time in the past that was positive, or a person who inspires them. If they have a particular emotion they want to feel or a time in the past that was positive, you would ask them to move like they imagine that emotion feels or the way they remember moving in the memory. If they want to invoke a person, they would move the way they imagine the inspiring person moves/moved or how they feel when they think about that person. An example from my (Terry's) life would be that, if I am particularly nervous getting ready to present at a conference, I tell myself to move like Cher, one of my heroes. I also often do a Tank Girl dance if I am feeling particularly anxious, based on the energy of a character played by Lori Petty in the movie *Tank Girl*. You could ask a client who was having difficulty trusting others to do an invoking dance to bring in the energy of his beloved grandmother who had passed away and can still inspire him to trust other people. Or with a client who is preparing to take an exam designed to get her into graduate school, you could ask her to move the same way she remembers moving right before passing her last final in college. Notice in these examples that sometimes you ask clients to move the way they remember moving at a specific time in their lives; sometimes you ask them to move the way a particular person moves; sometimes you ask them to move how they feel when they think about that person; and other times you ask them to move to the "energy" of a time or person. Even if they don't know how a particular person moves or remember how they moved in their memory, they can just make it up (if they are willing—some are and some aren't).

Practicing Dances

We use practicing dances to help clients to practice new behaviors and attitudes. They can be substituted in the place you would usually use role-playing with clients who are more body-oriented than word-oriented. This is one of those techniques that can be used to forward any number of therapeutic goals. You just have to use the "setup" (and any processing) to aim clients in the direction of the goal you want them to achieve. Our favorites involve the goals listed under the Interacting–Increase category.

Practicing dances are basically role-playing without words. You invite clients to move the way they would move if they were actually doing the new behavior or displaying the new attitude they want to adopt. For example, if you have Monica, a 6-year-old who is learning to walk away from an antagonistic person, rather than engaging in a fist fight, you would have her practice simply turning around and walking away. If you have Demetrius, a teen who wants to try out being more positive about school and school work, you would have him show you how he moves when he is being negative about school and then move like he would move if he was being more positive. (You would probably want to have him practice the positive version repeatedly since you don't really want him to lock into that negativity. [We both have had teenage children, so we are pretty vehement about that.]) With Cloe, a fifth grader who has a tendency to be a pleaser, you would have her do a "no-No-NO dance," getting louder and louder in her articulation of the word "no," accompanied by whole body gestures. With Chase, who wants to learn how to ask someone out on a date, you could have him practice how to physically approach the person he wants to ask out in an open and inviting way. (Based on the examples, you have probably already figured out that this is a strategy that works well with all ages.)

Sand Tray Activities

Problem-centered trays for clients to do

1. Tray about what it would take for the client to solve a problem (could be a specific problem or a generic problem)
2. Tray exploring potential alternative behaviors to replace a behavior that is causing difficulties
3. Tray showing how to solve a problem or resolve a conflict framed by the play therapist as a "consultation" with another client who has a similar problem
4. Tray on different strategies people use for solving problems
5. Tray on how client wishes the other people in his or her life would resolve conflicts
6. Tray on how client thinks someone else perceives a problem
7. Tray on how client thinks someone else feels about a problem
8. Tray on how the client wishes he or she would resolve interpersonal conflicts

Therapist sets up trays for demonstrating specific skills for client

1. Tray demonstrating problem solving or conflict resolution strategies
2. Trays to model demonstrating specific relationship skills, communication skills, anger management skills, assertiveness skills, negotiating skills, and so on

Therapist and client collaborate on trays so client can practice new behaviors

1. You set up a specific situation in a tray (e.g., a conflict, a situation that would invoke frustration or anxiety in the client, a situation

in which the client would need to set a boundary or be assertive, a situation in which the client would need to negotiate with someone else, a situation in which the client would need to apologize, etc.). The client adds other figures and proceeds to use them to practice the set of skills needed in the situation the play therapy has built in the sand tray.

Art Techniques

Mood Dude Drawings

Have you ever seen those small figures called Emotes (which seem almost impossible to find anywhere—trust us, we have looked, searching the Internet for a new source) or those stress ball heads called Mood Dudes? While you can use those figures for lots of different things, we have a drawing technique that uses them. You can also use sand tray figures for this activity if you have some sand tray figures that look like they are in the throes of strong emotions. We have used this technique with children, teens, and adults; individual clients, groups, and families. The primary goal is increasing awareness of feelings and acquiring and practicing skills for appropriately expressing feelings. Depending on how you explain the directive, you could also use it to increase feeling vocabulary, getting through strong emotions without getting stuck, learning to recognize the feelings of others, increasing frustration tolerance, learning to deal appropriately with frustration and anger, setting appropriate boundaries, developing assertiveness skills, and learning to be encouraging to others. If you emphasized cognitive patterns, you could also use it to help clients recognize discouraged self-talk and shift to more positive self-talk. Here's what you would need: sheets of paper (we like to use 12″ × 18″, but you can use smaller sheets if you wish), drawing materials, and either Emotes plastic figures, Mood Dude stress heads, or emotionally expressive sand tray figures. Invite the client to place the figure (or head) somewhere on the paper. Then tell the client something like, "This paper is the world where that figure lives" (or works, goes to school, hangs out—you get the idea). Invite the client to use the drawing material to make the world that surrounds him/her/it. Say, "As you draw, be sure you illustrate what is happening in that world (work, school, neighborhood, or planet) that would lead to the figure's feelings we can see." (Keep in mind that you can focus on attitudes, thoughts, or behaviors instead of emotions when you give the directive.) After the client has finished the drawing, ask him or her to tell a story about the figure and what happened before, during, and after the pose the figure is in for the drawing. You can ask the client to flesh out self-talk, feelings, coping strategies, and so on—either in the story or in the drawing.

Safety Shields

This activity is designed to give children tools for dealing with stress and setting personal boundaries. You could also use it to help child clients practice accepting responsibility in interpersonal interactions, recognizing and appropriately asking for personal needs to be met, realistically assessing the characteristics of other people, developing assertiveness skills, and assessing interpersonal risks, as well as skills for keeping themselves safe and protected. It is pretty basic, so it probably won't work well with most adolescents and adults; however, with lower functioning older clients, it might be useful. We have used it with families and groups as well as individual client sessions.

For this activity, you need a package of 12″ × 18″ thin foam sheets you can buy at a craft store and a collection of Sharpie pens of assorted colors. The first step is for clients to draw a shield on the foam sheet that takes up the entire sheet and cut it out. Then you would help them brainstorm actions that can keep them safe, thoughts that help them feel safe, people who can help them stay protected, things they need to say to themselves or to other people to ensure safety, and anything else that they can use to make sure they are "shielded." Then they would draw pictures or write words on the shield to remind them that they have many tools for keeping themselves safe. For clients who like processing, you could have a follow-up conversation about how they can bring the ideas they illustrated on their safety shield into practice in their lives outside of the playroom.

Map around _____

This is another art technique focused on recognition and coping strategies for any pattern that is contributing to clients' distress. You can do it about specific feelings (e.g., fear, anxiety, depression) and emotional, cognitive, or behavioral patterns—whatever is contributing to the clients' difficulties. We have used it with a wide range of ages and play therapy settings. For older clients, you would elaborate more on the extraneous details of the drawing before you ask them to start developing a path to get through and/or around their problem. Because it is a flexible technique, it can help your clients move toward a plethora of goals, including awareness of specific feelings, getting through and out of anger, sadness, and depression, recognizing the feelings of others. If you wanted to help your clients work on changing thinking patterns, you could set this activity up to help them recognize self-defeating self-talk and substitute positive self-talk, optimistically reframing situations and experiences, recognizing their own needs, and enhancing problem-solving skills.

The materials you need for this activity are paper and drawing materials. The first thing you have clients do is draw whatever problem they are having—be it an emotion, a cognitive pattern, an attitude, a relationship, or the like. Then have them describe the issue for you. After they have described the issue, suggest that they need to add a couple of other features to the page—a "swamp" area surrounding the problem that they could be sucked into, the place where they are starting on their journey, and the destination—where they want to go with their lives. Next invite them to devise a "map" that can take them around the issue—remind them that they can add people who can help them; coping strategies; shifts in thinking, feeling, behaving; resources; and so forth—whatever it would take to get them from where they are to where they want to go without getting stuck in the "problem swamp." As they draw, you can ask them questions about their process, or you can just be silent—depending on what works best for the particular client. You can also provide scaffolding for the drawing process, with suggestions about ways to incorporate changes in their journey. This is one of those activities that lends itself to staying in the metaphor of the journey and the map for clients who prefer the distance provided by a metaphor. Alternatively, you can help clients to determine ways they can bring what they have drawn into reality in their lives outside of sessions.

Energy Drawings

This might be a little "woo-woo" for some of your clients, but for the ones who like these kinds of things, it can be very helpful. The primary thing we use it for is helping clients learn to assess the characteristics of others, and we tend to use it with older elementary children, adolescents, and adults because the idea of different people having "energy" that you can draw is a bit abstract. We have used it with families with older kids and in groups of teens as well as with individual clients. If you "aim" your clients properly with your directive, you can also use it for helping them learn to assess interpersonal boundaries and set boundaries.

This is another drawing technique, so you need paper and drawing materials. (You can also do it as a painting if you have clients who prefer that medium.) Part of deciding how to go about doing this activity is to determine who it is clients want to examine for the types of energy they have and the impact of their energy on the client or the clients' energy. If your clients feel comfortable drawing human figures, you can ask them to draw people's body outlines; if they are not confident in their representational artistic abilities, you can have them use gingerbread people or even circles or squares to represent a person's body. Then, surrounding the body they have drawn (in whatever form), suggest that they use colors, textures, and shapes to depict that person's "energy." When they have finished the drawing and processing whatever they want to process verbally, you can further expand the activity by asking them to also draw themselves on the same page, draw their own energy, and draw the energy that exists between themselves and the other person. You can also ask them to draw someone else who is in a relationship with the first person as the second person on the page. After they have finished, if they are inclined to talk about what they have drawn, you can ask them what they have observed about the first person they drew that gives them the sense of that person's energy, what they have observed about the second person that gives them a sense of that person's energy, and what they have observed about their interactions that gives them a sense of the interactive energy between the two of them. You can also have them draw barriers or boundaries between the two people if the interactional energy is difficult for them. You can have them draw speech or thought bubbles over the figures to indicate things each of them say or think. If you are doing the activity as part of a group or family session, you can have the members draw a figure for each participant, for the interaction between the various members, and the energy for the group or family as a whole.

Problem Pass-Around

Like many of the techniques in this chapter, problem pass-around is one of those activities that you can use for a variety of different goals, depending on how you explain it to clients and how (if) you process it. Just as the name of the technique would imply, the usual goal is to help clients improve their problem-solving skills and cultivate the willingness to follow through with possible solutions to problems. It can also be used to enhance self-scaffolding, skills involved in learning to "reset" after a problem occurs, recognition of needs, skills required to optimistically reframe experiences, and proficiencies in taking the cognitive perspectives of others into account. We usually do it in groups or family sessions, and you can adapt the technique for working with individual clients. It is a technique that works best with clients 10 years of age and older. It is especially helpful in groups with teen clients, who think they are the only ones who experience difficulties and who tend to be more willing to listen to peers than adults.

In a group or family, each member needs a piece of paper and some drawing materials. To start, invite everyone to draw a problem they are having—we like to begin with a relatively simple difficulty that they are currently experiencing to give clients the idea of how this technique can work. Tell them that you are not going to give them a super-long time to sketch the difficulty and that they should not get too attached to their art work. Give them about 5 minutes to draw the problem, and then go around in a circle and ask each member to describe his or her difficulty. When everyone has explained, ask the members to pass their drawings around the circle so that everyone in the group (or family) can draw a "potential solution" to everyone else's problems. By the time each member's drawing comes back to the original artist, he or she should have a suggestion for a possible way to resolve the difficulty from every other member. Ask all of the members to take turns, holding up their drawing and giving a brief summary of their problem, followed by the other members explaining their proposals for a potential solution one at a time. When everyone has finished hearing all of the possible solutions, you can (if you think this would be helpful) ask each member to commit to following through with one of the proposals, either in the form that it was proposed or modified in some way.

If you are using this technique one-on-one with a client, you can still do it—you just need to be willing to self-disclose enough to draw a problem while the client is drawing a problem. Then you pass the drawings back and forth, drawing a potential solution each time; you draw one for the client while the client is drawing one for you, and then you draw one for your own problem while the client draws one for his or her own problem. We usually do this process three or four times so that each of you wind up with six or eight potential solutions—some generated by you and some generated by the client.

You can also do the technique with sand trays or as a sticker picture rather than as a drawing if that would work better for the particular client. To do either of those, have each client choose several sand tray figures (or stickers) to represent the problem; then the other members can use sand tray figures (or stickers) to represent potential solutions.

Insecurity/Security Blankets

When my (Terry's) son, Jacob, was in elementary school, I spent quite a bit of time at the school, fighting the good fight to get him the special education services he needed. I felt particularly unskilled in these battles, and one day, in my discouragement, I wrapped myself in a fleece blanket I had bought on the Internet. The blanket had things like "Do I smell, or is it this blanket?" "Am I too rude to telemarketers?"—it was billed as an "insecurity blanket." My friend, Andrea Christopher, the school counselor, suggested that we make similar blankets for all the sixth-grade students, who were feeling very nervous about going to junior high. This was the birth of this activity—I took Andrea's original idea and ran with it. So, the goal of this activity is to help clients examine their negative self-talk and pessimistic thinking and come up with ways to substitute positive self-talk and optimistic thinking. It can also help clients practice "owning" their own assets and cultivate positive feelings toward themselves, enhance their self-confidence, and increase their sense of self-efficacy. We have used it with all ages and with individual clients, groups, and families. It has spawned a multitude of variations—and now, (hopefully) it can inspire you to generate some of your own.

It does have very specific materials you need (though, in reality, you can even modify them if you choose not to purchase the materials we use): two lengths of fleece material that are different colors and several dark-colored Sharpie pens. To decide on the length of the fleece material you need, remember that you are making "blankets," so you want it to be long enough that your clients, whatever size they are, can wrap themselves in either of the blankets. (Here's a tip we learned to save a bit of money: you can buy fleece material in the spring when it goes on sale and then cut each piece lengthwise, so that every piece of fleece you buy makes two different blankets.)

Ask your clients to choose two different colors of fleece, making sure the length is sufficient for wrapping around them. Then make a list of things they ask themselves when they are feeling down or insecure—things like, "Will anyone ever ask me on a date?" "Will I ever pass second grade?" "Does my family really like me?" "Am I a good enough wife?" "Why can't I learn to read when everyone else has?" "Why did my dad leave me?" "Does my boss even think I am good at my job?" "Will I graduate from high school or am I stuck here forever?" (We usually go for about ten to twelve questions that represent negative self-talk and self-doubts; if you have spectacularly negative clients, you can even go up to fifteen or twenty if they write small.) Next, to create the insecurity blanket, ask clients to write those questions with the Sharpies on one of the fleece pieces (or draw things that represent those doubts if they can't write or you can write them for them while they make little pictures). (The other important "safety" tip is to watch out so that the Sharpie writing doesn't get smeared—there is nothing worse than a smudged insecurity blanket.) When they are finished writing their questions all over the insecurity blanket, ask them to make a list (either writing it or dictating it to you) of the things they tell themselves when they are feeling positive, optimistic, self-confident, and self-assured. This list can include things like "I am lovely." "I know that I am a good dad." "I am learning to read at my own pace." "Of course, my book will get written." "My mother loved me—she just wasn't great at showing it." Then (I bet you're already on top of what happens next), tell them to take the other piece of fleece and use the Sharpies to create a security blanket. What is lovely is that sometimes your clients will even say something like "Oh—I get it! I can choose whether to wrap myself in my insecurities or I can let go of them and wrap myself in my securities." (Okay, we admit it doesn't happen that often, and it has actually happened to us—it can happen to you.)

Fairy Godparents/Guardian Angels

When I (Terry) taught special education, there was a child in my school (not in my class) who had experienced a multitude of traumatic events. He was in fourth grade and had been in six different foster care placements—having had to switch foster homes a number of times due to circumstances beyond anyone's control. He seldom made eye contact, never smiled, and his teacher reported that he felt like he couldn't count on anyone caring about him. I remember thinking, "That little boy needs a fairy godparent or guardian angel to protect him and help him feel like somebody really cares about him." I originally developed this technique for him—I made him a fairy godparent and watched his face as his teacher gave it to him. He looked at the fairy, and his face lit up with the biggest smile I had ever observed on his face. Afterward, I kind of wished that I had talked to him about whether he would have preferred a guardian angel or a fairy godparent and that I had engaged him in making it, rather than making it for him. So . . . that is what we do now. Depending on what you want to accomplish, this technique would work with a variety of different kinds of clients. It seems especially effective with clients who do not believe that they count and believe that they cannot get their needs met. You could use this activity to convey the notion that clients "count"—they are important and significant, without having to earn affection or belonging. In this case, the function of the guardian angel/fairy godparent would be for them to always provide someone (besides you) in their lives who cares about them. It would also be helpful in helping to give clients someone (basically a physical imaginary friend) with whom they can connect—someone to confide in who will not have any expectations of them. Sometimes we use the fairy godparent/guardian angel as a transitional object to represent us in settings outside our offices. We also like to use this activity to help clients explore what it is that they need and how to get their needs met and/or help clients to prioritize their current needs. The "need" could be framed in a situation-specific way, depending on their circumstances; for instance, the need could be connected to what they need to feel safe, what they need to have fun, what they need to feel like they belong, and so on. We have used this technique with every age group, from very young children to very elderly clients, in groups and with individual clients. Sometimes if we want to do it with families and want to build in practice in cooperation and negotiation skills, we have them make a family fairy godparent or guardian angel, and other times, we have everyone make one of their own. (It, of course, depends.)

This is another activity that requires some specific materials: wooden clothespins (the old-fashioned kind that are one piece, with no metal) and pipe cleaners (a.k.a. chenille stems). It can also be helpful to have permanent markers, paints, feathers, yarn, and other craft materials, depending on how elaborate you want to be with the creation.

Before you start the activity, you will need to decide the purpose of this particular fairy/angel. When you explain the activity to the client, you will "pitch" it differently according to your purpose with this particular client (whether it is for conveying to clients that there is always someone with them/in their lives who cares about them, whether it is a transitional object for them, whether it is designed to help them think about their needs and getting them met, etc.). Next, it is helpful to determine which would work better for particular clients—a fairy godparent or a guardian angel. This may depend on clients' spiritual beliefs, their willingness to be whimsical, your practice setting, and so on. Sometimes you will already have a clear idea of what would be most appropriate, and sometimes it would be better to have a conversation with clients about their preferences. After it has been decided whether to have a guardian angel or a fairy godparent, it can also be important to have a discussion about whether to have the creation be a man or woman, a boy or girl. (This will vary from client to client.) Then, especially if you are targeting clients getting their needs met, you could decide to help them generate a list of their needs, followed by a brainstorming process to decide what powers the fairy/angel would need if he or she were going to help them get those needs met.

Now to get started (finally!), have the client take the clothes pin and decorate it with paint or marker if so desired. It can be painted or colored one color or multiple colors; the client can draw a face on it or leave the face blank. If the client wants wings, he or she will bend the pipe cleaners into the shape of wings—the wings can use one pipe cleaner or two. By twisting the pipe cleaner around the clothes pin, the client can attach the wings to the body of the fairy/angel. Other decorations (like yarn, feathers, and beads) can be added to enhance the looks of the creation. If desired, the client can name the angel/fairy, make a list of the powers wielded by the angel/fairy, generate a list of encouraging things the fairy/angel might say, and so on. With clients who like to process verbally, you can ask questions such as:

"What did you name your fairy godparent/guardian angel?"
"How did you decide on his or her name?"
"How did you decide whether you would rather have a guardian angel or a fairy godparent?"
"What powers would you want your guardian angel/fairy godparent to have?"
"How did you decide whether you wanted a man/woman/boy/girl?"
"What do you think you are going to get out of having a guardian angel/fairy godparent?"
"What kinds of things do you want your guardian angel/fairy godparent to say to you?"
"How did you decide what needs you would like to ask your angel/fairy to help you get met?"
"How will the angel/fairy's powers help you get those needs met?"

"How can you get your own needs met if there are some needs the fairy/angel can't affect?"

"Have you ever had another adult who helped you in the same way you might be helped by your guardian angel/fairy godparent? Who were they? How did they help you?"

"Have you ever acted like a guardian angel/fairy godparent for someone else?"

"Who were they? How did you help them?"

"If you had three wishes, what would you ask for?"

Foot-in-the-Mouth Faces

I (Terry) learned this technique in art class when I was in junior high. We love using it with clients who need to work on the social skill of gracefully apologizing, and could use help with taking responsibility for their own behavior. It is also helpful for practice in taking someone else's emotional (and maybe even cognitive) perspective. We don't know that it would work well with adults (I haven't actually tried it with adults), but it does work with adolescents who have a sense of humor about themselves and with younger children. We have done it with individual clients, in groups, and with families. It's one of those simple things to do that gains impact with verbal processing.

Start by instructing clients to take off their shoes and trace around one of their feet on a large piece of paper; then ask them to draw a face around the foot tracing, making the foot into the mouth of the face they draw. (Keep in mind the size of their feet when choosing the size of the paper—clients with long feet need a *big* piece of paper.) Next, have them make a speech bubble and write something they have said that might have hurt someone else's feelings. Then you could either have them make another speech bubble and write what they could say to apologize, or you could just engage them in brainstorming several different possible ways to phrase the apology, even going so far as role-playing an apology. (If you are working with a younger child who doesn't know how to write yet, dictating to you would also work, and you could write in the bubble or you can just let them talk about what they said and how they make amends.)

Love Language Drawings

Chapman (1992, 2000) and Chapman and Campbell (1997) posited that sometimes disconnections in relationships occur when people are speaking different "languages" to express love and caring for one another. The main idea, in all of Chapman's books, is that there are five ways love can be expressed and received: physical touch, acts of service, words of recognition, quality time, and gifts. Chapman actually has assessment tools that clients can use to determine the hierarchical order of how they prefer affection to be communicated to them, and lots of clients like filling them out. We tend to believe that the more fluent people are in every language of love, the better the world will be. We often use drawings to explore clients' love languages as a vehicle for working with them on asking for their needs to be met. Clients of every age seem responsive to this activity, even younger children, who do not really understand the underlying concept of the languages of love. We usually do it in individual sessions and with families.

Here's how you set it up. Give clients a big (12″ × 18″) sheet of paper, have them divide it into five sections, explain that different people show their love and caring in different ways called love languages, and ask them to label each section with a different language. (With clients who can't write, you can have them draw a symbol at the top of each section to represent the languages.) Then have them draw the things they like getting in each of the categories. (We usually give them examples, so I [Terry] would say, "Under Physical Touch, I would draw hugs and holding hands; under Acts of Service, I would draw washing my car and emptying the dishwasher; under Quality Time, I would draw doing puzzles together and going on walks; under Words of Recognition, I would draw speech bubbles that say 'I like your hair' and 'You inspire me'; and under Gifts, I would draw bracelets and earrings.") The drawings give clients something concrete to discuss with the other people in their lives when they want to practice asking to have their needs met.

You can also do this as a sand tray—it's the same kind of thing, just divide the tray into five sections and put a couple of things in each section—or you can do it as lists. This is something we often do with families. We give them the homework assignment to take a sheet of paper for each member of the family and come up with five different lists with about eight or ten items on each list of things the other members of the family could do that they would accept as being loving.

Structured Play Experiences

Gremlin/Evil Twin Puppets

Gremlin/evil twin puppets are a great way to work on getting rid of negative self-talk and pessimistic thinking. You can also use the variation (the "best self" puppet) to practice shifting to positive self-talk and optimistic thinking, as well as cultivating more positive feelings about self. We have done them with every age group and every configuration of play therapy. It might seem silly to ask adults to make paper bag puppets, but most of them seem to be willing.

It's a pretty simple procedure. You give clients a brown paper lunch bag and tell them they are going to make a puppet that represents their gremlin (or their evil twin)—that voices all of the things they don't like about themselves and all the negative ideas that occasionally float through their heads. Clients can use crayons or markers to draw a face (an "evil face") on the paper bag, using the bottom flap as the place where the mouth can open and close. Then have clients make a list (either in their minds, on a piece of paper, or on the body of the puppet) of all of their negative self-talk and their negative, pessimistic thoughts about self, others, and the world. Then ask them to imagine the voice that the gremlin/ evil twin would use to say those things and have them put the puppet on and have the puppet recite the litany of negativity. Once they have done this (sometimes it takes several times to get it out of their systems), ask them if they are ready to silence that voice. If they aren't yet, let them know that is okay too, and they can just take the gremlin/evil twin home with them and keep it around until they are ready to let go of that negativity. If they are ready, help them brainstorm ways they could either silence or destroy the puppet (e.g., putting it through a shredder, stapling the mouth shut, gluing the mouth closed, blowing into it until it is filled with air and then popping it). Depending on whether they really are ready to let go of the negativity, invite them to go ahead and follow through with one (or more) of the silencing/destroying ideas. If they want to practice more positive self-talk and positive, optimistic thoughts, they can make a second puppet—the "best self" puppet, one that represents their best self, the self that is confident and has positive feelings toward self, others, and the world—and have it recite counterthoughts (positive self-talk and thoughts that counter those negative ones spouted by the gremlin/evil twin).

Pocket Pals

I (Terry) had a fifth-grade boy client who was hugely struggling with social skills. He really wanted to have friends, and, despite all of my concerted efforts to help him learn social skills, both of us were discouraged because he could recite what he should do in our sessions (and even role-play appropriate social skills for making and maintaining friends), but when it came to execution in his interaction with peers at school and in his neighborhood, he was tanking—and he was feeling more and more lonely and discouraged. I decided we should just make him a friend. One goal for using this technique with clients (and it works best with elementary school-age children) is helping them think about the qualities they want in a friend and what they bring to friendships. This will lend itself to giving children a chance to learn to assess the characteristics of self and others, help them consider appropriate and positive roles in their peer group, and accept responsibility in interpersonal interactions. We have done this with individual clients and with groups.

You will need at least one popsicle stick or tongue depressor for each client and a ball point pen or skinny markers. The first step in the activity is to brainstorm with the child characteristics of the kind of friend he or she would want. Come up with a list of four to six traits that the child feels are desirable in a friend (e.g., good listener, big heart). Help the child figure out how to represent each of the chosen traits with a small drawing or symbol (e.g., good listener might be a picture of ears, big heart might be a picture of a heart), and have the child draw the symbol on the popsicle stick with a ball point pen or skinny markers. Explain to the child that the Pocket Pal can be carried in his or her pocket and brought out if the child is feeling lonely or discouraged or needs encouragement or companionship. If this is an issue, you can discuss whether doing this in public might bring on teasing and whether it might be better to confine interactions with the Pocket Pal to when the child is alone or with trusted others.

With clients who are willing to process verbally, you can invite the child to make a list of his or her characteristics that would be desirable in a friend. If the child is being unrealistic in his or her self-assessment, you can provide feedback about how you see his or her characteristics and how they are played out in relationships. Have the child make another Pocket Pal for himself or herself, with symbolic small drawings representing the friendship characteristics he or she would have to offer in a relationship if he or she were to make a lot of friends (or even one or two close friends). If you want, it is fun to make one for yourself. For instance, you could make a Pocket Pal that represents you and the characteristics you think make you a good friend. If the child struggles with making one that represents him or her, you can make one for the child, featuring the characteristics you think might make him or her a good friend. If you made one for yourself, your Pocket Pal could interact with the child's Pocket Pal to practice friendship skills. This can lead into a conversation about whether he or she demonstrates those traits he or she desires in potential friends. If the client doesn't think that he or she has the qualities that make a good friend, you can have a conversation about what it would take to change his or her attitudes and/or behavior to be able to exhibit those traits. In order to help develop the ability to assess friendship potential in others, have the child think of several other children with whom he or she would like a relationship and have him or her make Pocket Pals for them. Using the Pocket Pals, with one of you playing the other children and one of you playing the client, you can role-play interactions with those children, In this way, you can help the child explore whether or not those children would want to be friends.

If the child likes the Pocket Pal process, he or she can design Pocket Pals for specific situations (e.g., a Pocket Pal that helps with math problems, a Pocket Pal that reminds the child he or she is amazing even when he or she does not meet expectations in a race). (This way, the client can develop a whole stable of virtual friends just in case the skills you are trying to teach don't generalize into real life.)

Worry Boards

This is a technique developed by Rebecca Dickinson (personal communication, January 2017) for working with clients who are overly anxious, with the goal of providing them with a strategy for learning to manage or reduce their anxiety and self-created stress. Another goal for this technique would be to help clients take more responsibility for their own thinking and behaving. You could use it to increase clients' willingness to act on/follow through with possible solutions to problems. It can be helpful for clients age 7 and up, and can easily be transferred from an activity done in a play therapy session to an activity continued as a homework assignment. Adolescent and adult clients could do this assignment by themselves, and child clients would need help from parents to do this activity at home between play therapy sessions. With families who have multiple members with elevated levels of worry and stress, this tool could even be adapted for the whole family.

To set up this intervention, you will need a medium-sized poster board, post-it notes, manila envelope, and markers. If clients are younger elementary education students, you will have to help with part of the setup of the activity or invite parents or teachers into the session to help with the creation of the board and the post-it notes; older children, teens, and adults can usually set things up themselves. The poster board needs to be divided into three columns, one column labeled "I can control," the second column "I have some control," and the third "I can't control." Invite clients to make a post-it note for each of their worries (e.g., wetting pants on the school bus, tests, having no one to play with, being caught in a tornado, getting fired, having to go to the prom without a date). Younger clients can draw a picture on the post-it note of each of the things that worries them; older clients can write a description of each worry on the post-it note.

When this process is completed, help your clients identify the section of the board on which each post-it goes. After all of the post-it notes have been distributed, as a way to help clients become better at coping with worry or stress, practice taking responsibility, and increase their willingness to act on possible solutions to problems, you can engage them in brainstorming possible ways to take more control of the situations labeled "I can control" and "I have some control" (like going to the bathroom before getting on the school bus to avoid having wetting accidents, studying for tests, asking someone to go with you to the prom instead of waiting for an invitation). You can even help clients set a limit for how many things they can worry about at any one time, noting that the board looks overwhelming with all the post-it notes on it. Next, ask them to label the manila envelope "Trash" and attach it to the bottom of the poster board. Invite clients to choose the items to remain on the board and the ones to put in the trash with the knowledge that if they choose to resume worrying about something that has been put in the trash, they can trade out the post-it notes as long as they do not exceed the limit on the board.

Obviously, with younger clients, parents (or teachers) are going to have to help with the brainstorming of possible ways to gain more control and the limiting of the number of worries in the foreground at any one time. If you have an entire family of worry warts, they can all participate in this activity—either with a large family Worry Board or with smaller, individual Worry Boards.

Mad Scientist

This is a technique I (Terry) developed for the 5–12 age range. In the past, we would have suggested that mostly boys are interested in this one, but lately girls have been too. It is one of those techniques that you can use for a wide range of goals, spanning from taking personal responsibility to taking turns and being a good sport, to cooperating with others, to asking for help, to learning and practicing the skills to keep out of fights and use self-control in social situations . . . (you get the idea). We have done it with individual clients, with groups, and even with families.

It involves a bit of a weird procedure for gathering materials. Go around your house and get some baking soda, some vinegar, some cornstarch, some old bath oils, some bubble bath, some bath crystals—whatever is leftover in your bathroom cabinet that didn't work or you no longer want. You will also need a very large mixing bowl, some water, and a big stirring spoon. Before your session, it will be helpful to use construction paper and tape to make fake labels for your ingredients. (What the labels say depends on what you want to use the technique for. If you want to work on self-control, for example, use the baking soda and vinegar, labeling them as "temper" and "trigger"; if you want to work on self-esteem, use the bath salts, some bubble bath, and bath crystals and label them something like "helpful deeds," "pats on the back," and "kind words"—you get the idea.) Then you are basically going to give your client permission to make a big mess, creating a "potion" and then (eventually) take responsibility and clean up the mess. (You could probably even work in some practice for apologizing if it is a *huge* mess.) Then, of course, later, if you want and they are willing, you can process.

We offer a caution. Be sure that the combination of the ingredients you choose does not create an unwanted or even dangerous effect. It's our understanding that most bathing and hygiene materials are safe and that sometimes baking soda or other cleaning materials mixed together can be dangerous. If you're looking for a big, safe, bang, try Coke and Mentos! But have a sink or lots of towels nearby.

Detangling Your Thoughts

Detangling Your Thoughts was developed by Melissa Wehr (personal communication, December 2016) to work with children with anxiety who needed help with thinking more clearly so that they could focus and attend to what was important. However, it can be adapted and useful with adolescent and adult clients as well. This activity works with clients who have anxiety, are quick thinkers, get stuck in thinking patterns, have a hard time focusing, or feel overwhelmed with intense or multiple thoughts. The goal of this activity is to identify the multiple thoughts happening simultaneously, to separate them, and to give them individual attention or put them aside.

You will need a piece of paper with different shapes on the opposite ends: circles on one end, squares on the other end, and so on. You can draw the shapes or use felt or construction paper cut-outs. Ask clients to pick a few different colors and draw squiggly lines from one shape to another shape, being sure that the lines crisscross each other on the page. You could also use precut pieces of yarn of different colors and have the client connect the shapes. Ask the client to give a feeling or thought to each of the different colors (e.g., red = I'm scared of the dark; blue = I don't like to go to my mom's house; yellow = I get nervous before spelling tests; green = my new boss is a jerk).

Ask the client to pick one of the thoughts or feelings and trace the line or feel the yarn as he or she thinks about the thought or feeling. Practice deep breathing or relaxation (pretaught) as the client thinks and traces or feels. If you're using yarn or a tangible medium, the client could literally untangle the thoughts as he or she is doing this. Repeat this with each color. If you choose to continue to process this activity, you can do so between the different thoughts or feelings, or you can do it all at the end. Some potential processing prompts could be about the corresponding colors the client chose with the thought or feeling, the client's visceral reactions to the exercise, and the client's ability to stay focused on one thought during the activity. You could ask the client about the ratio of negative to positive thoughts identified. We're always curious if the overwhelming thoughts are positive, negative, within or beyond the client's control, rational, or irrational, and so on. You could practice and/or discuss with the client how this could be applied in real-life settings such as before a big test, during a work meeting, or before meeting new people. For clients who tend to get stuck in negative thought patterns, you could ask them to switch negative thinking to positive thinking during their meditation. There are countless ways to incorporate or alter this activity that will meet a variety of clients' concerns.

Responsibility Pie

This activity started out as a way to work with children who do not take responsibility for their behavior. Over time, however, we discovered that lots of adolescent and adult clients have difficulty with that same behavior, so we have expanded it to those populations. Although it can work with groups and families, we usually like to start out doing it with individual clients, just because we find that, especially when people are not in the habit of taking responsibility for their behavior, they often react more defensively if they have an audience. (Once, again, learn from our mistakes.) We also feel a need to acknowledge that this technique is bordering on talk therapy in the playroom—it does involve a lot of words.

The first thing you need is a circle. We actually like doing this activity on a dry erase board because the divisions of the circle tend to shift as the conversation unfolds, but if you don't have access to a dry erase board, you can just draw a circle on a piece of paper and use a pencil with an eraser to draw the lines for the pie chart. Next, you need to ask your client to tell you about a recent conflict or disputed incident. As the client lists the cast of characters involved in the situation, you need to write the names down next to the circle; then you will want the client to tell you step by step what happened. When the client is finished with the story, ask him or her to think about who started things, who kept things going, who tried to resolve things, and so on. At the end of this discussion, invite the client to think about the proportions of responsibility he or she would assign to each participant—you want to make it clear that you are not looking to "blame" anyone, that you are just trying to help the client figure out what part of the responsibility for the situation goes to each of the participants. It is often helpful to use the skill of confrontation in this process if the client is trying to avoid taking any responsibility. As you talk, either you or the client will make a pie chart in the circle, with a person's name in each wedge, along with the part of the situation that person created or was responsible for. (We like having a dry erase board because, as the story unfolds and you and the client get clearer about the responsibility of each party, many times things change with the divisions drawn in the pie chart). The end result is a pie chart that shows who had responsibility for each part of what happened—including the client. You can then use the chart as a jumping off place for talking about how each person could have handled things differently and what the outcome would have been if they had. You can also discuss how the client can handle similar situations differently in the future.

Hula Hoops

This technique can be used for all sorts of explorations of how to use social skills in a variety of situations. The two primary goals are to help clients (usually children or teens, but every once in a while, an adult) experiment with personal space and with the setting of limits and boundaries. It is especially useful with clients with social skills deficit and/or ADHD. It is fun to do in groups and families, and it works with individual clients as well. You can even extend it to help clients keep out of fights and use self-control in social situations.

You will need at least two hula hoops (more if you are doing the activity with groups or families). Tell the client that the hula hoops are personal space boundaries and that the two of you can use the hoops to tell each of you how close you can get to someone else and have them remain comfortable with the closeness. The two of you can play with getting closer and having your hula hoops overlap, and talking about how you both feel when that happens. It is also interesting to have the client practice watching nonverbal communication about whether or not the two of you are too close or just right, even without the hula hoops. You can use the personal space boundaries as a way to practice conversing in socially appropriate ways, letting someone know that he or she is too close, becoming more aware of personal space, considering that getting too close can be considered to be an aggressive move by many people, and so forth.

Encouragement Missionary Work

This technique is a way to teach encouragement skills and give clients practice having positive experiences with connection. You can use it with all ages of clients, but for us it has been an easier "sell" for children than for adolescents and adults. In some ways, it is an experience that works better with a group or a family, and you can certainly use it with individual clients.

You will need a supply of small, flat wooden pieces. You can get them at craft stores in different shapes—circles, stars, hearts, squares, and triangles—about 1 inch to 1½ inch across. The only other material you need for this activity is a ballpoint pen for each participant. Work with clients to brainstorm positive things they like to hear or things they like to tell other people. We try for comments like "You rock!" "I care about you." "You are special." "You know how to do a lot of things." "You are a star." "You are fun." "You tell funny stories." It is helpful if you can steer them away from evaluative words (like great, good, pretty), and sometimes that is impossible. After they have come up with a list, invite them to write those comments on the small wooden shapes. When they have accumulated a stockpile of encouraging shapes, explain that one of the best ways to feel better about yourself is to help others feel better about themselves and they now have the tools to do just that. Help your clients come up with a list of people to whom they could give the "encouragement shapes" in order to help spread encouragement. They can give them to people they know or they can give them to total strangers—whichever feels safer for them.

Self-Soothers

Self-soothers really aren't exactly a technique or an activity—they are more like tools you can teach clients. Over the years, we have learned or developed a number of them, and we use them with all our clients. They can help clients deal with specific feelings, manage anxiety and stress, develop positive feelings about themselves, share power, win and lose gracefully, keep out of fights, and increase self-control.

Here is a list of the self-soothers we use—we know you have some too.

1. Rocking—either in a rocking chair or standing and shifting your weight from side to side on your feet.
2. Giving yourself a hug—wrapping your arms around yourself, with one hand on your ribs and the other hand holding the outside of your opposing elbow.
3. Taking your hands and putting them gently on the bottom half of your face, cradling your face and head.
4. Doing a starfish meditation—tracing around the outside of your hand and fingers with the other hand.
5. Keeping a small flat piece of glass or rock in your pocket and rubbing it.
6. Counting your inhale and exhale, slowing your breathing down.
7. Carrying a small piece of satin or silk (like blanket edging) in your pocket and rubbing it with your thumb and forefinger.
8. Laying your entire hand across your forehead and slowing your breathing.
9. Wrapping yourself in your security blanket.

THEORETICAL CONSIDERATIONS IN HELPING CLIENTS MAKE CHANGES IN PLAY THERAPY

As we said at the beginning of this chapter, most child-centered play therapists do not target working with clients to make changes in their behaviors. As Virginia Axline, the originator of child-centered play therapy, has suggested: "The therapist maintains a deep respect for the child's ability to solve his own problems if given an opportunity to do so. The responsibility to make choices and institute change is the child's. The therapist does not attempt to direct the child's actions or conversations in any way. The child leads the way; the therapist follows" (Axline, 1947, p. 73). Because these therapists are vehemently nondirective, they would not use the techniques we have described in this chapter, though they might use the skills outlined except teaching, which they would adamantly not use.

Practitioners of the other approaches to play therapy featured in this book could all use the skills and techniques in this chapter. Quite often, the goals would differ depending on the approach. Adlerian play therapists would be open to using all of the techniques because they believe it is important to use any technique available to help clients change thinking, feeling, behaving, and interacting—all aspects of clients' lives that are possible to improve. Cognitive-behavioral play therapists are going to mainly focus on the techniques designed to help clients make changes in their thinking (like self-talk) and behaving (like social skills and assertiveness skills). Ecosystemic play therapists are goal-oriented and flexible about different techniques, so there is a good chance that they would be open to most of the activities described in this chapter, with specific clients working on selected goals. Gestalt play therapists would tend to focus more on the movement and art techniques designed to help people become more emotionally aware and expressive. Jungian play therapists, because most of them tend to be relatively nondirective, would probably be amenable to using the skills described in this chapter (except teaching) and perhaps they might be interested in some of the art or sand tray techniques. The metaphor techniques would certainly appeal to narrative play therapists, especially those strategies that target self-image thinking and behavior. Practitioners of psychodynamic play therapy would be working to help clients develop adaptive skills and more sophisticated defenses, so while they might possibly be willing to use some of the techniques in this chapter, they would probably phrase their goals differently than we have phrased them in the descriptions. Although there are no standard Theraplay intervention strategies in the chapter, we have noticed that Theraplay therapists tend to be open to considering the use of techniques if they can be adapted to helping clients' attachment; quite a few of the activities described in this chapter could be used for that purpose. And integrative/prescriptive play therapists are open to using everything at some time or another with some clients for some purpose.

MOVING ON . . .

Now it is up to you . . . we have uploaded (downloaded?) most of the skills and the techniques we currently use in play therapy to help clients make changes. The only ones we haven't included were those we either thought too difficult to explain how to do or those we thought we got from someone else and didn't remember who, so we could not give them credit or we haven't invented them yet. We are hoping that this list will inspire you to create your own techniques, either totally from scratch or through modification of techniques you have learned from other people or read in books. We hope we have accomplished the thing that was most important to us in writing this book: giving you permission to give yourself permission. (Have we said, "Go wild!"? Go wild!)

The last set of tools we want to convey in our quest to teach you how to do play therapy is related to working with parents, family members, teachers, and other important folks in the lives of children and adolescents (and sometimes even to our adult clients, depending on their developmental level). We know that lots of folks who are drawn to becoming play therapists are a little afraid to work with anyone who might be considered to be an authority figure. If you are one of those people who is a bit intimidated by the idea of working with parents (or teachers), we want to reassure you—they are only grownup kids. Often, they are scared too . . . and hurting and confused and feeling lost and a whole bunch of other things . . . and, in many cases, they need just as much help and support and compassion as our child clients do.

Interlude 7

Giving Yourself Permission

*Y*ou might have noticed that many of the techniques in this book were invented by one of us or one of our students. And many of the other techniques were modified from something someone else invented. One of the main things we want you to get out of this book is *permission*—permission to make "stuff" up; permission to change activities or techniques you learned from someone else; permission to pay enough attention to your clients that you know the kind of things they like to do and how they like to do them; permission to take yourself seriously as a play therapist; permission to have fun in the playroom; permission to remember what it was like to be a kid or a teenager; permission to have fun in the rest of your life; permission to take yourself lightly as a play therapist; permission to pretend to be someone else in the play room; permission to put yourself in the shoes of your clients; permission to hear and see your clients and their lives with your ears, your hearts, and your spirits; permission to hear and see your clients and their lives with their ears, their hearts, and their spirits; permission to set energetic boundaries to keep yourself and your clients safe in the playroom; permission to be yourself in the playroom (and everywhere else).

(Imagine us both waving ginormous magic wands.)

Permission to give yourself permission!

CHAPTER 8

Working with Parents, Teachers, and Families

You may have noticed that our chapters tend to start with us interrogating you with a bunch of questions. In the name of consistency, we'll do the same in this chapter. Here are some of the questions you should consider regarding including parents or teachers and families in the play therapy process. How do you define your client? Is it the child, is it the family, or is it the person who can give consent (i.e., the parent or guardian)? Do you believe it is necessary to include parents (and/or teachers) in the play therapy process when you are working with children or adolescents? How do you decide who to include? How do you decide whether to include them and how much? In what ways are parents and/or teachers helpful in the process? What is your goal with the parent and/or teacher? What does your guiding theory say about the inclusion of parents or teachers? Do you believe it is helpful to include the other members of the family in the process? If so, how often and to what degree do you include them? If a child or an adolescent is struggling in school, do you believe it is helpful to include other students in the process? If so, how often and to what degree do you include them? What is your goal with family members or classmates? What does your guiding theory say about the inclusion of family members or classmates? (We recognize that most theoretical orientations don't actually address the inclusion of family members and classmates in the therapy process, so you can decide what you think about it even if your guiding theory doesn't mention anything about including them.)

This chapter is unique in this book because throughout we've focused on helping you learn to do play therapy with people of all ages, not limiting our definition of play therapy to apply just to kids. Talking about including parents and/or teachers (and maybe even other members of the child's family or classmates) kind of assumes that the play therapy client is a child or an adolescent. We also believe that some of these skills and techniques can be applied to couples or adults and co-workers, and so forth. (Please give yourself permission to expand the borders of our descriptions and to use the points and ideas of this chapter in a variety of ways beyond child and adult relationships.)

Parents can be your most valuable ally when working with children and adolescents. We tend to think that the relationships and dynamics within the family influence the formation of the personality and the functioning of children, adolescents, and adults. (While we have seldom convinced the parents of our adult clients to come in to a play therapy session, it would be helpful if we would get them to come.) We try very hard to get parents of children and adolescents to participate in the play therapy process. Sometimes we work with parents without the client present, and other times we work with parents and the client or with the entire family. The client's presenting problem will help steer us initially. We also use what we learn (or what we want to learn) about the client as a guide for how and when we use family members in sessions, including family play therapy.

Teachers are also influential in a child's (and adolescent's) functioning. It's not uncommon for us to see children based on the recommendation of a teacher. Sometimes the presenting problem is a struggle in school, and sometimes teachers suspect that their students are struggling at home and need help from an outside professional. We do not expect teachers to come to counseling sessions with their students, especially outside of the school. However, we have found that having phone conversations with teachers, meeting teachers in their classrooms, or visiting during conferences can be a powerful tool in a number of ways.

It can also be helpful to include other members of the family (and other students as appropriate for children and adolescents struggling in school) as part of the therapeutic process. We tend to see things in the context of systems, so if children are struggling at home, it may likely enhance their movement toward positive mental health to include other members of the family in family play therapy. If children are struggling at school, it can often be beneficial to include other students in the process along with their teacher. (Of course, this is best carried out by the school counselor, school social worker, or a school-based mental health provider and will necessitate getting informed consent from the parents of the other students to include them in a play therapy group.) (This probably went without saying, and we're sorry—we felt compelled to say it anyway.)

INTERVIEWING PARENTS AND TEACHERS FOR INFORMATION

Parents provide a perspective that is different from, and yet related to, a child or an adolescent client's perspective on a problem or situation. Even when the entire family experiences the same event, each family member interprets the event differently. For instance, in the case of a divorce, one parent might be relieved and excited about the future, the other might be devastated and depressed, and their children are often just confused and conflicted, unsure of what the future holds and worried about whether they are going to have to choose a side or they are going to lose one or both parents. If there are multiple children, each one might interpret the divorce differently. It always helps the play therapist and the family to know how the different family members feel and think about a particular situation, person, relationship, or change if it is problematic for some of the members.

Parents can also provide the play therapist with information about child and adolescent clients' development (e.g., whether the child learned to crawl, walk, or talk within the typically expected time frame, child illness, birth abnormalities, learning disabilities), breaks in attachment (e.g., a deployed mother or father, adoption, foster care), family constellation (e.g., birth order and ages of children, sex of children, gaps between children), substance use in the family (e.g., sibling or parent, in utero), recent challenges or changes (e.g., death of a pet, divorce, or move), or experience of trauma. Parents might even share family secrets that are important to the play therapy process. In the context of the presenting problem, we also ask about cultural values and beliefs. For example, if a family comes to counseling because of a death in the family, we want to know what the family believes and teaches about death. Does the family believe in reincarnation? Do they believe the deceased goes to Heaven? Does the family celebrate the life or mourn the death of the deceased?

Teachers can also give information about child and adolescent clients' functioning. We ask teachers about how our clients build relationships with peers and adults, areas of strength or limitations, noted changes in clients' functioning, and academic ability and interest. Sometimes, when we visit schools, we take the opportunity to watch our clients "in action" as they move through the halls, do work in class, play at recess, and interact in the lunchroom. Each of these scenarios gives us valuable feedback about how our clients function in different areas, how they interact with others, and how others interact with them.

An important discussion we have with the adults in our child and adolescent clients' lives is how the adults feel and what they think about them. We want to know what the parent(s) and/or teacher likes best about the clients and what the adults dislike about them. (Unfortunately, many parents and teachers want to spend much more time on this last one.) Knowing this information helps us learn about clients. Asking about clients' assets sometimes reminds the adults in clients' lives that there are things they like about them, which is something that is often overlooked in times of stress.

Here are a few questions often asked of parents and/or teachers. How do you define or describe the presenting problem? When did it start? What else was going on in the child's/family's life when it began? When is the problem behavior (thinking, feelings, attitudes?) elevated or worse? When is it better? For whom is this a problem (parent, child, other kids/ adults, teachers, everyone)? What have you tried in the past? What seems to have worked, at least a little? Who is in charge of the discipline, and how is it done? How does the child respond to correction, redirection, punishment, or consequences? How does the child interact with other children? adults? authority figures?

RECRUITING PARENTS (AND TEACHERS) AS ALLIES

When you are working with child clients, parents (and sometimes teachers) can be your biggest allies in the play therapy process if you take the time to make a connection with them. Many times, parents will want to bring the child (or adolescent) in to your office, drop them off, and say, "Fix this kid. Don't try to get me to change though." (We're not trying to be cynical—you can't imagine how many times this happens.) If you believe it is important to include parents and/or teachers as part of your play therapy process through consultation or participation in family play therapy or in a small group with students, you will need to acquire some expertise in "pitching" play therapy in order to enlist them as willing collaborators. We use a couple of different tactics to enlist these important adults as our partners in supporting children. Our favorite strategies in this process are (1) building and maintaining a relationship with them, (2) making sure they understand what an important role they have in the play therapy process, (3) front-loading the idea that play therapy often takes a long time and doesn't provide a miracle cure, (4) tailoring the way we speak to them to maximize the possibility they hear what we have to say, and (5) explaining the system approach for thinking about shared responsibility in creating and solving problems.

Your first step in engaging parents and teachers in working with you as a play therapy team is to use your counseling skills to build a relationship with them. As they feel heard and understood, supported and cared for, these adults are much more likely to listen to what you have to say because you listened to their story. They are going to be much more likely to care about asking for insight and guidance from you and following through with your recommendations if you have conveyed caring about them to them.

Because we believe including parents (teachers, and often other members of child and adolescent clients' families) is essential, we talk to them about how important they are in children's lives—that they live with them 24/7 (or they have them in class five days a week), whereas we only get to interact with them for an hour (or so) a week. We emphasize that they will have ideas about the best way to build a relationship with the children. We talk to parents about how they know things we will never find out directly from them; they know the developmental history; they know the history of the problem and what they have tried to make things better; they know the impact on their children of their culture; and so forth that will help us explore children's interpersonal and intrapersonal dynamics. Teachers know about communication skills, learning styles, problem-solving strategies, learning difficulties, peer relationships, and so forth. Because of the closeness of the relationship and the time spent with children, parents and teachers are in a special position to help support children/adolescents, gaining insight into their patterns and into changes to be made in behaving, thinking, feeling, and interacting. From your very first contact with parents (and teachers when you are working with them), it is helpful to emphasize the idea that you and the child (adolescent) will need their help and that they play a crucial part in making sure that progress is being made. You will want to remind them that their support and encouragement will be critical in fostering positive growth in the child. Indeed, they are much more important in this process than you will ever be. You should also work to assure them that they will not be alone. You will be with them and the client on the journey, coaching, encouraging, giving feedback, and so forth.

We also remind parents (and teachers) that play therapy is a gradual process. It isn't quick and easy, it isn't "just playing," and (although we do both have magic wands) it isn't magical. It is often useful to present some preliminary education about what play therapy is (and is not), even before you start seeing the client. That way, you make a preemptive strike designed to prevent later difficulties with parents (and teachers) who think you are playing tiddlywinks and eating bonbons in the playroom with the client.

We also use what we know about parent (and teacher) intrapersonal and interpersonal dynamics as we communicate with them. The way we do this is using the Adlerian concept of their personality priorities, but you do not have to be Adlerian to make use of this strategy. Personality priorities are patterns of behavior and reactions based on individuals' convictions about how they gain belonging, significance, and a sense of mastery (Kfir, 2011). There are four personality priorities: comfort, pleasing, control, and superiority. Because personality priorities are a major influence on their style of parenting and their relationship with their children and how teachers interact with their students (Kottman & Ashby, 1999; Kottman & Meany-Walen, 2016), we use our understanding of the personality priorities to customize our "pitch" to parents and teachers. As you listen to parents (and teachers) describe their own lives and problems exhibited by their children, their personality priorities are often evident, as there are patterns of complaints described by each of the personality priorities. You can take what you believe about personality priorities and custom-design how you interact with them as a way to enhance the possibility that they will want to work with you. The tactic here is to listen to the adults and to develop a hypothesis about their personality priorities, after which you can tailor how you talk about the play therapy process and how it will make life better for them and their children, paving the path to a maximally cooperative relationship.

The primary complaint of comfort-oriented parents (and teachers) is that being a parent (or a teacher) is difficult and is causing them stress and discomfort. The best way to approach them is to explain how being a part of your care team can help make their lives easier, less stressful, and more comfortable. Pleasing parents (and teachers) struggle with believing in their own abilities as they repeatedly fail in their attempts to make everyone else happy. The way to invite their collaboration is to remind them that, while it is impossible to make everyone happy, you will give them support and some recommendations for helping everyone get along better. Parents (and teachers) whose personality priority is control try to make sure that they have control over others (e.g., children, spouse, the play therapist), over situations (e.g., how things go for the child at school), or over themselves, and they feel out of control. It is often helpful to suggest to them that working with you will help them feel more in control (notice we don't say "be" more in control) and you will have some ideas for them that might be helpful in interacting with the child. Because parents (and teachers) whose personality priority is superiority have such high standards for themselves and for their children, they are often locked into how the child simply does not live up to these standards in some way. To make a cooperative connection with these adults, it will be essential for you to acknowledge how hard they work, how dedicated they are to the welfare of the child, and how impressed you are with all of their efforts and knowledge. Because they feel acknowledged by you, they are more likely to be willing to enter into a collaborative partnership with you in working with the child. (Ta Da!! We just summarized an entire fifty-page chapter from *Partners in Play: An Adlerian Approach to Play Therapy* [Kottman & Meany-Walen, 2016] in two paragraphs! Who said play therapists don't perform miracles.)

One other thing we do in conversations with important people in the client's life is to point out that the difficulty the client is experiencing is not just the client's. (This is even the case when we are working with adults. We often ask the client to bring in a spouse, a sibling, parents, and any other people in the client's system.) You can explain that the way you see client struggles is that everybody in the client's life has a part in creating and maintaining the problem; therefore, everyone in the family (or the classroom) needs to have a part in making things better—for the identified client and for everyone else in the family/classroom. As part of this discussion, it is helpful to stress that you are going to be asking everyone in the system to make some changes—sometimes in their attitudes toward the client and one another; sometimes in their interactions with the client; sometimes in their parenting strategies, family relationships, or marital interactions. We also emphasize our belief that, if they are willing to work with us to support the changes their children are making, things will get better for the family faster than if they choose not to participate in the process. By saying this at the very beginning of our relationship with these important people in child clients' lives, we often save ourselves from later criticism from these adults that we are "just playing."

FAMILY PLAY THERAPY

In addition to consultation with parents (and teachers), you may also want to initiate some family play therapy. Family play therapy "invites family members to engage with one another in ways that are mutually satisfying and relationally edifying" (Czyszczon, Riviere, Lowman, & Stewart, 2015, p. 186). It is a way to build relationships between family members; explore interpersonal dynamics among family members; help clients to gain insight into their own issues and into issues related to other members of their families; and give clients opportunities to learn and practice new, more appropriate ways to get along with other family members. Many of the techniques described in this chapter will work well with families in play therapy.

In a recent book focused on family play therapy (Green, Baggerly, & Myrick, 2015), the editors suggested that many therapists are uncertain about how to include all members of a family in a play therapy session. A likely explanation for therapists' uncertainty is not knowing how to engage adults and children simultaneously. Yet, because family issues are a major reason children come to play therapy, including the family in the process is an important and logical practice. Family play therapy meets the developmental needs of children and adults, keeps everyone engaged, and helps to create solutions to family problems. Not every approach to play therapy has published information about family play therapy. We have included all of the theoretical approaches to family play therapy we could find: Adlerian family play therapy, child-centered family play therapy, cognitive-behavioral family play therapy, Jungian family play therapy, narrative family play therapy, and Theraplay.

In Adlerian family play therapy, Kottman and Meany-Walen (2015) described the importance of including all members of a family in the counseling process because of the influence members have on one another. In Adlerian family play therapy, the therapist would use activities and questioning strategies to explore family rules, expectations, and functioning. As the therapist developed a clear understanding about how the family operates, he or she would use play therapy strategies to help family members gain insight into the patterns of the family and of individual members. The play therapist would design activities to help them understand one another better, teach new ways of relating and interacting with one another, and give members opportunities to practice those new patterns of working, together with good will and kindness.

Child-centered play therapists underscore the importance of the parent–child relationship (Landreth & Bratton, 2006) and its effectiveness at reducing the symptoms of children who receive counseling services (Bratton et al., 2005). Typically, family play therapy sessions are not conducted beyond gathering information and assessing progress. Rather, parents are encouraged to participate in filial training or child–parent relationship therapy in order to learn child-centered play therapy skills and improve the parent–child relationship. Filial therapy (Guerney, 1964; VanFleet & Topham, 2016) uses group or individual teaching of empathic understanding and acceptance. Parents meet for an unspecified number of sessions (sometimes up to several years) in which they are given support from other group members and leaders/therapists. Parents are taught nondirective play therapy skills they can use with their children in at-home play sessions. Parents discuss their experiences with the therapist and/or group members during weekly sessions in order to strengthen their skills and process their experiences. Child–parent relationship therapy (Landreth & Bratton, 2006) is a ten-session filial model developed from the work of Bernard and Louise Guerney. In this manualized model, a group of parents meet weekly to learn play therapy strategies. Like the filial model, they use those skills in weekly at-home play sessions with their child. Parents are expected to video record their sessions, bring recordings back to the group, and receive feedback from the members and leader during group meetings. This model has a rich body of research to support its effectiveness.

Shelby's (2015) description of cognitive-behavioral family play therapy emphasizes the use of interactive and play-based activities in which parents and children can work together to help understand one another's perspectives. The therapist works to help parents make decisions and set expectations that are reasonable and attainable. In cognitive-behavioral family play therapy, family members are typically given information and instruction as well as homework assignments. Family members return to counseling to discuss progress and questions.

The Jungian family play therapist interweaves the symbolic languages of talk and play to understand the influence of member roles, personal beliefs, family values, and personal and family history on the presenting problem (Paré, 2015). Using Jungian and family systems concepts, the therapist offers hypotheses about the problems of individual family members, family subsystems, and the entire family, shadows, personal roles, and dynamics (e.g., scapegoat, princess, wicked step mother, etc.) to determine how to work with the family and its members. Different subsets of the family might be involved in sessions at different points, with all members being included to some degree across the therapeutic process. The ultimate goal is for the family members to strengthen their relationships with one another, relying less on the therapist and more on the family for problem solving, supporting one another, being playful, and enhancing their family life.

The underlying belief in narrative family play therapy is that each member of the family has his or her own life story and the roles other family members play in creating that story (Taylor de Faoite, 2011). Through metaphor and other storytelling techniques, the play therapist works to understand the uniqueness of each person's story. Then, together as a family, they help each other to adjust, correct, add to, alter, better understand, and retell their stories in ways that improve interpersonal and intrapersonal dynamics. It is believed that by including families in the narrative play therapy process, counseling can be more efficient and effective.

Munns and Munns (2015) asserted that a significant component of Theraplay is helping parents become sensitive and responsive to the basic relationship needs of children. It could be argued that all Theraplay sessions are family sessions because of the active involvement of parent (or caretaker) and child in each session. The relationship between adult and child is the center of the therapy. Parents are taught fun, playful, and interactive techniques, such as songs and dances and play activities that include nurturing touch. They practice these activities in session and are assigned tasks to complete during the week between sessions in order to improve the parent–child relationship and secure the child's attachment.

SKILLS FOR PARENT AND/OR TEACHER CONSULTATION AND FAMILY PLAY THERAPY

Generally, we use our basic counseling skills when we work with parents and/or teachers in consultation and when we do family play therapy. We paraphrase, reflect feelings, ask open-ended questions, listen actively, and practice other relationship building skills outlined in Chapter 4; we ask questions and observe in line with the skills outlined in Chapter 5; we interpret, use metaphors, and confront discrepancies just like we discussed in Chapter 6; and we may even do some teaching like we outlined in Chapter 7. While the goal of consulting with parents and teachers is to *consult*—meaning that we are checking in, gathering information, and imparting information that might help them in their relationships with the child or adolescent clients—we still need to build and maintain a therapeutic relationship built upon trust with them. Additional skills and attitudes that we've found to be helpful when working with these stakeholders and in doing family play therapy are reframing and helping them define their "stake in the ground."

Reframing

The goal of reframing is to help parents, teachers, and other family members to look at the client or the problem from a different perspective. In order to do this, you will need to hear the other person's perspective on the client and his or her behavior or attitude and recognize that it is problematic (e.g., irritating, discouraging, challenging) for the other person in some way. Then you would work to come up with some other ways to frame the client or the problem that might be more positive and optimistic. Sometimes that would be asking parents or teachers to take someone else's perspective on the client (e.g., "I can tell you are worried about George, and I have noticed that the other children in his class seem to like him. What do you think other kids would say about him?" "I hear you saying that Gretel was a great little kid, and now that she is 13, it feels much harder to figure out how to parent her. Would it help to tell you that, compared to the other teens with whom I work, Gretel is a delight?" "It sounds like you are annoyed with Joaquin for asking a lot of questions in class. Often experts talk about gifted teens as being likely to challenge the adults in their lives, trying to figure out what they, themselves, think about things. Could Joaquin be doing that?"). Other times, giving parents, other family members, and/or teachers an alternate way of thinking about the problem helps to reframe the client or the difficulty. For instance, you could say things like, "You describe Aisling as being very competitive with her siblings. While I can certainly see how that might create some challenges, I also wonder if there might be any assets associated with being competitive?" "I get how you see Aaron as being stubborn. An alternative way to describe him would be 'determined and self-confident.' What are your thoughts?" "I know that it is frustrating when Sybil makes jokes in your class, and I am guessing the other kids give her a lot of attention for being funny. Might this be a problem for the whole class and not just for Sybil?" It also sometimes helps to reframe things for parents, other family members, and/or teachers by asking them to consider the child's perspective, like inquiring: "I know you feel that Chelsea's homework is a big problem for her and for you. How do you think Chelsea would describe or interpret the problem?" Notice that in reframing the client or problem, we are not attempting to disregard the other person's opinions or feelings. Rather, we want to acknowledge their thoughts and emotions and help them to consider alternative perspectives. By doing this, we let them know we heard their concerns, which often softens their stance and opens them to the possibility that there is another, more positive way to think or feel about things.

Helping Define "Stake in the Ground"

Another key skill in consulting with parents and/or teachers and doing family play therapy is helping everyone involved define their "stake in the ground" for the course of treatment and for the changes they desire (in the client and maybe even for themselves—we can always dream). A "stake in the ground" is sometimes the "hill you are willing to die on," and sometimes it is just something that is important to the client and the other people in his or her life that they want to have change. Now, usually, the process of defining their stake in the ground will start with parents, other family members, and teachers wanting you to change the client's behavior. A big part of your job is to get them to clearly define in concrete terms what they would like to be different—not just in the client, but also in the client's interactions with the rest of the family (or classmates), in the rest of the family's (or classmates') interactions with the client, in their own behavior management philosophy and strategies, in their attitudes toward the client and other members of the family or classroom system, and so forth.

Defining the stake in the ground is often our way of helping parents, other family members, and teachers figure out how to pick their battles and explore who actually "owns" the problem. We often use scaling to get them to consider just how important each of the changes they desire is. Using a one (not really that important) to ten (absolutely necessary) scale can help them prioritize their goals for the play therapy process, and it can help us teach them to choose which things are important enough to focus on in their interactions with the client and which can probably be put on the back burner. By asking parents, other family members, and teachers who are bothered by difficulties with the client, we can help them explore who actually "owns" the problem. In many cases, if the client is not bothered by things in their life, he or she is going to lack motivation to change. When the client is not concerned enough to make an effort to shift his or her behavior, it may be better to work with the adults to figure out ways to make changes themselves (or let go of the things they want to change). (We often use the story about trying to teach a pig to sing . . . if the pig doesn't want to sing, it probably isn't going to learn how.)

While parents (and teachers) often come in to the consultation and family members start family play therapy with a list of things they want to have you eliminate, it is more helpful to aim for something positive, rather than focusing on taking something away. We try to get them to focus on moving toward specific desired changes in something they want to improve or enhance.

It is also essential to help clients, parents, family members, and teachers define stakes in the ground that are reasonable (not a miracle cure) and reachable through the play therapy process. For instance, a teacher who wants you to take the child with ADHD from his classroom and transform him into a child who always listens, obeys, thinks before he acts, and stays in his seat all day; or a parent whose child is on the autism spectrum who wants you to wave your magic wand and turn the child into a social butterfly is setting a near impossible goal. You would have to help with a bit of reality testing, helping the client and the other people in the client's life become more realistic about what is possible.

TECHNIQUES FOR PARENT AND TEACHER CONSULTATION AND FAMILY PLAY THERAPY (AND MAYBE EVEN SMALL GROUPS)

We have many different ways of interacting with parents, families, and teachers (and sometimes even classmates) that are playful and valuable. These techniques are intended to be easily adaptable and can even be spontaneously introduced in sessions. It is incredibly important to remember that, in many cases, parents, other family members, teachers, and students who share classrooms with identified clients are often discouraged because the things they have tried in the past haven't managed to make things better. Quite often the family members (or other students) are feeling pretty depleted of positive energy and needing an infusion of positive energy to move toward getting insight and making changes. Some of these techniques are simply fun things to do with other people as a vehicle for building up the positive emotions in the family/group positive energy bank because the only way to get through hard times is to have some positive emotions in the positive energy bank from which to draw.

The previous chapters outlined techniques for the specific goals related to a specific phase of therapy. This section is a bit different because you might work with parents, family members, teachers, and/or classmates at any point during the treatment process. Remember, be creative and flexible. Adapt any of these in ways that work best for your goals within the therapeutic process, with whom you're working, and the specific goals of your clients. You can use some of these techniques as a part of your consultation with parents or teachers. Most of these techniques are applicable for your work with families in family play therapy sessions (or classmates in small-group sessions).

Adventure Therapy Techniques

Although you can use adventure therapy techniques with individual clients, we prefer to do adventure therapy activities with a group. We might include both parents, parent(s) and other family members, the teacher and child, child or adolescent with a classmate, a husband and wife, or other configurations of people. Ashby et al. (2008) and Kottman et al. (2001) have lots of helpful and easy-to-implement active and fun interventions to use with children, adolescents, and adults.

Everybody Up

This is an adventure technique that can be done with as few as two people and up to an entire family or classroom. The goal of this intervention is for clients (and the other people in their lives) to improve communication, increase self-awareness and self-acceptance, demonstrate responsible behavior, and practice problem-solving skills.

Instruct people to partner-up. If you have an odd number of people in the session, you can ask one person to sit out or you can participate. If you have someone sit out, still make sure that person has a job of some kind (e.g., observing, noticing positive qualities and giving feedback, serving as an "outside consultant" who provides helpful suggestions for solving problems) so that everyone is involved. The two people in each pairing sit on the floor, facing each other, their knees bent, their toes touching, and holding hands. To complete the task, both pairs must get to a standing position with their toes and hands still connected to one another. Some twosomes get this right away, whereas others take a while and might need some suggestions from you or their helpful observer. (Hint from your helpful observer: it works best if you keep your bottom close to your heels.) If you have more than two people, after folks are successful in standing up, you can expand the group to four people—everybody in the group needs to hold hands with someone else—and then they all stand up at the same time. In groups with odd numbers, you can join to even the teams or you can have them attempt to stand up with three people holding hands in a circle. This will be harder, but it is possible.

Like all interventions we've described, you don't need to verbally process the activity. However, because you're working with adults (adult clients, parents, and teachers), verbalized processing can be an added benefit. We often ask participants how they contributed to the success of the task, whether they cooperated or created a roadblock in completing the task, how they communicated with one another, and whether that communication was helpful. If they could not manage to stand up, how did they handle not completing the task? If there are significant size differences (i.e., adult and child), what was that like for both participants? This activity can be completed with a large adult and small child as long as there is cooperation, communication, and a desire to complete the task successfully. It can be particularly helpful to process as you focus on how people can contribute in ways that they (and the other people in the process) don't expect. If you added difficulty by increasing the number of people involved, you can process the changes in difficulty as more people were added. If you want to make a bridge to other situations, you can ask how this activity was similar to or different from challenges in other areas (i.e., home or school). Most of the time, we hear laughter and feel an energy of fun from the participants. We process this and brainstorm ways that they can do fun challenges at home. Maybe they could teach this activity to other family members or use it in the classroom.

Balloon Carry

Although this technique can be used to foster cooperation and communication just between you and a parent or teacher as part of the consultation process or between a client and his or her parent(s) or teacher to strengthen their relationship, we usually use it in family play therapy or in a small group of students as a method of encouraging cooperation and communication between family members or members of a classroom. So, you do need some supplies—you need as many balloons (or beach balls) as you have people who are going to participate, minus one. (So, if it is just you and the client, you need one balloon; if you have eight family members, you need seven balloons, or if you are doing it with all of the first graders in a class or all the members of the student council at the high school, you might need thirty balloons). Here are the instructions: "Get in a straight line, with everyone facing the same way. Put a balloon between your body and the body of the person in front of you. Once the balloon is placed in between the bodies, you can't touch the balloon with your hands. Walk all the way around the room (or the block or the office building—whatever works in your location). If the balloon falls down, you have to go back to where you started and begin again." The person at the front of the line will not have a balloon in front of him or her and will have to pay close attention to pacing because if he or she goes too fast, the balloon will fall. About halfway through the walk they are taking or if they drop the balloon and have to start over again at the beginning, it is often helpful to have them stop and have a conversation about what is working and what is not—how they could do the assignment with greater levels of communication and cooperation. (Obviously, if it is just you and the client, you might want to let the client lead the discussion, rather than you just talking about what you think would work better.)

Beach Ball Bounce

This is another technique you could do just with you and a parent or teacher, with the parent (or teacher) and the client, or you could do it with the entire family (or small group). If you wanted to, you could do it with members of a class or school organization—with more than about eight participants, you will need to divide the group up into subgroups and get more materials. Again, the primary focus with this activity is on practicing cooperation and communication. You will need a large (54″ × 108″ rectangular plastic table cloth (like the ones you use for outdoor picnics) cut in half (so that you wind up with a square table cloth—54″ × 54″) and a beach ball. Have your participants blow up the beach ball, position themselves around the table cloth holding on to the edges with both hands, and put the beach ball in the middle of the table cloth. Tell them their job is to bounce the beach ball as many times as they can, without letting go of the edge of the table cloth with either hand. (In other words, they can't hit the beach ball with their hands to keep it on the table cloth.) We add another rule (based on Terry's extensive adventure therapy experiences) that no one can "head" the ball (we promise that this helps avoid injuries from when two people try to "head" at the same time and wind up crashing heads with one another). Then we ask them to count how many times they can bounce the beach ball without it escaping from their circle and the table cloth. If the beach ball does escape, they just have to replace it on the table cloth and start counting from zero again. After they have been doing the activity for about 5 or 6 minutes, you can ask them to stop (tell them they can just start the count from where they left off and don't have to start over again or you will have a rebellion on your hands) and have a brief conversation about what is working, what is not, and how they could improve their performance. We usually give them a couple of minutes to talk this over and then have them start bouncing again. You can do this several times if you want . . . you can also make suggestions if you have any, but we try to let the participants figure it out by themselves.

Positive Energy Bank

The goal for this technique is to help a parent and child or the members of a family (or small group or even members of a class) to recognize that many things can contribute to the positive energy present in the relationship. It is pretty simple—you have the family members (or students in the class or group members) stand in a circle, and, as they think of things (e.g., events, relationships, situations, experiences) that contribute to people in the family (class, group) feeling better, more optimistic, encouraged, more alive, and so forth, they step into the middle of the circle and tell the rest of the family (class, group) what it is. Any of the other members of the family (class, group) who feel that same way about whatever the first person mentioned join him or her in the middle of the circle. After everyone who feels that same way has met in the middle of the circle, everybody steps back into the circle. Then someone else suggests something that could contribute to the positive feelings in the family (class, group) and steps into the middle to be joined by the other members who agree with that suggestion. You will be sitting on the sidelines, making a list of the events, relationships, situations, experiences that can be added to the possibilities for adding positive energy to their positive energy bank. They can take this list home (or back to their classroom) and post it somewhere so they can have a kind of menu they can consult when the energy bank needs a deposit (or you can ask them to do at least one of these things every week as a homework assignment).

If you think that the family (class, group) is so discouraged that the members cannot come up with anything, you can prime the pump by saying things like, warm cookies coming out of the oven, blowing bubbles together, sitting and cuddling in front of a fire on a winter day, someone giving you a compliment, getting a shoulder rub from someone, sledding down a really cool hill, lemonade on a hot summer day . . . whatever you think will get folks to join you in the middle and serve as a model for the kinds of things people could say. ("Is that it?" you ask. Yes—that's it. Sometimes the most powerful things are the simplest. Not all play therapy is rocket science.)

Storytelling and Creating Therapeutic Metaphors

Puppet Introductions

This is a technique you would most likely use with a family (or small group) to work on building positive relationship skills, such as active listening, taking turns, and cooperating with other people. If you are using it with just a parent (or teacher) and a child client, it can help them learn and practice skills for interacting in positive and socially appropriate ways.

This activity works best if you have a variety of puppets. (This is not a challenge for us as we have a purchasing problem and puppets are so very cute!) Have animal puppets, people puppets, happy puppets, angry or sad puppets, occupation puppets (i.e., police officers, wizards, fire fighters, teachers, or circus masters), princess or prince puppets, trees, birds in nests, different colored and sized puppets . . . you get the point. You can make puppets with socks or oven mitts if you want to expand your collection or you can work with clients to create a specific puppet. I (Kristin) make an effort to purchase at least one puppet a year that I do not particularly like (i.e., the three-headed dragon). This way, I'm not only purchasing cute unicorns and kittens. (Terry likes those ugly three-headed dragons, so she doesn't have a problem with just having "nice" puppets.)

To start this activity, ask each person in the session (parent, teacher, child, or other family members) to pick one puppet and introduce that puppet to the others. Sometimes we ask the identified client to go first, sometimes we ask the most or least powerful person in the group to go first, and other times we allow the people in the session to decide. When we do this, we can process how the decision was made and how members felt about the decision and the order of presentation. If you have an actual puppet theater or setup that allows the presenter to hide, that works best. This way, only the puppet is visible. The child, parent, or teacher is not the focus of the introduction. If you don't have a puppet theater, no worries, it can work fine with each person just sitting in a circle holding on to his or her puppet.

Be clear in your instructions that the introduction should be about the puppet, not the person wielding the puppet. We often have to give examples of how this works and sounds because parents can feel a bit awkward at first. An example of a wizard introduction could be, "I am a wizard. I have a pointy hat and long gown. I can make magical things happen. Usually, I grant people's wishes, but sometimes I misunderstand or make mistakes and people get upset with me. I get so mad at myself when I make mistakes that I make myself disappear." You can have people discuss specific things such as what they like best about being that puppet or what they like least. You can ask questions as people introduce themselves and use your therapeutic skills of summarizing, paraphrasing, or reflecting to bring about particular points and guide the introductions. It is important that each person in the room gets a chance to share.

Variations of this activity include asking the puppets to tell the other puppets what they like best about each other, things they have noticed about one another that folks haven't mentioned, things their puppet would like to do with other puppets, and so forth. In a family or parent session, you can ask the puppets to describe a habitat or home in which all puppets would feel safe and valued and get their needs met. With teachers or parents, you could ask the puppets to describe to one another what they need from the other puppets. The important thing is to stay in the metaphor while you're discussing these things. With older children or with only the adults, after the puppet introductions you could have a consultation in which you might make connections between what happened in the metaphor and what might be helpful in real life, such as in the classroom or at home. Depending on the questions you ask and the topics you want the clients to discuss, you can use this activity to build relationships, help the clients understand their interpersonal and intrapersonal dynamics, increase clients' understanding of their own dynamics and the dynamics of one another, or generate alternative ways of thinking or behaving.

Family Timeline Story

The goal of this family play therapy technique is to give children in a family a sense of the history of the family. (Or if you are using it in a parent consultation session, it can be a way for the parent to give you a sense of the family life cycle.) It is helpful with foster and adopted children to give them a context of how things work in the family; sometimes it is important when you are working with teens, who forget that their parents were adolescents at one point and actually do understand what it is like to be a teen; it is often significant for families in which the focus is on "the problem" to the exclusion of remembering that there have been problems before that the family has overcome. If you are working with families, consider this technique as a possible family play therapy intervention just to build a sense of shared history and connection among family members. As they build the timeline, they are developing a story of the history of the family that they can tell together.

Here's how it works—you give the family members a long sheet of white (or butcher) paper (we are beginning to wish we owned stock in a company that manufactures it), have them put it on the ground or hang it on the wall, and draw a timeline. It is often fun to have folks take turns writing or drawing on the timeline so that the responsibility is shared and interest is maintained for all members.

We always suggest that they start with several generations before the parents (like the parents' grandparents or even great grandparents). You can recommend different milestones for recording on the timeline. We like to include the country or state where people lived; in what kind of environment they grew up; when and how they met a partner or spouse; when they had children (and how many, what gender they were, and their names); what they did for work; what kinds of cultural traditions they had; when they died (and of what); and where they were buried (if they were). The things we ask them to record are, of course, rather arbitrary, so use milestones that you think will be helpful or meaningful for the family to record and discuss. It is also fun for many families to have a reason to interview extended family members to get more information to add to the timeline . . . either in subsequent sessions or as a homework assignment that could involve the whole family.

I Could Talk About . . .

This is a technique I (Terry) learned at an InterPlay conference in San Francisco about 10 years ago. I have, of course, changed it quite a bit, so

I am not sure anyone from the conference would recognize it. We use it to get folks talking—kind of to prime the pump—especially adolescent clients, parents, teachers, and family members. You can use it in your parent/teacher consultation, in family play therapy, and in small groups of students. It is helpful for you to get a "feel" for what might be going on with someone who is extremely guarded and unwilling to tell you anything deeper than what is on the surface to talk about something connected to family functioning other than the presenting problem or to reveal something that they might think is shameful or embarrassing. We also use it for exactly the opposite goal, with folks who want to tell story after story; it can get folks to distill things down to only important things. You need to use it judiciously and not violate the basic premise, though, because otherwise it won't work twice with the same client(s). (Learn from our mistakes.)

Here's how it works: if you are doing it as part of parent/teacher consultation, you ask the parent (or teacher) to share a series of one-sentence headlines, starting each one with "I could talk about . . ." or "I could tell you about . . ." using a single short sentence without any details for each thing they *could* tell you about. Your job is to just create the space for the parent (or teacher) to give you the headlines, without responding verbally. If you are including this activity in a family play session or a small play therapy group, you will ask each participant (one at a time) to tell the group their one-sentence headlines, prefacing each one with "I could talk about . . ." or "I could tell you about. . . ." The job of the other participants is to quietly create the space, taking in the headlines without making any kind of comment or responding in any way—just being open and listening.

As you give the instructions, you will want to emphasize that you are not actually asking participants to tell you about anything—you are just asking them to tell you what they could tell you about . . . (if they wanted to, if you had time, if they thought you cared, if it felt safe, and so on—but you are not going to mention that—just that you want them to give you lots of things they could tell you about . . .). You can do this without giving clients a specific topic, just asking them what they could talk about in general, or you can have them give you a list of things they could talk about on a selected topic (your choice or theirs). Your job is to listen to the list, noting things you might later (not in that session—have we mentioned we want you to learn from our mistakes?) ask clients to discuss in more detail, or sometimes you can ask them if there is one of the things they listed about which they would like to elaborate. If you are doing this with a family, another way you can do it is to set it up by telling folks to talk about the things they could talk about if they thought someone was interested, then ask the other members of the family to pick one of the topics and ask questions about it. This gives the family a way to connect positively.

What Did It Teach 'Em?

I (Terry) developed this activity based on a session taught by Jane Nelson, an amazing parent educator, I attended at the North American Society for Adlerian Psychology. At one point during the workshop, she said something like, "Have you ever asked parents what they are trying to teach their kids?" Her question actually spurred a series of conversations between my husband and myself about what we wanted to teach our son, Jacob. The goal of this technique is to get parents (and teachers) in the consultation process to think about what they would like to teach their children and (maybe) help them generate ways to teach them the things they want them to learn. In our experience, it works best in consultation sessions with individual parents or couples (or with individual teachers or a team of teachers), rather than in family sessions (or small-group sessions with students).

In preparation for the activity, it is helpful for you to generate a list of ways that parents (or teachers) interact with the kids—both positive and negative. We use things like yelling at them, hugging them, ignoring them, giving them a compliment, smiling, turning their back on them, doing activities that the kids like, doing activities the kids don't like but the parents do, and so on. We put each one of the things we have listed on a strip of paper (2" by 5" or so), and we show up to our consultation session with a little pile of them, along with some blank strips of paper. Then we have the parent(s) (or teachers) list things they do when they interact with kids (sometimes we say "When you are trying to get kids to do what you want," but most of the time we leave it open-ended), and we write those down on the strips of paper. Next, one at a time, we ask the parent(s) (or teachers) to draw one of the strips of paper and have kind of a guessing game about what that behavior could teach children (and adolescents), followed by speculation about what that behavior might be teaching their kids. This can lead to a fruitful conversation about what the parents (or teachers) want to teach their children, along with further discussion about the best ways to teach them what the adults want them to learn.

Movement/Dance/Music Experiences

Simon Says

This activity is designed to build relationships between parent–child and teacher–child. It can also be used to help change behaviors or attitudes of children and/or adults. It could be used in a one-on-one session with just the adult and the identified client or in a family or small-group session. (It isn't something you would use in your parent/teacher consultation—we don't think parents or teachers would think it was fun if no kids were involved in the exercise.) Start by reminding or teaching the clients how to play Simon Says. That is, there is one person at a time leading the activity (Simon), and the other participant(s) are supposed to follow the leaders' instructions. The leader chooses activities or tasks for the followers to complete. To begin with, the leader says "Simon says" before all of the instructions. For example, "Simon says to pat your head." The followers complete the instruction. Eventually, the leader starts intermittently adding instructions that are not prefaced with "Simon says." If the leader does not say "Simon says" and only gives the directive, followers don't have to complete the task. If a follower completes a task without the leader saying "Simon says," that person is "out" until he or she completes some fun activity to rejoin the game. Remember that people are never out for the rest of the game. We always find some strategy for people to rejoin the fun. You can invite participants to help generate ideas for how "out" players can get back "in." They may even decide that people don't get out, which might be particularly helpful for people (children or adults) who are perfectionists or "too tight."

Ultimately, we want participants to have fun and to increase opportunities for positive interactions. We take note of leaders' willingness and attitudes toward leadership. We take note of the followers' willingness and attitudes toward following. How do participants exchange roles? How are mistakes addressed and handled? How do participants encourage or discourage each other? If decisions about the game were made, how did that happen, and in what ways did each participant have input?

Flock Dancing

Flock dancing (Dan Leven, personal communication, February 2015) is like a follow-the-leader movement game that lets people practice watching others and matching what they are doing. It is also a way to share leadership and practice taking turns and communicating with one another. It works best in a family play therapy or group session because it is difficult to have a two-person flock. The first thing you do is to have your family (or class) form up into a flock (which can look like a line or a V shape like a flock of geese). Tell the person in the front that he or she is the "temporary leader" (this is a strategy to avoid temper tantrums with clients who only want to be the leader) and the other people are the "temporary flock." Explain that it is the leader's job to lead the other members of the flock in movement or dance steps that they can all do. (This is an essential component of the instructions because you want to also encourage empathy and paying attention to the capacity of others in a compassionate way.) Tell the group that, when you change the music, they need to shift things around so that there is a new leader. Usually what happens is the person next in line (or to one side or other of the V) takes over being the leader and the person who has been serving in that capacity moves to the back of the flock. Give them a chance to have a conversation to figure out how they are going to manage the changing of the leader. Start some music and play about a minute or two of music; then switch the music to a different tune, signaling the changing of the guard. Do this enough times so that everyone in the family/group gets to be the leader two or three times. One variation would be to play the same music and let the leader decide when he or she wants to give up the power to lead and pass it on to someone else, letting the group/family pass the reins without interference/guidance from you. After they are done dancing, you can decide if you want to process with them, asking things like the following:

> "Who liked being the leader of the flock? What did you like about it?"
> "Who didn't like being the leader? What didn't you like about it?"
> "Who sometimes liked it and sometimes didn't? What did you like and dislike about it?"
> "How did you figure out what everyone in the flock could do to make sure that everybody was included?"
> "Were there some things you would have liked to try but decided not to do because you thought other people in the flock couldn't do them? How did that feel?"
> "What did you do if you weren't sure whether folks in the flock could do the things you were thinking about doing?"
> If they were managing the role shifting themselves, "how did you decide to change from being a leader to being one of the flock or from being one of the flock to being a leader?"

Family Dancing

(Semiobviously, this is an activity for family play therapy rather than parent and teacher consultation.) There are a couple of ways we have done family dancing, and we want to share all of them. Your goal for family dancing will determine which format you use for family dancing. If you want to work on solidifying positive connections in the family, you should usually just do a free-form family dance—either to music you bring or music various family members bring. If you use music family members bring, be sure you let everybody have at least one song of their choosing. This activity can put positive energy in the family's positive emotions bank if the members are willing to just have fun with it—and with families who won't have fun with it, don't do it. (That might have been obvious, and we weren't sure, so we thought we would just say it. We aren't even going to give you directions for the free-form family dance—you are smart, you can figure it out.)

You can also do a more structured family dance if you want to see the various members' impressions of how the family moves/works together. This can be an exploratory-type activity, getting a feel for the different perceptions of the interpersonal family dynamics, and/or it can be a way to help family members gain a greater sense of how other people perceive what happens in the family. With this one, what we usually do is let all the members move or dance their impressions of the family. You can also have the members turn their backs to one another and dance. Either of these versions will give you a chance to observe and see the differences in the individual perceptions, but they do limit the members' ability to observe one another. If you want the members to get an increased awareness of how others see the family and the members are willing to take psychological risks, you can ask the members of the family to sit in a circle, while one member at a time takes turns being in the middle using dance or movement to demonstrate what happens in the family and the other members observe. (If you do this version, you need to make a rule that no one gets to give feedback or voice disagreement about the perception of others—the idea is to increase awareness, not start a fight.)

Toning

Years ago, I (Terry) went to a conference—I don't even remember what organization was doing the meeting, and I don't remember anything else I learned there. This technique was worth whatever it was that I spent to get there because I use it all the time—with clients (in individual play therapy sessions, in parent/teacher consultation, and in family and group play therapy session) and with my own family. The universal goal of this technique is to create a physical resonance or at least remind people that they have a connection with one another. It is a great thing to assign as homework, for when things are getting tense or conflicted—it builds a bridge of reconnection and can be used as a reminder to begin working together or to restore communication. (My husband and I hold hands and tone together, quite often stopping in the middle of an argument; I know it sounds crazy, but it really works.) You can do it with individual parents or teachers during consultation sessions to cement the relationship with them; we usually do it to teach it to them so they can use it in their family or classroom. We also do it with families in family play therapy and in group play therapy. It is easier to demonstrate than it is to explain because it is musical, and we are going to do our best to explain it.

The usual way of starting it is to ask folks to face one another (if there are only two people) or to get in a circle, facing one another. Then you will need to get one person to start and lead the tone. That person (if you are showing someone how to do it, you should start) sets down a musical base by singing (chanting?) (toning?) a single note. We recommend starting with a long vowel sound (so *eeeeeee, aaaaaaa, ooooooo, iiiiiiii*) because, for some reason, that is easier to match and easier to sustain. Then that person continues making that sound, joined by the other person/people, who match that note. Obviously, the original person will have to breathe some time—that's okay . . . the other people can continue to tone the note while the first person takes a breath, then rotate, as people need to stop and take a breath and then rejoin the tone. When the original person is ready to be done with that note, he or she can signal somehow. I always make a grand gesture, kind of like a conductor because I feel special when I do that, but it certainly isn't part of the activity. It usually works best to do the same tone for about 3 or 4 minutes, and you can do it for a shorter time if that is what works for clients. You can also try a couple of different notes—we like to do short vowels sometimes too.

Something else that is super fun for families or small groups is a variation on this activity. Sometimes I call it a voice symphony, and I am not at all musical, so I am pretty sure that is not a legitimate title. I quite often give it as a homework assignment because it is so fun that, for the families that like it, it is a sure-fire way to contribute positive energy to the family's positive energy bank. Here's what you do: one person (usually the one who has the best breath control) uses his or her voice to set down a tone that serves as the foundation for the "symphony." That person becomes the "conductor." He or she points to other members, inviting them to add a sound they can sustain to the symphony (it can be the same tone, a different tone, or just a sound he or she likes making) until the conductor has included everyone in the family (or group) as part of the symphony and signals to everyone that it is time to end the music. (Okay, sometimes it is more a cacophony than music, and it is really fun.)

Sand Tray Activities

Chapter 3 provided an overview of sand tray play therapy and outlined the procedures to follow to set up sand trays. We also provided suggestions about processing and additional resources that can help you develop your sand tray play therapy skills. We use sand tray play therapy techniques with parents, families, and teachers in any of the stages of therapy. You can do trays in your parent/teacher consultation, with a parent and a child, with a teacher and a child, or with a family or group.

Building a Relationship with Parents/Teachers in Consultation

1. Tray about "my family" or "my class"
2. Tray about things he or she likes about the child/family/classroom
3. Tray about what it's like to be a parent/teacher of this child

4. Tray that depicts how the person feels about the child being in play therapy
5. Tray about what they know/think about play therapy
6. A general tray about "my world"

Exploring Parents'/Teachers' Interpersonal and Intrapersonal Dynamics in Consultation Sessions

Parent or teacher does a . . .

1. Tray about what gets the child in trouble
2. Tray about how he or she feels/what he or she thinks when the child _____ (whatever brings them to counseling or something that the parent/teacher really appreciates about the child)
3. Tray on what he or she wishes the child could do better or differently.
4. Tray on what he or she wishes he or she could do better or differently
5. Tray about a time when he or she felt particularly connected to the child
6. Tray on a time when he or she felt particularly disconnected with the child
7. Tray on what being a parent/teacher means to him or her
8. Tray on parenting/teaching strategies (ones that work well and ones that don't)
9. Tray on rules the child does and does not follow
10. Tray on how he or she connects with others
11. Tray on how the child connects with others

Helping Parent/Teacher Gain Insight into His or Her Patterns of Thinking, Feeling, and Behaving in Consultation Sessions

Because the goal is to help the parent or teacher gain insight and develop a deeper level of understanding of himself or herself and/or the child, sometimes you would create a tray for or with the parent/teacher. You can also make a tray for the parent or teacher and invite him or her to make changes or consider other alternatives to the tray that you have created.

1. Therapist does a tray showing his or her perception of parent's, teacher's, and/or child's assets
2. Therapist does tray to depict his or her understanding of how the parent/teacher/child sees self, others, and the world
3. Therapist creates a tray of his or her perception of the parent–child or teacher–child relationship

4. Therapist informs parent/teacher that he or she will bring in a "wise" character who comes into the tray to help tray characters to think differently about some aspect of the tray
5. Therapist or parent/teacher creates a tray that depicts the "problem" from a different perspective.
6. Parent/teacher creates a tray that represents how life would be different if the "problem" were resolved
7. Parent/teacher creates a tray of the problem from the perspective of the child
8. Therapist and parent/teacher depict a picture of the problem and then take turns creating additional trays of solutions to the problem

Facilitating Parent/Teacher Making Desired Changes in Thoughts, Emotions, and Behavior in Consultation Sessions

Parent/teacher creates a tray about what he or she needs in order to solve the problem.

1. Parent/teacher does a tray on how he or she can collaborate with the child to solve a specific problem
2. Parent/teacher depicts how to resolve a problem that is getting in the way of him or her feeling successful as a parent/teacher
3. Therapist does a tray to model specific parenting/teaching skills (e.g. encouraging, determining problem ownership, communicating, etc.)
4. Parent/teacher and child create a tray together about what they want in the future
5. Parent/teacher and child create a tray about how their relationship has changed

Art Techniques

Quick Draws

Wait for it . . . Yep! You guessed it. This is where the clients draw quickly, just like the ones described in Chapter 6, but these are focused on parents and teachers and would be used in your consultation sessions with them. This activity can be used to help the therapist build a relationship with parents or teachers. It can also be used to help with exploration of interpersonal and intrapersonal dynamics or help parents (or teachers) become more aware of those dynamics.

This intervention requires parents (or teachers) to give a quick response to a prompt (determined by your goal for the session or activity). (Think Freud's free associations, but with pictures.) Like all of the art techniques in this book, emphasize that artistic ability will not be evaluated. Tell parents (or teachers) they have one minute to draw a picture based on your prompt. If you think it's helpful, you can tell them that the picture can be representative or abstract. You want them to start drawing quickly without thinking (or overthinking) their response to a prompt starting with, "In 60 seconds or less, draw a picture of . . ." Some prompts that are applicable with many parents or teachers are "the last time you were mad at the child," "the last time you were proud of your parenting/teaching," "the thing you worry most about your child/student," "the part of parenting/teaching you think you're worst at," "the thing you like best about the child," "the thing that irritates you most about the child," "the last time you enjoyed the child," "something the child is good at," "your relationship with the child." You might have tailored quick-draw prompts related to specific circumstances such as, "In less than one minute draw a picture of how you felt when you found out your daughter was pregnant," "when the child kicked the family/class pet," "when the child goes to his mother's home/a different classroom," "when you were a teen and felt like no one was listening to you."

With parents and/or teachers who like to verbally process, you can ask about the size, shape, colors, or proximity of the different features of the pictures. You might also consider the implications of *how* they approached the drawing (i.e., nervously, excitedly, slowly, or self-consciously) and engage them in talking about those factors as well. You can process the drawing with statements such as "I notice . . ." or asking the parent or teacher to expand more on the picture(s). You could ask how drawing the problem is different from talking about the problem.

Ideal Family/Classroom Drawings

This activity is for individual parents in parent consultation or individual teachers in teacher consultation, though you could use it with an entire family or an entire classroom. You would have several different goals with this technique, depending on where you were in the consultation. You can use it to explore what is important to parents/teachers, to help them gain insight into what is working and not working in their family/classroom, and to motivate and guide making changes to move closer to the "ideal."

We are beginning to think lots of our techniques are pretty obvious—this one certainly is. You give clients two large pieces of paper (or even a small one, I guess) and some drawing utensils (or stickers) and on one, ask them to make a picture of the way their family (or classroom) is currently, and on the other, ask them to make a picture of their ideal family (or classroom if you are working with a teacher). After they are done, you can ask them to describe both pictures and to detail how the ideal is different from the reality. If you think they are ready for this, you can follow that up with asking them what they are willing to change in order to move closer to the ideal.

With a family or a class, just have members do the two drawings and then invite them all to participate in a conversation designed to come to some kind of consensus about what the members can agree that they want. When you have finished that process, you can follow it with a conversation about what each member is willing to take responsibility for changing in terms of behavior, cognitions, attitudes, problem solving, and communication in order to have what they all agree would be closer to their ideal.

Family Art Assessment

The family art assessment is adapted from Landgarten (1981). The term implies that this is done with families, and that's true. It can also be done with subsets of families such as one parent and child, two parents, just children, and so on. You can also do this activity with teacher and child or with parts of a class. And you can do it with small groups if you are doing group play therapy. It is usually done with the goal of exploring interpersonal dynamics, and it can also be used to help clients (and the other important people in their lives) to gain insight into their dynamics.

To do the activity with a family or small group, you will need four large sheets of paper (such as poster board or butcher paper) and enough markers or crayons for each person in the family to have a different color. Tell the participants that there are going to be three procedures for this technique. Instruct each member to select a different color of marker or crayon and explain that each person will use that same color throughout the activity.

For Procedure 1, ask the participants to divide into two teams. (They can use any method they wish to decide on the teams.) When they have decided on the teams, give the participants two sheets of paper or hang them on a wall where everyone can reach them and tell them that they are to draw something. Tell the teams that they are not permitted to speak or write notes to each other when working on the art. Inevitably, someone will ask if they are to draw *together* or *separately*. We avoid answering that question by returning responsibility, saying something like "You can decide" or "I do not have a rule about that." When they are finished, they stop. To signal that they are done, they put down their marker/crayon. The ban on talking continues until both teams have completed the task. Then ask each team to title their artwork and write the name on their piece of paper somewhere.

For Procedure 2, lay out or hang up another sheet of butcher paper. Tell the participants to dissolve the teams. This time, give the entire family (or group) one sheet of paper. Ask them to draw something on the paper, again without verbal or written communication. When they finish with the artwork, they again choose a title and add it to the sheet of paper.

For Procedure 3, give participants another sheet of paper, ask them to draw something, but this time they can talk or communicate any way they want. When they are done, they should choose a title and write it on the paper somewhere.

If you are doing this technique with a subgroup of a family or a teacher and student, you obviously can't divide into two teams, so you would just do procedures 2 and 3. (And you would only need two sheets of paper.)

You will want to observe the entire process without giving feedback until the very end of the process. You might note who initiated the drawing in the first picture and how that process unfolded—who was a leader and who was a follower? Who was respectful of the other members' drawings and who drew on top of other people's drawings? Who followed the rules and who ignored them? What was the level of involvement of each member? Pay attention to how they divided up into teams. Were the teams what you expected based on what you already know about family dynamics, or were they different? How did the various members react to having to divide into teams? How did they handle having the teams dissolved during the second procedure and moving into having the whole family share one piece of paper? Notice who took up the most room on the picture and who the least; who drew in a corner, on the side, or in the middle. Who listened to who? Which member's suggestions were heeded, and which member's suggestions were ignored? Who functioned independently? Who asked for help even though they didn't really need it? Who didn't ask for help even when they did need it? How did people arrange themselves (who sat/stood by whom)? How did they communicate even when they could not talk or write notes? How was it different when they were allowed to talk? Did people have fun and use humor?

Mouthpiece Puppets

This is an activity you could do with an individual play therapy client, an individual parent or teacher in a consultation session, an entire family, or a small group. I (Terry) developed it when I was teaching in Ireland. I wanted to come up with something I could give the adults in my class as a way to say some things that they had never been allowed to say to family members and friends. (And an important safety tip: I actually didn't ask them to say those things to actual family members or friends—just to me and/or other members of the class. If you do this kind of a setup, you want to be sure you are not setting your client up to do something that will come back and bite them later when you are not around to protect them.) The goal for this activity can be adapted to whatever you are working on.

We usually use it to help people give themselves permission to give voice to things that would usually be hidden or forbidden. You could also use it to have folks in a family or group give one another compliments or encouragement; you could use it to ask them to take responsibility for behaviors they would usually deny; you could use it to help them practice setting boundaries they would usually be afraid to set. (And those are just some examples of things we have used this activity for in the past—insert our usual exhortation to use your imagination.)

Obviously, you could make the puppets with paper bags, paper plates, paper mache, ice-pop sticks, or any other material, and we like to make these puppets from something a little more substantial, like socks or wooden spoons. Because we want clients to be able to keep them and use them at home, we don't want them to be flimsy or insubstantial. So, you need a sock or a wooden spoon (preferably a clean sock or a new wooden spoon), some markers, some yarn, chenille stems (a.k.a. pipe cleaners), hot glue, glitter glue, and any other craft materials you or your clients prefer. Then you let your participants go crazy and make an amazing puppet. (You can have them make the puppet be themselves, their best self, their future self, their positive self, their loving grandmother, their honest twin, their imaginary friend . . .) Then you let them say (through the puppet) what they want or need to say (to themselves, to you, to other family members, to classmates, to their spouse, etc.).

Most of the time, if you do this with individual clients or in parent/ teacher consultation sessions, you will guide folks to saying those things to you or to themselves (even if it needs to be in the privacy of their own bedroom with the door closed when they are by themselves, it will relieve some of the pressure). The only restriction for this activity is that if they are going to say things to other members of the family or other members of a small group, you want to make sure that whatever they want/need to say is either not hurtful or not delivered in a vindictive way. Clients who cannot or will not agree to having the puppet give feedback that is constructive are probably not good candidates for this activity.

Solutions

This is an activity I (Terry) developed for parent and teacher consultation sessions after a workshop I attended led by Jane Nelson at a North American Society for Adlerian Psychology, and it can be used whether or not you are Adlerian. Traditionally, Adlerians are very invested in helping parents and teachers apply logical consequences when children are misbehaving. This technique is in service to a paradigm shift away toward the generation of solutions to children's problematic behaviors. It is based on the idea that many times children misbehave because they have a need that is not being met, and their misbehavior is a misguided attempt to get that need met. In order to meet that need, parents (and teachers) would change their behavior as a way of helping children learn to meet those needs in other, more appropriate ways. Instead of setting consequences, they would develop potential solutions to try to meet the needs of the children with the idea that in doing this, the children's inappropriate behaviors will be unnecessary. It is a technique we use in parent or teacher consultation, without the child present. (We're not actually sure why. It might be interesting to use it with the child present; if you do, let us know how it works.)

It's a drawing activity, so you will need paper and drawing materials (though, of course, you could also do it with stickers if you have an adult who doesn't like to draw). The first thing you will want to do is to have the adult close his or her eyes and remember the last time there was a power struggle with the child or the child was misbehaving. It is helpful to have the adult step through the entire situation from start to finish—from whatever triggered the difficulty through whatever the child did that was upsetting to what the adult did in response. Next, have the adult draw a picture of what happened, including all the players—they can use stick figures if they want. Then have the parent (or teacher) make a thought bubble over each person involved and fill it with a list of what he or she surmises that person needed in the situation. For example, Jason might be acting out when the family had company with a baby because he felt upstaged and needed a little extra attention from his parents to remind him that he was still important to them. Jessimane might refuse to stay in her bedroom after a nightmare because she needs more comforting than her parents provide. In order to help parents and teachers generate ideas of what they can do in response to these needs, you could have them draw another picture just of the child, expressing his or her needs, and then add a picture of themselves applying solutions that help the child get that need met. You could also just help the adults brainstorm ways to meet the child's needs by either changing their behavior, the family system, the classroom interactions, or the circumstances.

Structured Play Experiences

Role Reversal

This is a technique you would use when the child is present in the session with the parent or teacher. We have several goals in mind when we ask clients to do role reversal. We want the child and adult to have fun, laugh, and connect. We also look for feelings, attitudes, or behaviors that emerge that might be indicative of typical patterns between the two people or reveal underlying thoughts, emotions, or areas of discouragement. It can also be used for practicing simple social skills, like taking turns and listening; for helping clients recognize and accurately interpret social information, for assessing characteristics of self and others, and for recognizing roles in the family or classroom. We would also love for the dyad to practice taking one another's emotional and cognitive perspective, though this may be thwarted depending on the child client's level of development. (Remember, the younger the child, the less capacity the child has to take another person's perspective.) Even if the child cannot take the adult's perspective, however, the adult may be able to have a conversation with you about how it might feel to be the child or what the child's role-play revealed about his or her perceptions of the adult.

You can instruct them that they are going to do a role reversal where the teacher is going to "become" the student and the child is going to "become" the teacher, or the child "becomes" the parent and the parent "becomes" the child. We start with this as the only instruction and see if the participants will run with it. If so, we observe the process and use our routine play therapy skills. For people who need additional instruction, you might brainstorm with the child and adult a specific "scene" they would like to act out. It could be spelling or reading instruction with teachers, or it could be supper time or bedtime routines with parents. During or after the role play, you might ask them to ask the other person what they need, what they think, or how they feel from the perspective of their role plays.

Hero/Victim/Villain

This is usually a family play therapy activity, though it can work with individual parents (or teachers) in consultation. It is more appropriate for families that have older elementary children and/or adolescents (or upper elementary classrooms) because the concepts are probably too abstract for younger children. The goal of this technique is to teach participants about the Karpman Drama Triangle (Karpman, 1968), how people can frequently get stuck on it, and how people can get themselves off the triangle. Karpman, a student of Eric Berne, the founder of Transactional Analysis, posited that quite frequently people in relationships get stuck on what he called the Drama Triangle—where people take the role of the Victim, the Persecutor (or Villain), and the Rescuer (or Hero).

In preparation for the activity, you will need to have a way to make a large (about 4 or 5 feet on each side) triangle on the floor of your office. We use masking tape to mark out a triangle and then make signs for each of the three angles—one with Victim written on it, one with Villain written on it, and one with Hero written on it. We then ask participants to generate a list of times when there is conflict in the family (or among classmates). It is helpful to take notes as you have them give a brief summary of who is involved in the conflict and how it plays out between members. After you have explained the dynamics of each role on your triangle, read back their descriptions of the conflict situations and have the various members of the family (or group) go and stand on the angle that describes the part they played in that particular drama. When you have done a couple of these, you can introduce the idea that it is possible to step off the triangle if they would like to have less drama between members. If they are interested, you can lead them in a brainstorming session for strategies they can use to get off the triangle.

In parent/teacher consultation, you can use the same triangle and explanation of the Karpman Drama Triangle and get them to generate different scenarios in which they have interacted with other people in these patterns. Or you can invite them to describe situations in which they have observed other people participating in the triangle. Then you can help the parent (or teacher) to generate ideas for keeping off the triangle or helping others avoid participating in the triangle.

Reset Button

I (Terry) developed this technique for my family. My husband (Rick) and son (Jacob) have had a pattern of escalating power struggles from the time Jacob was 2 years old. In order to nip these power struggles in the bud, I thought I would suggest to them that each of them had a "reset button"—an imaginary button that could be pressed to shift the conversation between the two of them to a more constructive note. I use it with individual clients (children, teens, and adults); I teach it to parents and teachers in consultation sessions; and I use it in family play therapy sessions. The goal is to help children and parents (and teachers) develop the skills to recognize when they are in a power struggle and give them a tool for getting themselves out of the power struggle and into a more productive, socially appropriate interaction. You can use it in your own sessions when you are working with kids who try to get you into power struggles. (This is not to say that we ever get into power struggles with clients! "The sand needs to stay in the sand box," anyone??)

If anyone is involved in a power struggle in your session (a parent, a sibling, a peer—no matter who), it is a perfect time to teach this technique. The first thing you do is to label what is happening as a power struggle by saying something like, "This seems like it is a power struggle." Next, you ask the combatants to stop for a moment and take a big, slow, deep breath, hopefully in synch with one another. Ask both participants in the power struggle if they know what a "reset button" is on a computer or other electronic tool. If the answer is affirmative, go on to the next step. If neither one knows what it is, explain what a reset button is and how it works. Tell the power strugglers that the next step in this process is for each of them to imagine what their own reset button looks like and ask them to describe it to you (and to their power struggle buddy). Get them to be very specific in describing their reset button, including how big the button is, what color it is, what texture the surface is, where it is located, how they would press it (e.g., with their pinky finger, with their elbow, with their entire body, etc.), and how hard it would have to be pressed in this particular instance in order to be effective in resetting. Next ask them to look at one another, making eye contact, and take a couple of deep, slow breaths together before you bring them to the next step.

Invite them to come to an agreement that if either of them (or anyone in their family or class) "invokes the resetting," they will actually follow the resetting procedure. (A conversation/power struggle may follow this statement wherein they might not want to agree to this; if they don't, this technique really won't work, and you should probably abort the process.) Tell them that the way to "invoke the resetting" is to say "It's time to hit our reset buttons." Remind them that it is not "You need to hit your reset button" or any other similar phrase that opens the way for a different power struggle about who started it or who needs to step back. The idea of this technique is that both parties have had a part in getting the power struggle going and both parties need to have a part in getting themselves out of it.

Now ask them if either of them would like to practice "invoking the resetting" by saying to the other person, "It's time to hit our reset button." Once you get a volunteer, give them the go ahead to "invoke." In response to the "invoking," each party simultaneously is to press his or her imaginary button, take three deep breaths together (we just made that number up—you can have them take as many breaths as you want), let themselves relax, and the person who didn't get to invoke gets to start the conversation over—in a more respectful and constructive way—maybe even with an I message or a reflection of the other person's feelings. (Okay, that might be too much to ask for, and, if you are one of the combatants, that could totally happen—hopefully.)

You can also teach the technique in the abstract without an actual power struggle happening in your session by asking people to describe the last time they got into a power struggle and then asking if they would like to learn a strategy for getting themselves out of future power struggles. Then you can role-play the process with an individual child or adolescent client, with a parent or teacher in a consultation session, or with members of the group, family, class—re-creating their engagement in a power struggle in the session.

My Strengths/Family Strengths

This technique was developed by Jill Thomas (personal communication, December 2016), who taught it to us. It is usually used in family play therapy as a vehicle for helping family members focus on personal and interpersonal strengths, though you could also use it with clients who have a poor self-concept, with the goal of helping them learn to "own" their assets.

To begin, you need index cards, a large piece of paper or poster board, and thin markers or colored pencils. Invite clients to brainstorm a list of positive qualities they possess and write one of them on each card. (If the client or a member of the family is artistic, you can even ask him or her to illustrate the cards.) Some examples of positive qualities could be things like "I am able to see the good in every situation." "I am cheerful." "I see the bright side of things." "I like to help others." "I am special." "I keep trying, even when things get difficult." "I am smart." "I can make people laugh." "I am hard-working." "I love animals." "I appreciate nature." "I know how to find solutions to problems." "I try hard." "I like to talk about feelings." "I admit when I make mistakes." "I am artistic." "I am fun to be around." "I am positive." "I can cheer other people up." Have clients pick out a few cards to describe themselves and a few cards to describe each family member as well. If the parents or other family members are present, have them do this step too, picking out characteristics to describe each family member. Next, invite clients to share at least one of the characteristics they chose to describe themselves and explain how they manifest that characteristic. Later, have them pick at least one of the traits they chose to describe other members of the family and share examples of times the members of the family have displayed this quality—for example: "My sister was positive when our car broke down, and she focused on being glad that at least it wasn't really cold outside."

Draw circles around the perimeter of the large piece of paper (or poster board)—one to represent each family member, with a larger circle in the middle of the paper labeled "family." Write all of the family members' names on the top of their circle, choose a "scribe" to write things down on the paper, and invite members of the family to remind the scribe of all the strengths and positive qualities listed for each person inside of his or her circle. Draw a line from each person's circle to the center "family" circle to show how each family member contributes and is connected even though everyone has different strengths and positive qualities. Facilitate a brainstorming session, writing a list of family strengths in the center "family" circle. This should illustrate the positive qualities that the family possesses due to the individual members that contribute to it. Invite the client and other family members to share examples of times they have noticed their family displaying that strength and what that meant to them.

Some clients or family members may struggle to identify strengths in themselves or in others if they have significantly poor self-esteem or severe relationship issues within the family and, therefore, may need more assistance and involvement from you to help identify strengths and offer examples of times you have witnessed this characteristic being displayed. To maintain clients' trust in your input, it's imperative to be genuine and sincere in choosing these traits. (If you have clients or families whom you perceive as only having a few positive qualities, you might want to skip doing this activity with them.)

In a later session, if you think it would be helpful to the family members, revisit the "my strengths/family strengths" board and invite the family members to discuss other positive qualities that the family could use in order to make improvements and better meet the needs of the members. For example, maybe the original drawing highlighted family strengths as being hard working, determined, and having lots of rules, and the family members identified needing more "togetherness" or "fun" in the family circle in order to improve family functioning.

Fake Pokémon Go

I (Terry) have recently had a lot of clients who either were playing Pokémon Go religiously or wanted to play and were too young or didn't have a smartphone, which precluded them from getting to play. I invented this activity as a way to bring Pokémon Go out of the virtual world into the physical world. We usually use it with children in individual sessions, in family sessions, or in small groups with students. (In other words, it isn't something we would use just with a parent or teacher for a consultation.) We often use it with families (or small groups) who have members needing to build their belief that they are capable and/or members who have difficulty connecting with others. Because the game can be a bit challenging at times, families (or groups) with members who need to work on anger management and frustration tolerance could also be good candidates for this activity. For families that enjoy it in session, you can assign it for homework as a way to put positive energy in their positive energy bank.

To play, you will need some small (1-inch) Pokémon figures (your best bet for getting them relatively inexpensively is to order them from Amazon, Walmart, or eBay) and a tossing ring (you can actually use a ring from a ring toss game, but those are kind of small and would make the activity more difficult. We got the ring we use at a sporting goods store in the section where they have Frisbees). Place the small Pokémon figures on the floor all around your office/playroom. (Don't put them on your desk or by your computer—learn from our mistakes! Have we said that before now? Just trying to save you money and aggravation and clients guilt.) To start the play, first demonstrate how to throw the ring to try and "capture" the figures by gently tossing the ring and having it land so that one of the Pokémon figures is inside the ring. Give the ring to one participant and tell him or her to toss the ring toward the figures to try to capture them. Have members take turns tossing the ring and capturing the figures. (You can decide how many tries each person gets per turn. We let them have three, but you can do it with one try per turn if you have family members who are low on patience.) (You can decide whether you want to let clients keep any of the figures they catch. You probably don't want to let them keep them all, as that could be too expensive. We like to let each participant keep the one they like the best.) After you are done playing, for families (or groups) with members who like to verbally process, you can ask questions such as the following.

> "How is this game like the game of Pokémon Go you would play on a phone?"
> "What did you like about the game?"
> "What did you do well playing the game?"
> "What was frustrating about the game?"
> "How did you deal with being frustrated?"
> "What are some other methods you could have used when you were frustrated?"
> "When you were missing the figure with your toss, what were you telling yourself about your abilities?"
> "How can you use the frustration tolerance tools you practiced in this game in other situations in your life?"

THEORETICAL CONSIDERATIONS IN WORKING WITH PARENTS (AND TEACHERS) IN PLAY THERAPY

As you'll remember from Chapter 2, different theoretical approaches have different philosophies about the degree to which and how parents or teachers are used in the therapeutic process. All of the theories we've described in this book acknowledge that working with parents and/or teachers is an important part of the process. To a greater or lesser extent, all of these approaches suggest that the play therapist provides support, gives information, consults with these stakeholders, and offers referrals for personal counseling when necessary.

In addition to those strategies, therapists who identify as Adlerian, ecosystemic, psychodynamic, and integrative/prescriptive play therapists frequently include parents, and/or teachers, in the therapeutic process because they believe these adults significantly influence the child's functioning. They will conduct family play therapy sessions in which all members of the family participate in play therapy activities in order to witness or attempt to help change interactional patterns. Child-centered and Jungian play therapists work with parents and teachers every three to five sessions with the primary focus on providing consultation and support. Cognitive-behavioral play therapists emphasize modifying parents' and teachers' interactions with child clients and coaching them on how to reinforce therapy in other areas of the children's lives. Gestalt play therapists work with parents and teachers primarily with the goal of gathering information about the child to help the therapist better understand children's unfinished business and contact boundaries. Narrative play therapists work with parents and teachers initially to gather information and provide support. As therapy is nearing its end, the parents and teachers are given more direction in how to help the child sustain the changes made in counseling. Unlike other approaches, Theraplay play therapists depend on the interactions between parent/caregiver and the child to conduct therapy. Not only are caretakers always included in the process, they are the primary "object" of interaction for the child in the therapy room.

MOVING ON . . .

So, now that you are an expert on individual play therapy, parent/teacher consultation, and family play therapy (along with a little group play therapy), are you ready to tackle tricky situations in the play room? We are, so we hope you are too.

Interlude 8

Avoiding Judgment

*W*hile most play therapists respond with empathy toward children without much effort, avoiding judgment when dealing with parents, teachers, and other family members is often difficult. Sometimes it feels easier to blame the parent(s), teacher, other family member, or classmate for the child's behaviors or problems, whether or not these other people have any part of the responsibility for the genesis or maintenance of the problem. However, blame and judgment seldom help parents, teachers, other family members, or children to function better.

You will need to be aware of and avoid indulging your own triggers when they stir up negative feelings toward your client's parent, guardian, family members, classmates, or teacher. Maybe it's the parent who says he cannot purchase new shoes for his child but can manage to buy cigarettes. It might be the teacher who complains about a student's wild and rowdy behavior and continues to withhold recess from her. Maybe it's the "golden child" who scapegoats and blames your client when things go awry in the family. Become familiar with behaviors or attitudes from others that really grind your gears, or get under your skin. When you better understand your own triggers, you are more likely to be able to be fully present and accepting of your clients and their parents, other family members, teachers, and classmates.

It is essential in your relationship with the other people in child clients' lives to remind yourself that they are doing the best they can and to acknowledge to them that you believe this. It is pretty easy to get sucked into blame and/or judgment about parents (or other family members, teachers, or classmates) of children who come to play therapy because, after all, if they were perfect parents (or perfect teachers, family members, or classmates), there would be no need for play therapy, because the children would be perfect. Now, we all know this is not true (especially those of us who realize how hard it is to be a parent or a teacher, family member, or classmate). Another crucial thing for you to remember is that parents (and to a certain extent, teachers) of children who come to play therapy often feel badly about their skills related to parenting (and skills related to classroom management for teachers). They are often "down" on themselves and, in many cases, feel like failures. As a result, they may blame themselves for the struggles of the child or blame the child. This makes it even more vital that, in your work with them in consultation sessions and in your thinking about them outside your sessions, you keep your focus on the notion that they are doing the best they can.

CHAPTER 9

Challenging Situations in the Playroom

So . . . now you are eager and ready to hop into the playroom and get going on your playing (and telling stories and having adventures and dancing and hearing stories and making up songs and building worlds in the sand and doing art). Before you jump in, we thought it might be good to give you some information (and maybe a little advice) to help you prepare to handle some of the possible challenging situations that happen in the playroom. We don't want to scare you—you will probably not encounter all of these situations—in fact, you might not have to deal with any of them in your entire career. (Though that is possibly pretty optimistic—you *will* probably have to deal with a couple of them at the very least.) We also want to acknowledge that we are pretty sure we haven't included every single possible problematic situation that could come up in the playroom. These are just the ones we brainstormed sitting around the coffee shop where we write, generating a list of challenges that have come up in our playrooms that were difficult for us to handle. Here is the list we created:

- A client who doesn't talk
- A client who doesn't do anything
  - A client who doesn't want a relationship with you (or anyone, sometimes)
  - A client who says he or she is not interested in playing
- A client who doesn't know how to play

- A client who keeps deliberately breaking the rules
  - A client who wants to take and keep something from the playroom
  - A client who starts to trash the room or breaks a toy on purpose
  - A client who wants/tries to leave early before the end of the session
  - A client who wants to bring his or her toys to a play therapy session
- A client who asks to sit on your lap
- A client who has a temper tantrum during a session
- A client who refuses to leave the waiting room to come into the playroom
- A child client who wants the parent or someone else (friend, sibling, spouse) to come to the room with him or her
- A child or adolescent client who says he or she wants you to be his or her mom/dad
- A client who asks uncomfortable questions
- A child or adolescent client who poses a challenge regarding confidentiality, such as a youngster who is cutting classes but insists you don't share with parents
- A parent who wants to come into the room with the client
- A parent/teacher who doesn't follow through with your recommendations
- A parent/teacher who wants to know everything that happens in a session
- A parent/teacher who is complaining about lack of progress or a parent/teacher who says he or she doesn't see progress even though you do
- A family where you must make a Child Protective Service (CPS) call
- An adolescent or adult client who is sexually attracted to you

So, here is what we are going to do in this chapter. We are going to describe each of the challenging situations, explain how we think most play therapists would handle that situation, and then tell you how we think the various approaches to play therapy would handle it (if they would do something specific or special—something different than the "usual" way of handling it). In many circumstances, our answer to "what do I do when . . . ?" is "It depends! It depends on the exact nature of the situation (e.g., the stage of therapy, how long the situation lasts, your setting, the interpersonal and intrapersonal dynamics of the client, the age of the client, and your theoretical orientation), so in some cases we may not be able to definitively answer how to handle each of these situations. (And we will give it our best shot . . .)

THE CLIENT WHO DOESN'T TALK

We thought we would start with something simple and build our way up to some situations that are more troublesome. Although having a client (whether the client is a child, an adolescent, or an adult) who doesn't talk is very disconcerting to our students (who tend to come out of a session in which the client isn't talking, being freaked out), this one is easy. Remember when, in Chapter 1 (and kind of every other chapter afterward), we discussed the paradigm shift you have to make from "talk therapy" to "play therapy"? Remember when we said the foundational premise of play therapy is that the play (and the rest of the "doing" that happens in the playroom) is the communication that happens in the playroom? That the play is the therapy? This means that the client who doesn't talk isn't a problem because communication (and therapy) is happening, whether or not the client is verbalizing. So, as long as you can make that paradigm shift, there is nothing to worry you—the client *is* communicating even when he or she is silent.

So . . . since there really isn't a problem, there is nothing you need to do differently than what you would already be doing. The key is to focus on watching what the client is doing—paying close attention to the themes of the play, the client's body language, shifts in the action, shifts in intensity of the play—and respond to that. You can (this one is the most obvious one) track the behavior of the client, so that he or she can tell that you are paying attention to what is happening. You can ask questions (and watch for the answers in what the client does in reaction to your questions), and you can make interpretations (and watch for confirmation or contradictions of your guesses in the play).

Most theoretical approaches to play therapy would do exactly the same thing. However, in many cases, the play therapist might be thinking about different things (and maybe even asking questions or making interpretations based on the meaning of his or her theoretical orientation). Child-centered play therapists are just going to go along tracking behavior, reflecting the feelings that are communicated through the client's nonverbal behavior, returning responsibility to any nonverbal requests for help or decision making, limiting in passive voice when clients start to silently violate playroom rules, and so on. Adlerian play therapists are going to be thinking about (and probably doing some limited metacommunication about) the purpose of the client's silence, especially with clients who usually talk while they play. Gestalt play therapists are going to be wondering if the client's silence indicates that the client is in contact with his or her own internal process, or if it is some kind of disconnection to the environment of the playroom. Jungian and psychodynamic play therapists will consider if the silence is actually some kind of resistance to the therapeutic process or if it is just the client's level of absorption in and comfort with the playing and the therapist. Narrative play therapists are going to look to the client's play for a story that is emerging without words, and if there doesn't seem to be one, they might make up a story to go along with the play and speak it for the child. Most of the time, Theraplay therapists and ecosystemic play therapists are going to be actively engaged with the client, so they would seldom feel the need to do anything with the silence. Integrative/prescriptive play therapists would . . . well, you know . . . it depends.

One thing we believe is essential in dealing with a client who doesn't talk, no matter your theory: you must avoid doing anything to suggest that there is anything wrong with not talking. This means you need to avoid suggesting that the client "should" talk or ask questions designed to trick the client into talking. It is also important to look at your own "stuff" if you are uncomfortable with a client who doesn't talk in a session. There are many play therapists (and other therapists too) who are uncomfortable with silence. We want to remind you that silence is perfectly acceptable. Your job is to convey acceptance to the client—if the client is silent and you are uncomfortable with that silence, that is your problem, not the client's, so be careful to avoid taking care of your own needs to the detriment of the client.

THE CLIENT WHO DOESN'T DO ANYTHING

This one is much harder to figure out what to do and is often even more intimidating to new play therapists than a client who plays but doesn't talk. A client who doesn't talk, doesn't play, doesn't move, doesn't do anything—just sits or stands there in your playroom—is daunting, even to experienced play therapists. The first response that comes to our minds is . . . be patient with the client. Don't nudge this client into doing anything—because (maybe) doing nothing is exactly what he or she needs to happen in that moment in that session. If you can manage your own anxiety about the client not doing anything and convey acceptance through both your verbal and your nonverbal communication, this acceptance may be enough to free the client up to be more expressive.

The first thing we always consider is, "what is the purpose of the behavior?" Now, we know this is an Adlerian approach (not surprisingly, given that we are both Adlerian), and it can work for you even if you are not Adlerian. Our response is going to be dependent on what we think the purpose of the behavior is—and there are a lot of possibilities of what it could be. If we think the client is trying to avoid building a relationship and we guess that if we are patient, it might foster trust and lead to an increased level of openness, we rest in the patience while continuing to choose to be present. (We know that it is difficult if you don't get anything back from the client.) If we think the client is trying to show us that we (and whoever sent/brought the client to therapy) can't tell him or her what to do—with the underlying message of "I am in control of myself and you can't make me do anything"—we are also patient, rather than getting into a power struggle about whether the client needs to play or talk. If we think the client is afraid of trying anything because he or she is worried about doing something wrong or making a mistake, we might expand on our opening salvo of "here in the playroom, you can do many of the things you want to do—you can play by yourself, you can ask me to play, you can talk, you can be quiet . . ." as a vehicle to suggest we will be patient and let the client warm up to us and the space. We might do a little tracking, or we might go ahead and play by ourselves in the room, even when the client is not playing (or doing anything else). (Are you getting the general theme that we think the best response to this situation is being patient?)

We recognize that this answer isn't a one-size-fits all, though because there are many factors to take into account, this sitting and being patient plan is totally possible to do if the not-doing-anything lasts part of a session, a whole session, or even a couple of sessions. However, if it lasts session after session after session, you may want to rethink your strategy. The first thing we would consider is whether the form of therapy you are offering is the best option for this particular client. Perhaps the free-form nature of most approaches to play therapy is anxiety-provoking for this particular client, and he or she would be better served by a more directive approach to play therapy (like Theraplay or ecosystemic play therapy). Perhaps this client has experienced so much trauma that a completely different approach to working with clients, like trauma-focused cognitive-behavioral therapy (trauma-focused CBT) or eye movement desensitization and reprocessing (EMDR) might be more appropriate. Perhaps the client is one *who doesn't want a relationship with you (or anyone else)*. Usually, this would be either a client on the autism spectrum, a client who has reactive attachment disorder (RAD), or an adolescent or adult client with borderline personality disorder. When this is the case, sometimes it is better to refer the client to a specialized form of therapy like Autplay (Grant, 2016) or sociodramatic affective-relational intervention (Lerner, Mikami, & Levine, 2011) for clients who fall on the autism spectrum, Theraplay (Booth & Winstead, 2015) for clients with attachment disorder, or dialectical behavior therapy for adolescent or adult clients with borderline personality disorder (Robins & Rosenthal, 2011). If the client was sent to counseling and doesn't want to be there and is refusing to do anything as a form of protest, sometimes a better first step is working with the entire family (rather than the individual client) or with the parents (if the client is a child or teen). If it is an adult client (or a resistant adolescent or older elementary child), it could be that the client is offended by our using play as the therapeutic modality and/or we haven't done a good enough job of explaining why we think play therapy is the best path for his or her healing. If the client feels as though you are being condescending by doing play therapy, not taking his or her struggles seriously enough because you are "just playing," you can either re-explain your reasoning/motivation for doing play therapy or regroup and try another modality first before play. This can also apply to *the client who says he or she is not interested in playing*. With this client, it also might help you to explore whether any of the many exciting resources and fun activities that the client would like to do are at your disposal. Remember, many people have no idea of the vast expanse of possibilities that constitute the repertoire of a play therapist who has read this book. We also want to mention that neither of us has ever had a child client under the age of 10 who said he or she wasn't interested in playing . . . and if you are inventive and allow the possibility of making up activities connected to video games, you probably won't have a client under the age of 15 who declines to consider playing as a viable modality for therapy. Therefore, a client who persists in saying he or she doesn't want to play after all your blandishments of fun things to do as part of the therapeutic process is probably an older adolescent or an adult. It could be that this particular client is not a great candidate for play therapy. (All of us make an occasional error in judging regarding who to introduce to play therapy and who to suggest doing talk therapy.) So, you can always reset your own course and go back to the talking cure with this particular client. If you are locked into doing play therapy with all of your clients, you can always refer.

THE CLIENT WHO DOESN'T KNOW HOW TO PLAY

Every once in a while, you will come across a client who doesn't know how to play. The client may tell you he or she doesn't know how to play; just sit around not doing anything, looking at you expectantly, wondering what to do; refuse to make eye contact; or insist on doing talk therapy despite your offerings of play possibilities. While usually these are adolescents or adults who never learned to play when they were children, sometimes even small children who have lived in restricted circumstances don't know how to play. When you encounter a client who hasn't learned or has forgotten how to play, you can model how to play by playing by yourself in the playroom with the client as your witness; you can invite the client to play with you; you can even have the client watch a video of children or other adults or adolescents playing. Now, if you are nondirective (e.g., child-centered, Jungian, psychodynamic), you will have to consider whether this form of orientation to play is acceptable to you or if it violates your rules about avoiding directing the client. If you follow one of the very directive theories (e.g., ecosystemic or Theraplay), working on teaching the client to play can just be incorporated into the beginning sessions. For the theoretical approaches that make use of teaching as part of the orientation, working with the client on learning to play will come naturally. For the most part, play therapists who come from those approaches would probably invite the client to play with them as a way of teaching the client to play; this is probably the least psychologically risky way to ease into playing would-be board games, followed by perhaps making sand trays. Younger children might be willing to start playing with things that resemble real things they might have seen outside the playroom—like the kitchen area, a tool chest, or the doll house.

THE CLIENT WHO KEEPS DELIBERATELY BREAKING THE RULES

There are lots of different rules in the playroom (depending on your approach to play therapy), and the answer to "how do I deal with a client who keeps deliberately breaking the playroom rules?" is inevitably going to be (*of course*) "It depends." "On what does it depend?" you ask. Part of what it depends on is the kind of rules the client is breaking. There are some absolute rules that we believe you must be strict in enforcing. These are the rules designed to keep clients (and you) safe. It is essential that clients know that it is against the playroom rules to hurt themselves, to hurt you, or to hurt anyone else. This would almost always be the case, no matter what your theory. If you have clients who are not willing to abide by this limit, their difficulties may be too severe for a regular play therapy practice. If it is not possible to keep yourself and a specific client safe, that client might need to be in a hospital or residential setting. We also believe in the absolute rule that the client is not to break toys or deliberately damage the playroom (or trash the room). We consider this issue very important for several reasons. It helps to ground the play therapy setting and relationship in reality (in most settings and relationships, it would not be okay to break things or deliberately destroy things). In addition, it helps to limit the number of possibilities for your countertransference to be activated by a client's destructive tendencies (it is almost impossible to continue to be fully present and unconditionally positively regarding someone who is wreaking havoc on your stuff). And finally, it is demoralizing to clients to have been allowed to physically hurt the play therapist (if the client has a relationship with you and then hurts you, the client will then have to deal with guilt in addition to any of his or her other issues).

However, some aspects of these rules about not hurting self or others and not damaging the play therapy materials and props might be relative in some approaches to play therapy. This is because different schools of thought about play therapy have different rules about what is and what is not okay to do in a playroom (and what constitutes danger to self and others and disrespect to the playroom or the play therapists). It also depends on how the clinician defines harm to self and/or others and damage to the playroom and the things in it. We have both gone to play therapy training sessions and witnessed recordings from other play therapy teachers who let a child client do things (like sweeping everything from every shelf in the room and slamming it onto the floor or using markers to draw on the walls) that we would not allow to occur. You must examine what works for you in the playroom and what you believe you should limit by examining your own rules and values.

We believe it is important to be as consistent and fair in applying rules as you can possibly be—including what you say and how you say it—so that there isn't any question about what the rules in the playroom are. We also think it is a mistake to confuse tolerating behaviors that are not appropriate and being accepting of the child as a person. I (Terry) can convey acceptance to a client at the same time that I set a limit and tell the client that the behavior he or she is about to exhibit is not acceptable in the playroom without any blame or judgment in my nonverbal communication.

If you think that the client is about to do something that should be against the rules, you must initiate some form of limit setting (Gonsher, 2016). No matter what form you use to limit (see Chapter 1), you are going to want to set things up so that the rules are reasonable, respectful, and relevant. The main goal would be to let the client know that he or she is about to do something that is against the rules in your playroom and to use some form of limit-setting—whether it be the passive voice version of child-centered therapy ("The mirror is not for hitting. I can tell you want to hit the mirror, but it is not for hitting. You can hit the chair or the floor, but not the mirror."); the more direct and active voices of cognitive-behavioral play therapy ("I do not allow clients to hit the mirror in the playroom."); or Adlerian play therapy ("It's against the playroom rules to hit the mirror. I can tell you were trying to figure out what I was going to say when you threatened to hit the mirror. I bet you can figure out something that would not be against the playroom rules that you could hit with the hammer.").

Some other, less serious infractions of the rules would include situations in which a client wants to take something from the playroom and keep it, a client who *wants* to leave before the end of his or her session, a client who *tries* to leave the session early, or a client who wants to bring his or her toys into the playroom. (We would like to tell you to "just say no." And there are times when you need to be more flexible about the rules than you are at other times.) Some of these situations that often invoke playroom rules might not bother you in the least. When this is the case, although that behavior might be against the overall rules in the playroom, you can decide to make an exception to the rule. You could either comment that you decided to let the client take the object home, or you could comment that this is one example of a situation in which the rule doesn't apply. For instance, if a client has made something in the session or we have gifted him or her with something small that might have meaning to him or her or a transitional object, it is perfectly acceptable to let the client take it home. There are other situations in which it is important that you set a limit and stick to it. For instance, if the client wants to take and keep one of your very expensive sand tray figures or wants a CD of a song you played in the session, it is probably more appropriate to stick with the general rule that the toys and other things in the playroom stay in the playroom.

With a client who expresses a desire to leave the session early, we both tend to just tell the client how much more time we have left and then restate the limit defining the length of time for the session. Because we are Adlerian (and you don't have to be Adlerian to use this tool), we ask ourselves (and sometimes with older clients we might even ask the client) what the purpose of the behavior is. Sometimes all it takes to settle the client is to acknowledge that you heard that he or she would like to leave early and that it isn't time to leave yet, followed by a guess or tentative hypothesis about the goal of the client's behavior. If the client feels you have heard and understood him or her, many times that is all the client wanted or needed.

If the client escalates a bit and actually tries to leave after you have cycled through these steps, it is often helpful to acknowledge the intensity of the client's urge to leave or even to make a guess about the intensity or purpose of the behavior so that the client feels heard and understands. That might defuse the situation—watch the client's nonverbal communication to figure out what is going on with him or her. It is also a way to assess whether the client really needs to leave (for instance, to go to the bathroom in an emergency situation) or just wants to leave (for instance, because she is bored or doesn't want to be there). If you think the situation does warrant stopping the session early (option 1), you can choose to make the exception to the rule of not leaving the session and escort the client to your waiting room. This can be a great opportunity to have a longer consultation with the client's parent. You can also decide that you really need a respite and let the client leave early just to give yourself a break (option 2). (This is not exactly professional, but it is sometimes the best option if the client is driving you crazy.). With option 3, you can just decide to sit in front of the door to your playroom to make sure that the client won't get out. (Now, if you are as slight as Kristin, this strategy may prove problematic if the client decides to just pick you up and move you out of the way. However, if you are as heavy as Terry, it is very effective—pretty much so, no one is going to move Terry unless she wants to move.)

As for the client bringing toys into the playroom, we have no problem with it, and clients (especially child clients) should be able to bring whatever they want to the session. Having said that, if they bring in things that would distract them from doing the "work" of play therapy, we might limit it. For instance, if clients brought a violent video game on an iPad, we would not let them play that in the session—though we probably would let them bring the toy into the session, with the caveat that we are not going to play the game. You could also decide that you are willing to let clients play with the toys if they bring toys that could be therapeutic into the room. There are other approaches to play therapy, though, that would not let clients bring their own toys to the playroom. Child-centered, Jungian, Theraplay, psychodynamic, and ecosystemic play therapists would not usually allow clients to bring "stuff" into the session in order not to distract from the carefully selected toys they have in the room already.

THE CLIENT WHO WANTS TO SIT ON YOUR LAP

A client who wants to sit on your lap presents a challenge that is often confusing to play therapists. On the one hand, we all know that touch is one way to convey caring and support to another human being. On the other hand, touch can also be retraumatizing for clients who have experienced physical or sexual abuse or frightening to clients when it is unwelcome or unanticipated. Because touch can be a very sensitive topic, the Association for Play Therapy published a position paper on touch (APT, 2015) to help guide play therapists in making decisions about whether to use touch in play therapy sessions. (See Appendix C for specific quotes from the position paper relevant to this topic.)

So, we would take the individual client's history into account and the context of the situation when the client was asking to sit on one of our laps. We would also take into account the client's age ("no one over 6 in my lap") and what we believe are the current needs of the client. We ask ourselves questions such as: "Does the client need special nurturing at this time?" "Does the client need comforting at this moment?" "Is this a tactile/kinesthetic child whose love language is touch?" We often give hugs and high fives. We even occasionally allow younger children to sit on our laps, but we don't let them sit facing us, only with their backs to us. We usually direct these children to sit next to us rather than on our laps. And we would completely limit older elementary (and teen and adult) clients from sitting on laps or any other form of cuddling. If we have a child who needs this closeness, it is often better to include a parent or other family member in your sessions so that the child can get the touch he or she needs in the context of family relationship, which is what you want to foster anyway.

You really have to decide this yourself and consult with the guidelines your particular theoretical orientation has about touch, if it does. For instance, Theraplay therapists and Gestalt play therapists often use touch as part of their therapeutic interventions. It is always essential to talk to parents and guardians (or teachers if you work in a school) if you do occasionally allow touch as a part of building and maintaining the relationship with specific clients.

THE CLIENT WHO HAS A TEMPER TANTRUM DURING YOUR SESSION

This may seem a bit weird to you (and we don't blame you—it is a bit weird), but we kind of like it when a client has a temper tantrum during our sessions. In many cases, the presenting problem for child clients who come to play therapy (and sometimes for teen clients who come too) is some kind of issue with anger or temper. Because, in many cases, the client is getting so much attention in our sessions and is feeling empowered by the play therapy process, we rarely see an example of how tantrums or other forms of the decay of self-regulation unfold, so it is good to be able to actually witness a tantrum and the circumstances that provoked it. (Having said this, we don't deliberately provoke our child clients to get them to throw a tantrum or otherwise lose their ability to self-regulate.) So, sometimes we just reflect feelings, track, and restate content, especially if the tantrum doesn't involve self-harming, threatening to harm someone else, breaking toys, or damaging the property—in order to observe the unfolding of the tantrum and experience something similar to what parents, siblings, and teachers endure. We think you can learn a great deal about the client and interactions with others in his or her world if you get a chance to observe some of the behaviors that are part of the presenting problem. If we want to interrupt a tantrum, we like using a technique I (Terry) learned at a conference from Jane Nelson (personal communication, May 2012). When a child is having a tantrum, we approach the child and say, "Hey, can I have a hug?" In many cases, this request will actually interrupt the tantrum and help the client reset his or her behavior. (This strategy, of course, is predicated by your having decided in the previous challenging situation you are okay with physical touch being part of your play therapy sessions.) If, however, we don't do anything to interrupt the tantrum and the child does not regain self-regulation and the tantrum gets out of control, we would set a limit on any destructive or threatening behavior (after making a guess about the purpose of the behavior). Sometimes it is even necessary to end the session if the client is really out of control. We might even ask a parent to come in and intervene if we think this would be productive. We would also use future sessions to work on the client's self-regulation and deescalation skills.

Other approaches to play therapy might handle this differently, even ending the session early and asking parents to come and retrieve the child so that the play therapist does not have to physically intervene. For Gestalt play therapists, a tantrum would be a chance to observe the layers of personality and the client's contact with the environment; for cognitive-behavioral play therapists, a tantrum would be an opportunity to observe triggering antecedents and to use behavioral intervention strategies to stop the client's behavior or change his or her thinking patterns. Child-centered play therapists would continue to track, restate content, and reflect feelings, limiting if they needed to do so to prevent damage to the playroom or harm to the client or themselves. Narrative therapists would consider the story that the child has made up or is making up about anger or tantrums.

THE CLIENT WHO REFUSES TO LEAVE THE WAITING ROOM TO COME INTO THE PLAYROOM

This is an interesting situation that we both encountered several times in our early years of practice, and it was pretty daunting. We had several ineffective ways of inviting clients back to the playroom, and we both had multiple ways of getting into power struggles about going back to the playroom. We sometimes said things like, "Are you ready to go back?" or "Do you want to go back?" Neither of these works because, with these questions, you are pretending that it is up to them whether to go back to the playroom. If you ask them if they are ready or if they want to go back and they refuse, you are kind of up a creek because if you then try to over-ride their decision, you have already lost credibility with them and their parents. If they don't really have much of a choice whether to go to the playroom, don't ask as if they do. Once they refuse to go, you are stuck with a power struggle. For a time, we were both grappling with this phenomenon. We tried all sorts of things to try to get these clients back to the playroom—bribing, begging, enlisting the parents' help, and so on. None of these things were particularly helpful.

And then both of us (yes, simultaneously and without consulting one another since we started out at very different times) figured out that if we avoided getting into this power struggle in the first place, we would not have to work so hard to get out of it. The first step in the process of dealing with this challenging situation is to reframe for ourselves (and sometimes for the parent) the interaction in the waiting room as part of the process of building a relationship with the client. We playfully inter-act with the client in the waiting room, having fun with the client and his or her parents. We might ask about the weather, we might comment on the child's apparel, we might ask how a favorite team's baseball game went, how the parent's business trip went, how the client did on a spelling test . . . We might even sit and do a puzzle or play tic-tac-toe on some paper in the waiting room. We often talk about all the cool things we have in the playroom, describing our anticipation of how much fun we are going to have there. As we interact in the waiting room, we pay close attention to the client's nonverbal communication so that we can time our suggestion that it is time to go to the playroom in a way that optimizes the chances of compliance with the suggestion. When we believe that the client is likely to be willing to go to the playroom, we use a method we evolved as a different way of delivering the plan for going back to the playroom. It goes something like, "It's time to go back to the playroom." Making a statement of fact based on the assumption that the client is ready to go back is a way to telegraph our conviction that the client is going to be willing to go back to the playroom without a power struggle . . . and that telegraphing works 90% of the time. If you don't think the child is predisposed to consent to go to the playroom, it is often helpful to request that the child's parents accompany you to the playroom. The other thing you can do to circumvent a power struggle about going back to the playroom is to make the journey to the playroom fun—challenge a competitive client to a race, invite the client to skip back to the room, offer to play pitch and catch together as you walk down the hallway, and the like. These strategies will work no matter what your theory is.

THE CLIENT WANTS SOMEONE ELSE TO COME TO THE PLAYROOM

When clients want to bring someone else into the playroom, it is extremely helpful to consider the circumstances and the motivation for this request before you decide how to handle the situation. For a plethora of potential reasons, clients might want to invite someone else into the playroom. The client might be anxious about the play therapy process or about going to an unknown place with an unknown person and want a parent or spouse to accompany him or her. The client could be into control and want to control you and/or the person he or she is proposing join him or her in the playroom. There might be conditions happening in the family that have evoked a clingy response in the client so that he or she wants a parent or sibling to come along. The client might be having such a great time in the playroom that he or she wants to share the experience with someone important. The client might be tired of serving as the symptom-bearer for the family and hope that someone else in the family (or the entire family) will join in the therapeutic process. The client could be tired of just playing alone or with you and want to expand the possible play partners by inviting someone else to come too. Your playroom might be the coolest place the client has ever visited, and so he or she might want to show it off to a friend, sibling, spouse, or parent. (As you can probably guess, a client might have many other reasons to invite someone else into the playroom. These are the ones we thought of off the tops of our somewhat pointy heads; we know you can come up with some of your own if you think about it.)

Unfortunately for our ability to give you concrete suggestions on how to handle this situation, your response should reflect the reason the client has made this request (along with your own rules about this and the guidance of your theoretical approach). (Once again, "It depends!") So, our general guideline for answering such a request is first to make a guess about the purpose of the request and then decide what we want to do with it—this would be the Adlerian play therapy response, and it could work for you even if your approach is not Adlerian. If we have a client who is feeling anxious, we often let him or her invite a family member (usually a parent) to the room to scope it out. Depending on the severity of the anxiety, we may even let the family member stay in the room with us. We are likely to set a timer for a reasonable amount of time the invited guest can stay (usually 10 minutes); then we ask the guest to leave. If the client is still anxious, we often ask the guest to bring a chair into the hallway outside our playroom and sit there so that the anxious client has the ability to check to make sure the visitor is still there. We would also do this when the client is feeling a bit clingy (even when we don't know exactly why the clinginess is occurring). This is often a cue for us to explore what is going on that has resulted in the client feeling insecure. If we suspect the client is trying to control us, control the person being invited to join us in the playroom, or control the situation, we usually decline to let a visitation occur. This way we avoid getting into a power struggle later about when the visitor will leave. In situations in which the client is having a great time and wants to show an important person one of the toys in the playroom, show someone something he or she can do in the playroom, or share how much fun the playroom is with someone else, we will often let the visitor come into the playroom for a predetermined short amount of time. When we believe that the designated client is just a symptom-bearer, we usually suggest (rather strongly) family therapy, in which case we say "Yes!" to lots of someone else's joining us in the playroom. This is also true if we think the client is getting bored or needs a different companion other than just one of us in the room—or we might decide to do group play therapy. This depends on whether or not including someone else in the process is the best therapeutic practice at that particular time with that specific client.

Some of what you decide about this request will depend on your own reaction to the request and your comfort level with having one or more extra people in the playroom. Several of the approaches to play therapy routinely include people in addition to the client in the room. In

Theraplay, the parents and an interpreting therapist will be in the play-room from the very beginning. For an ecosystemic play therapist, having a second (or more) person in the room may be an important part of the therapy process, especially when the client needs to work on social skills and social interactions. Play therapists who subscribe to narrative play therapy sometimes invite other family members or peers into the room for telling the client stories and hearing the client's stories. If a child-centered play therapist believes the family needs filial therapy and the parents are amenable to learning it, he or she will often include parents in sessions in order to have them observe how the therapist interacts with the child. Before an Adlerian play therapist is done with the course of therapy, he or she might include another child (a sibling or friend) in ses-sions as a way to practice skills the child has acquired in the process of the therapeutic relationship.

THE CLIENT WHO SAYS HE OR SHE WANTS YOU TO BE HIS OR HER PARENT

When a client says he or she wants you to be his or her mom or dad (assuming the client is a child or an adolescent), it is heaven for psycho-dynamic and Jungian play therapists and "a challenging situation" for the rest of us. For the psychodynamic play therapist and the Jungian play therapist, when a client expresses a desire to have him or her as a par-ent, it means that the transference process (one of the core therapeutic forces according to these theories) is working. Most of the time, the psy-chodynamic and Jungian play therapist would simply restate the content of the client's statement and reflect the feelings that might underlie this desire. They might also do some interpretation of why the client wants to become their child. Those of us who subscribe to the other approaches to play therapy would probably use those very same skills with a young play therapy client, but it wouldn't usually mean the same thing to us. We would be likely to want to understand what lay beneath the child's desire to adopt us as a parent, but we might or might not ask some ques-tions or make some guesses about it. Adlerian, cognitive-behavioral, and Gestalt play therapists would probably ask a question or make a guess about it. Theraplay therapists would probably ignore the statement or use the statement as a way to build a bridge between the child and his or her own parent(s) by pointing out that the parent(s) are engaged in learning the kinds of interactional skills demonstrated by the therapist in their sessions. Child-centered play therapists would usually simply restate the content and reflect a feeling without making an interpretation, though sometimes they might try to enlarge the meaning of the statement.

If you were a psychodynamic play therapist working with an adoles-cent who made this kind of comment, this would still probably be an indication of transference successfully happening and the therapist would either reflect feelings or make some interpretations related to the transference process. With the other approaches to play therapy, this kind of comment could easily lead the therapist to suggest that the client engage in a role play, an art project, a sand tray experiment, a movement activity, or a conversation about what the adolescent wants in a parent and other topics related to the desire to have the therapist become his or her parent. If you have an adult client who says something like this, you could do the same kind of activity, though it would be relatively unusual for an adult to make such a comment.

THE CLIENT WHO ASKS
UNCOMFORTABLE QUESTIONS

Clients ask several different types of questions: ongoing process questions, personal questions, practical questions, and relationship questions (Kottman, 2011). For the most part, ongoing process questions and practical questions would not usually be uncomfortable for you. These are questions like "How long does play therapy usually take?" "Do you have any more paint?" "What time is it?" "Do you have other teens as play therapy clients?" Most play therapists (with the exception of child-centered play therapists who tend to avoid answering questions by reflecting the feeling of curiosity or returning responsibility to the child) simply answer those types of questions.

It is more personal questions (such as "Do you have any children?" "Are you married?" "Do you have sex with your husband?" "Where do you live?" "How much money do you make?") and relationship questions (such as "Do you like me better than your other clients?" "Do you love me?" "Do you think about me when I am not here?" "Would you like to have sex with me?") that are sometimes uncomfortable for play therapists. Clients who ask the therapist uncomfortable personal and relationship questions present a dilemma for most play therapists. On the one hand, it makes sense for clients to be curious about the life of someone who is learning a great deal about them, and it makes an equal amount of sense for them to ask questions about how the play therapist feels about their relationship. On the other hand, it is important to be professional and avoid letting the client cross boundaries by expecting answers about personal matters. Lots of times questions about the relationship just reflect clients' insecurities and, although they might be uncomfortable for the play therapist to answer, they can often be addressed in a way that is both therapeutic and nonthreatening.

No matter what your theory, it is important to set limits for inappropriate questions. However, each of you will have to decide for yourself what you think is appropriate and inappropriate. Part of the process of figuring this out is to consider different factors that might move a question into the "inappropriate" territory. We tend to think about the age of the client, the nonverbals that accompany a question, and the context in which the question is asked. When young children ask personal questions or questions about the relationship, this is usually more innocent and less likely to be inappropriate than personal questions from teen and adult clients. It could easily be kind of creepy for an adult or adolescent client to ask if we were married or about our sex lives. If a client asks a question with a leer and a wink, even if it is a younger child, that would feel more inappropriate than if they ask it with a straight face. If you were processing sexual abuse with a child client (or an adult or adolescent client, for that matter) or difficulty in sexual relationships with a teen or adult client, the context of a super-personal question would move it into the realm of "inappropriate." Regardless of your theory, you will want to firmly (but without nonverbals that imply judgment or blame) set a limit on these kinds of questions by saying something like, "That is a question I do not feel comfortable answering." "That's private." or "I always choose not to answer that kind of question." If you think the client's purpose in asking the question is to embarrass or create discomfort, it might also be helpful to make a guess about it by saying something like, "I am thinking that you wanted to embarrass me so you asked a question you knew I would feel uncomfortable about" or something like that.

For the psychodynamic and Jungian play therapist, if the client wants to learn more about his or her therapist's life or asks about their relationship, this may be another sign that transference is happening. Therapists from those approaches almost always choose to avoid answering questions because knowing the answers might interfere with the client's transference. Once again, the therapist would restate content, reflect a feeling, and then set a limit by informing the client that he or she would choose not to answer the question. They might answer appropriate questions about the relationship though, usually with a simple reassurance that they have warm feelings toward the client.

Most other approaches to play therapy would do something similar in response to uncomfortable personal questions—acknowledge that the client asked a question, reflect a feeling, then set a limit by communicating that inappropriate personal questions will not be answered. It might also be important in some cases (especially with older elementary-age children, adolescents, and adult clients) to use immediacy to communicate that the question was too personal and/or uncomfortable. It is a bit tricky to point out that the question was inappropriate without conveying blame, shame, or judgment. This is essential so that your choosing not to answer the question will not damage the relationship you have worked to build. In Adlerian play therapy, we would do the same things as play therapists from other schools of thought, and we would also make a guess about the purpose of the question (e.g., finding out more about us, shocking us with the nature of the query, working to make a connection).

With appropriate personal questions and with most relationship-oriented questions, most play therapists, other than those who use transference as a major part of the therapeutic process, would just go ahead and answer them. With questions such as "What's your favorite color?" "Do you live here in town?" Do you like me?" "Am I important to you?" "Do you miss me when I am not here?" most play therapists (again, with the exception of many child-centered play therapists, who tend not to answer any questions) would simply give the client the information requested. The trickier questions about the relationships that are not inappropriate but often are uncomfortable are those queries (at least for us they are) that ask for information that would probably not be helpful for the client to know. Queries like "Do you like my dad?" "Am I your favorite kid that you work with?" "Do you think my sister is cuter than I am?" might be more effectively answered with a reflection of a feeling and/or a guess about the purpose of the behavior and a rather vague comment that might (or might not) really answer the question (e.g., "You are curious about how I feel about your dad. You want me to like him." "You want to be my very favorite client. I really care about you." "You would like to be better than your sister in the looks department. You are both very cute." (Sometimes redirection or even deflection can be your friend.)

THE CLIENT WHO POSES A CHALLENGE TO CONFIDENTIALITY

Once in a while a client will challenge the expectations of confidentiality. It's fairly common practice to start play therapy relationships explaining rules and exceptions to confidentiality with parents and child and adolescent clients. Then, several weeks into therapy, the client (usually a teenager) discloses something that makes you go, "Hmmm. Does this disclosure warrant breaking confidentiality?" Sure, there are some obvious ones such as abuse, neglect, and risk of suicide where the answer is, "*Yes,* I do need to break confidentiality and tell the parents." If a situation with a minor client involves clear and imminent danger to the client (such as suicide threats), there is a clear path of action for you to take. This is one of those "safety issues" you would have discussed with the client and his or her parents as a limitation to confidentiality. Working with the child or adolescent client to tell his or her parents (with or without you present) is probably the best course of action because it preserves the chance that the client will not feel betrayed by you and continue to trust you.

We are talking about *"challenging* situations," so, let's think about examples that are less clear cut—like a child who reports or has evidence of self-harm; a teenager who is using prescription medication, alcohol, or illegal drugs; or a teenager who is engaging in sexual intercourse. And, of course, the client doesn't want you to talk to his or her parent about the situation. These situations seem to be one of "the many of the activities adolescents engage in [that] do not rise to the level of reportable behavior" (Behnke & Warner, 2002), so it is going to require a judgment call on your part whether to breach confidentiality and tell the client's parent.

You likely have your own gut reaction about what you "should" do as the therapist in these situations. Both of us have our ideas of what we would want to know if our own children or adolescents disclosed such things in a therapy session. Yet, what we want isn't always what our ethics or laws allow. For instance, while the law varies from state to state, most of the time minor clients do not have the right to consent to treatment. Therefore, they do not have the legal right to restrict their parents' access to information about their treatment, and the legal course of action would be to inform the parents (Behnke & Warner, 2002). What the law says, though, sometimes contradicts what codes of ethics (which stress that the client has the right to confidentiality) say. This puts you on the horns of a dilemma.

So, how do you proceed? Drum roll please . . . it depends. The first thing to do is to clearly identify the problem or dilemma and the potential issues involved. Next, review the relevant ethical guidelines and find out about the applicable laws and regulations. Here are some things we think you should consider: (1) the severity of the disclosure—what is the likelihood someone will become seriously injured or die from the activity? (2) what is the age (chronological and developmental) of the client? (3) what does your professional code of ethics have to say about the issue? and (4) what guidance do state or federal laws provide? Different jurisdictions have different rules about what constitutes an "adult" when it comes to a person's ability to "consent" to sex or engage in substance use. In order to be certain you are complying with the law, it is essential for you to keep informed of both the federal laws and the state laws related to minors, consent for treatment, and confidentiality (Behnke & Warner, 2002; Corey, Corey, & Callanan, 2011).

You should also seek supervision and/or consultation when you are unsure of how to proceed in cases such as these. (We work really hard to avoid using the word "should," *and* this is a time when we are choosing to use it and really mean it.) Talk with a professional therapist in your community or an expert on the particular issue who can help you brainstorm potential courses of action. A child or family lawyer or child advocate will also be able to provide you with legal information about what needs to be reported and what is left to therapists' discretion. Check with your professional organizations about ethics and any perspective they might be able to give about your particular case. Some organizations provide legal services or ethics committees that you can use if you are a member, to help with such dilemmas. Supervision is also a helpful strategy as you differentiate your beliefs and morals from professional standards and laws (Behnke & Warner, 2002; Corey et al., 2011).

Play therapists come from several different disciplines and adhere to the distinct codes of ethics for their particular discipline. To help play therapists with the particular ethical challenges inherent in working with minors, the Association for Play Therapy developed a document that describes best practices for play therapy related to clinical, professional, and legal issues (APT, 2016). (See Appendix C for an excerpt for the best practices document related to this topic.)

All these particular challenging situations seem to be connected to confidentiality and informed consent. Whether you decide to override the wishes of the client in regard to sharing this kind of information with the parent basically depends on what you communicated to both the client and the client's parent in the discussion about confidentiality and the process of obtaining informed consent from the client and the parent. The Best Practices document from APT (2016) has some helpful guidelines when you are considering what to do in these situations. (See Appendix C for excerpts from that document relevant to this challenging situation.)

Obviously, the best way to resolve this type of challenging situation would be to work with the client to talk about the situation with his or her parent directly, which would extricate you from the horns of the dilemma. You can volunteer to participate in this conversation in order to provide a buffer between the client and his or her parents if you think it would help to make the conversation more productive. This resolution would allow you to stay true to your code of ethics, the best practices set out by the APT and the laws of your particular region. These responses are not going to be particularly affected by your theoretical orientation; for this challenging situation other factors trump theory.

THE PARENT WHO WANTS TO JOIN YOU AND THE CHILD IN THE PLAYROOM

Once again, there is no one-size-fits-all answer to this question. Believe it or not, the parent who wants to join you and the child in the playroom is also invoking some legal and ethical issues. A parent who wants to come into the room with a young child client actually has the legal right to do so (and in most states, even an adolescent client has few rights for privacy since the parents are usually the ones who get to give informed consent).

While this is the case, for many child clients (and certainly for most adolescent clients), having a parent in the room will inhibit their ability to be fully themselves, so you will want to consider how you want to handle this situation. According to most codes of ethics, your primary responsibility is to the child client, who has the right to your support for his or her journey toward autonomy. Part of your decision-making process should follow the same model as the previous situation (even though this instance doesn't seem quite so fraught with strong emotions as the client who was cutting).

Before we decide how we want to respond to this request (which is sometimes actually a demand), we always ponder the purpose of the parent's behavior. There are myriad reasons why a parent would want to join you in the playroom. The parent could be enmeshed with the child client and reluctant to part from him or her; the parent could be overprotective and want to hover to make sure you don't do any harm to the child; the parent could be extremely controlling and want to have power over what the child does and says in the playroom; the parent might be anxious about you discovering something from the child during a play session that he or she wants to keep secret. (Again, there could be any number of motives for this particular parental behavior. We came up with this list off the tops of our heads, and depending on your theory, you might come up with a whole plethora of reasons other than those we have generated.)

We tend to tailor our response to the specific parent and child at least partly based on our guesses about the underlying issues that lead to the request. If we think the child would not mind having the parent join us and having the parent in the playroom would not inhibit the process in any way (this is often the case with younger children), we just say yes. Sometimes we even turn this into an opportunity for family play therapy sessions. If we already have the parent in the room, it is a good time to work on the relationship between the child and the parent, to model the way we want parents to interact with the child, and so forth.

With an older elementary child or a teenager, having the parent join a session can be challenging because the client may not want the parent there. Every once in a while, you will even have a younger child who objects to the parent coming into the playroom. Our first line of defense with this issue is to invite the parent to consult with us even before we meet the child client to begin to build a relationship with the parent and to communicate how important the parent is in the process. In that first meeting with the parent, we explain that it is easier to build trust with an individual client without an audience because sometimes the child or adolescent client might need privacy to share things that are difficult to share. It sometimes helps to mention the possibility that a client might be more likely to act out and be uncooperative when there is an audience, and sessions where that happens are a waste of the parent's time and money.

(Remember this whole parent consultation thing? We talked about it in depth in Chapter 8.) We also regularly consult with the parent—usually every time the client comes in. Our firmness about involving the parent often (about 75% if the time, even with super-controlling parents) serves as a preemptive strike, and the parent doesn't even ask to join us in the playroom. If the parent insists on joining us, we may try to finesse his or her intention by asking the child to give the parent a tour of the room before the parent goes into the waiting room as we remind the parent about confidentiality and our intention to share important information with him or her during the consultation. At the end of the day, the parent does have the legal right to be in your sessions (depending on the age of the child and the laws in your state—some teens in some states do have the right of refusal; check your state laws). (Have we mentioned turning this challenging situation into the possibility of family sessions? We still think that might be the best approach in this situation.)

THE PARENT (OR TEACHER) WHO DOESN'T FOLLOW THROUGH WITH YOUR RECOMMENDATIONS

This problem is almost exactly the opposite from that of the parent who wants to participate in every session—the parent who not only doesn't follow through with your suggestions for improved ways of dealing with his or her child, but also drops the child off and says (either implicitly or explicitly) "Fix my kid. Don't jack with me." You already know how to engage parents in the process. (We talked about this at great length in Chapter 8.) This challenging situation is more focused on how to handle parents who say they want to make a difference with their children, are willing to make some changes in their interactions with them, and then do not act in accordance with your suggestions. A similar problem is deciding how to respond to parents who hear what you have to say and then vehemently disagree with you—disparaging your advice and expertise.

After years (literally) of experimentation, we have decided that the best way to handle the situation with parents saying they are going to follow through with your suggestion and then not doing it is the good old-fashioned counseling confrontation: "you say this, and you are doing this . . . and they don't match up." By pointing out the discrepancy in what parents are doing and saying, you can sometimes spur them into compliance.

There are times when this approach works and times when it doesn't. With those who don't then jump on the bandwagon and abide by their agreement to make changes, you have several choices. One path would be to continue to work with the child client, knowing that the parents (and/or the family) are probably not going to make the changes you have suggested—doing the best you can to help the child without support from home. Another path would be to suggest to the parents that, if they are not going to be on board with making the changes you suggest, then perhaps you are not the best therapist for the child and you should move toward termination. An alternative route would be to suggest family play therapy. (Yes, that again—it really does work well.) Another path would be to up the ante and make predictions to the parent about the future course of the child's life (and the life of the family) if conditions in the family persist in the way they have been going. (There are certainly other ways to handle this situation, but these are our best offerings.)

You would probably start with the confrontation regardless of your theory, but your theoretical orientation might impact what else you would do. If you are child-centered, you would probably focus on the feelings of the parent. Gestalt play therapists might do this, or they could focus on the bodily sensations or physical reactions of the parent as he or she listens to their recommendations. A cognitive-behavioral play therapist would use some kind of reinforcement schedule to work with the parents on increasing their compliance with suggestions. Getting the story of the parent from the parent (about being a parent, making changes, and so forth) would be important if you were a narrative play therapist. Adlerian play therapists would be trying to figure out the lifestyle of the parent and making guesses about the purpose of their refusal to cooperate with recommendations. If you are a Jungian or psychodynamic therapist, you would be considering the intrapersonal and interpersonal dynamics of the parent and the impact of transference on his or her response to you. Eco-systemic play and Theraplay therapists would reiterate their explanations of the necessity of parent involvement in successful therapeutic processes.

If you have parents who are actively hostile toward your suggestions or defensive in response to parenting recommendations or advice, this is a horse of a different color—even more challenging to those of you (like both of us) who assiduously avoid situations in which people are angry with you. Again (we know you must be tired of this, but it really is the key to so many of these difficult situations), the first thing for you to consider would be the intrapersonal and interpersonal dynamics of the parents, especially if you are following the Adlerian, Jungian, psychodynamic, Gestalt, or ecosystemic paths. We tend to lead with reflecting feelings with this kind of reaction from parents, use active listening to convey that we are interested in their thoughts and attitudes, and only then do we move into making guesses about what is "underneath" the reaction. It is also helpful to explore what they do not like about our suggestions as a bridge to coming up with some proposals they might think were more acceptable. We like to give parents several different recommendations at the same time so that they don't feel trapped or pressured into doing something that is uncomfortable for them.

Often you have less leverage with teachers than you do with parents because teachers are generally less invested in the child making changes. Again, we use confrontation with those who say they are going to follow through with our suggestions and then don't, and we reflect feelings and use active listening skills with teachers who are angry or defensive. Sometimes the best way to handle this situation is to report to the client's parents that the teacher is not willing to cooperate with you, and to ask the parents to handle things with the school to pressure the teacher to join in the efforts to help the child.

THE TEACHER/PARENT WHO WANTS TO KNOW WHAT HAPPENS IN YOUR SESSIONS

The first part of this is easy to answer . . . teachers do not have the right to know anything other than what you choose to share with them. (And in order to share anything at all with them, you need a release of information from the parent or guardian.) When we do teacher consultation (which we do fairly often with teachers of child clients who are struggling in school), we tend to talk about patterns we see and we ask the teacher about patterns at school (Kottman & Meany-Walen, 2016). In addition, we make suggestions about how teachers can be more encouraging and supportive of the child. (Many times, when working with adolescent clients who are struggling in school because they have so many different teachers, we get permission to consult with the school counselor or with specific teachers whom the client and/or parent thinks could be helpful.)

Working with parents who want to know everything that happens in your sessions is a bit trickier. Because, again, parents are the ones with the legal right to give consent, they also have the legal right to know what happens in your sessions, depending on the age of the client (Association for Play Therapy, 2016; Behnke & Warner, 2002; Corey et al., 2011). We handle this situation in a similar fashion to how we handle the situation in which the parent wants to join us in the playroom. As we said in Chapter 1, we usually start our time with child and adolescent clients by telling them that we will not talk to parents about exactly what happens (the things they say and do) in their sessions, but that we will consult with parents about patterns we observe and we will have suggestions for parents about better ways to understand and support them. If warranted, we often find it helpful to tell clients that if they have something they specifically want us to tell parents, we will be happy to be their advocates. (Notice we said this is what we usually do because sometimes we have to adjust to the personalities and demands of parents.)

If in a first session, parents telegraph that they aren't going to fall for our preemptive strike of explaining that it takes a trained professional to understand what play means and that we would love to talk to them about patterns in the child's behavior, thinking, feelings, and attitudes, help them understand why their child acts that way, teach them more constructive ways of communicating and interacting with their child, and so forth and so on, we might have to tell them what they want to know. Since we try really hard not to lie to our child and adolescent clients, if we have a premonition that these are parents who are going to insist on the truth, the whole truth, and nothing but the truth, we don't tell these clients we won't tell their parents what they say and do in a session. And sometimes we misjudge, and we have to go back to a client and confess that we have to tell the parents everything that happens, even though we said we wouldn't. (It stinks when this happens, and it is unavoidable because, after all, parents have the legal right to demand any information about our sessions that they want.) And remember the option of turning sessions into family therapy sessions: that way the parent will know exactly what happened because he or she was a participant.

THE PARENT/TEACHER COMPLAINING ABOUT LACK OF PROGRESS OR THE PARENT/TEACHER WHO DOESN'T SEE PROGRESS EVEN THOUGH YOU DO

Because these two dilemmas are similar, we've wrapped them into one section. We also acknowledge that they can be a bit different, and they might evoke different feelings from the therapist (and the clients). When parents or teachers tell us that they do not notice changes at home, we consider the evidence we know and try to gather other data. Here are some questions we suggest you answer for yourself when this happens:

How long have you been working with the child?
What are the presenting issues and contributing factors?
What are the parent's or teacher's expectations?
Are the expectations reasonable?
Have you explained reasonable expectations to the adult?
Is the child coming to therapy as scheduled?
If the child has not been coming to therapy as scheduled, why not (illness, transportation issues, conflict of schedule, forgetfulness)?
What is the relationship between you and the adult?
Does the adult trust you and like you?
Are you meeting regularly with the parent or teacher?
Have you given suggestions or information for the parent or teacher to use outside of session?
Are you following up with those suggestions and the information?
Is the parent or teacher trying the suggestions and employing the information?

Therapists know (or have learned over time) that therapy is not a quick fix. Clients don't always know this. It is also very helpful in this situation to do some teaching of the parent or teacher so that he or she knows what to consider in thinking about whether the client is making progress. Often these adults are looking for miracle cures, and really what they are going to get is often slow, slow, slow (and perhaps steady or perhaps one step forward followed by a half step backwards). You'll also want to educate parents and teachers about your guesses about the length of therapy. Different presenting issues have different challenges that influence the length of therapy. Trauma (single episode or ongoing), family dynamics, family and personal resources or resiliency, among many, many other factors, contribute to the length of treatment. Explore the expectations of the person who reports not seeing changes. It is often helpful to talk to parents about how important it is to come to therapy on a regular basis. Explain to them that disruption in therapy services can create significant delays in progress or lead to ineffective therapy. Inconsistent attendance may also be a sign of new or ongoing stressors at home that need to be explored and addressed.

As we've harped on before in this book, the relationship with the significant adults in a child or adolescent client's life is essential. Belief and hope in the counseling process often influences the effectiveness of therapy. In addition to building a relationship with the client, building a relationship with caregivers is crucial. In our experience, when a parent doesn't feel connected to the therapist, the parent discontinues therapy or complains a great deal. However, if parents are court-ordered to take a child or adolescent client to therapy, they have little recourse but to continue in therapy with a therapist they don't particularly like or trust. We recommend assessing the adult–therapist relationship and building, rebuilding, or improving this relationship in order to better help the child, family, and classroom.

A slightly more complicated, but not completely different, issue arises when the therapist notices changes in the playroom but the adult reports no changes. This is not unusual, and we start by asking the questions we've already outlined. We also suggest that the therapist take a look at what might be unique in the therapy room that isn't or can't happen at home or school. For example, a client gets one-on-one attention with the therapist. Is this possible, even in short bursts, outside of the therapy? We also consider what is contributing to the in-session change that could help out-of-session. Therapists might notice that a client responds really well to choices and encouragement but does not respond well to demands. It could be that a client is able to follow through on single- or double-order tasks but cannot manage tasks with three or more directives at a time. Maybe a client has a unique perspective and ways of going about an activity that is atypical for other children his or her age. It will be helpful to educate the parent or teacher about these things in order to help make things go better at home and in the classroom. Once the adult has made some of these shifts, there is a good chance that he or she will start noticing progress too.

The other thing that can help boost the parent's or teacher's perception of progress is to revisit the goals you set up at the beginning (and of course, in an ongoing way throughout the therapeutic process). Does the adult remember what these goals were? Were those goals reasonable? Has the adult changed the scope of the goals without telling you about it? Sometimes adults involved in a child or adolescent client's life forget what the original goals were or changed the goals along the way, sometimes without sharing those shifts with you. If this is the case, the parent or teacher might be measuring progress against a standard that is radically different from the standard you are using. When this happens, you might want to work to realign goals with them to make sure you are all evaluating the growth of the client with the same yardstick.

Adults also might need alternative perspectives about a client's behaviors. A child or adolescent described as demanding might be reframed as showing leadership potential or being self-determined. An adolescent who is messy might be creative. A child who is rambunctious could be a future athlete. Sharing your professional opinions and observations about the client and what you notice in session can be the turning point needed to help the parent and teacher perceive the client differently, interact with the client differently, and help the client be successful in the home or classroom.

THE FAMILY WHERE YOU MUST MAKE A CHILD PROTECTIVE SERVICE CALL

Many counselors agree that making a call to CPS is not the most pleasant part of their job, especially when the alleged offender is a client's family member. Counselors will also agree that it's necessary and important. Every state in the United States has laws about reporting child abuse and neglect. You should know the laws in your state and follow the guidelines set out by CPS. Ultimately, this is an ethical and legal decision, as you have a duty to protect *and* you are compromising rights to confidentiality. A few things to remember as you make the call: (1) if you suspect the possibility of abuse or neglect, you *must* make the call and (2) it is not your job to investigate. Leave the investigation to the investigators; that's their job. Regardless of if you tell (or don't tell) the parents that you're making a report, you might need to work with the child and/or other supports to create a safety plan to avoid continued abuse.

Okay, so you've made the call to CPS, and now you have to consider what this means for the client, the family, and your relationship with both. You have several options. You can tell the family that you are making the call, *and* you can decide to not tell the family that you are making the call. You will make this determination based on what you believe is in the best interest of the child. For some clients we have told families, and for other clients we have not told families (sometimes making the right decision and sometimes not). We consider the following questions as part of making our decision:

1. What is the evidence that triggered my suspicion?
2. How will it help the child if I do (or don't) tell the family that I'm making the report?
3. Is the child in more danger if I tell the parents that I'm making a report?
4. What is my reasoning for telling (or not telling) the family?
5. Who is the alleged offender (parent, sibling, relative)? And, does that make a difference in my decision to tell the family?
6. Might the family withdraw from counseling if I disclose that I am making a report?
7. How might I respond when/if the parents or child asks if I made a report?

Supervision or consultation is a wise idea during these circumstances. Processing with and receiving feedback from other professionals can help determine a safe course of action for both you and your client. Supervision helps you to consider the best course of action for your client and to see areas that you might not have considered otherwise. It also provides you with support in the event you are called to court or questioned about your decision to report *or* you decide not to report because you believe that what happened did not meet the standards for reporting set out by CPS in your location.

THE ADOLESCENT OR ADULT CLIENT WHO WANTS TO WOO YOU

Imagine your current or future line of work for a moment. You devote an uninterrupted, regular period of time to clients (either as individuals or as members of a family) on a regular basis. You communicate your understanding of their unique assets and challenges. You completely accept them as they are and help them to be the best version of themselves. You provide encouragement and empathy as they become vulnerable. What an amazing (and potentially seductive) relationship. No wonder that sometimes clients want to woo you.

By creating this kind of a relationship, it's not surprising that a client could develop an attraction to you. As flattering as it may be for a young adult, adult, or parent of a child client to express a romantic or sexual interest in you, it is completely, unequivocally, certainly, undoubtedly, positively, always inappropriate to reciprocate or encourage romantic or sexual attention from a client. (Do not do it!)

How to handle such a situation is not as clear-cut to figure out as it is to know not to respond positively to a client's sexual or romantic interest. There are a few ways to go about this that we'll discuss here. (And there are many more ways that we don't address here—use your imagination and creativity in saying "absolutely not.") In the spirit of preventing the development of this kind of challenging situation, we advise you to initially consider your boundaries and what you're willing to share with your clients and to be intentional in your interactions with your clients. For example, we usually give out our cell phone numbers to clients in case of emergency or to make last-minute appointment changes. However, we put firm boundaries in place during our first conversation with adolescent and adult clients and parents of clients that we do not do phone sessions and we do not respond to texts or calls in the evening or weekends. Both of us are fairly charismatic, and our natural behavior could be interpreted as being flirtatious at times, but we are not: we work hard to be kind, relational, fun, playful, *and* professional with clients without flirting with them.

Even though you may lay all of the necessary groundwork, things can still happen. Let's say a teen or an adult client or a client's parent still pursues you despite your clear boundaries. It is important that you are direct and firm about your position to not engage in a romantic or sexual relationship. You can explain your code of ethics or state laws about the rules that clearly outline the prohibition of engaging in such relationships. Even if the client seems to respect your limits connected to the code of ethics, you might have additional issues to consider regarding this challenging situation. You need to consider how this revelation impacts the therapeutic relationship between you and the client; if and how this attraction could be a part of the presenting issue (e.g., unfaithful relationships, dependency on others, dissatisfaction in marriage or partnership, low self-esteem or self-concept, sexually disruptive behaviors, inability/ unwillingness to navigate appropriate social relationships); your feelings toward your client (e.g., are you also interested in his or her proposal? Are you flattered by this attention? Are you repelled by his or her attraction?); and the age and maturity of the client. In the case of a parent coming on to you, you will also want to consider the relationship you've developed with the child. (Not that any of these factors will sway your decision to not engage, but they can help you determine how to respond.)

In most cases, it is helpful to have a very direct conversation with the client or parent about the inappropriateness of a relationship outside of counseling. In this conversation, your ethics and the law can provide the structure for turning down the invitation, but they do not speak to the dynamics that need to be addressed. You will need to develop a way to talk about those dynamics based on the particular client or parent. We suggest starting by reflecting the client's feelings or making a guess about the goals of his or her behavior. You can even normalize the client's feelings (because if you are creating all of the elements of the relationship described in the first paragraph of this section, who wouldn't be attracted to you?) It is often helpful to succinctly explain your reasons for turning him or her down (ethics, relationship, mental health, manipulation, respect for client, etc.). It is probably not necessary to speculate about whether or not you'd reconsider under other circumstances. (Actually, don't do that either; it's not important and it doesn't matter!). Follow up by having a conversation with the client about what to do next. Does your client need a referral to a different therapist? Can the two of you overcome this awkwardness? Do each of you need time to consider what to do next? Does anyone else need to be informed (spouse or partner, child, parent)? Perhaps this sounds familiar. It's a lot like limit-setting. State the rule, reflect feelings or metacommunicate about the goal of behavior; generate an alternative or a next plan of action. In the event you choose to continue to work together, you might or might not need to bring up this conversation again in the future. (You know . . . it depends.)

MOVING ON . . .

So . . . we know there is lots more to say, but we need to stop or else this book would never get finished. Here's what we have been trying to say throughout the book . . .

- Remember that choosing to truly be present with your play therapy clients is the most important thing you can do to make a difference for them and their lives.
- Let your theory guide your use and the timing of the skills and techniques described in this book.
- Have fun with the skills and the techniques in this book, *and* have fun with your clients.
- Give yourself permission to adapt techniques to meet the needs and interests of your clients.
- Be clear about why you are using specific interventions with particular clients and keep on being intentional with your interventions.
- Keep learning . . . we have barely skimmed the surface of how to do play therapy.
- Always remember that the real essence of being a play therapist is honoring the joy of telling stories and having adventures and dancing and hearing stories and making up songs and building worlds in the sand and doing art and *playing*.

Interlude 9

The Continuing Journey

*A*nd after Zan had learned the stuff about play therapy we had to teach her (at least the stuff in this book), she knew she needed to keep on learning—so she could be with kids (and teens and grown-ups) who were hurting, who were angry, who were sad, who were lonely, who needed to be seen and heard in a language that made sense to them . . . the language of play . . . the language of doing.

APPENDIX A

Theory and Play Therapy Resources

The following list contains our suggested additional resources for you to learn more about the application of the theories we briefly described in Chapter 2. This is not a complete list of resources available. We have attempted to create a list of classic works from the original theorists or other respected experts. The play therapy theory resources are from professionals who created the play therapy application to the specific theory and/or other leaders and experts in that treatment.

ADLERIAN THEORY/ADLERIAN PLAY THERAPY

Adlerian Theory

Adler, A. (1954). *Understanding human nature* (W. B. Wolf, Trans.). New York: Fawcett Premier. (Original work published 1927)

Adler, A. (1958). *What life should mean to you.* New York: Capricorn. (Original work published 1931)

Ansbacher, H., & Ansbacher, R. (Eds.). (1956). *The individual psychology of Alfred Adler: A systemic presentation in selections from his writings.* San Francisco: Harper & Row.

Carlson, J., & Englar-Carson, M. (2017). *Adlerian psychotherapy.* Washington, DC: American Psychological Association.

Maniacci, M. P., Sackett-Maniacci, L., & Mosak, H. H. (2014). Adlerian psychotherapy. In D. Wedding & R. Corsini (Eds.), *Current psychotherapies* (10th ed., pp. 55–94). Belmont, CA: Brooks/Cole.

Mosak, H., & Maniacci, M. (1999). *A primer of Adlerian psychology.* Philadelphia: Brunner/Mazel.

Mosak, H., & Maniacci, M. (2010). The case of Roger. In D. Wedding & R. J. Corsini (Eds.), *Case studies in psychotherapy* (7th ed., pp. 12–31). Belmont, CA: Brooks/Cole.

Sweeney, T. (2105). *Adlerian counseling and psychotherapy* (5th ed.). New York: Routledge.

Watts, R. (2013). Adlerian counseling. In B. Irby, G. Brown, & S. Jackson (Eds.), *The handbook of educational theories for theoretical frameworks* (pp. 459–472). Charlotte, NC: Information Age.

Adlerian Play Therapy

Kottman, T. (1993). The king of rock and roll. In T. Kottman & C. Schaefer (Eds.), *Play therapy in action: A casebook for practitioners* (pp. 133–167). Northvale, NJ: Jason Aronson.

Kottman, T. (2009). Adlerian play therapy. In K. O'Connor & L. Braverman (Eds.), *Play therapy theory and practice: Comparing theories and techniques* (2nd ed., pp. 237–282). New York: Wiley.

Kottman, T. (2011). Adlerian play therapy. In C. Schaefer (Ed.), *Foundations of play therapy* (2nd ed., pp. 87–104). New York: Wiley.

Kottman, T., & Ashby, J. (2015). Adlerian play therapy. In D. Crenshaw & A. Stewart (Eds.), *Play therapy: A comprehensive guide to theory and practice* (pp. 32–47). New York: Guilford Press.

Kottman, T., & Meany-Walen, K. (2016). *Partners in play: An Adlerian approach to play therapy* (3rd ed.). Alexandria, VA: American Counseling Association.

PERSON-CENTERED THEORY/CHILD-CENTERED PLAY THERAPY

Person-Centered Theory

Raskin, N., Rogers, C., & Witty, M. (2014). Client-centered therapy. In D. Wedding & R. Corsini (Eds.), *Current psychotherapies* (10th ed., pp. 95–145). Belmont, CA: Brooks/Cole.

Rogers, C. (1951). *Client-centered therapy: Its current practice, implications and theory.* London: Constable.

Rogers, C. (1959). A theory of therapy, personality and interpersonal relationships as developed in the client-centered framework. In S. Koch (Ed.), *Psychology: A study of a science: Vol. 3. Formulations of the person and the social context.* New York: McGraw-Hill.

Rogers, C. R. (1961). *On becoming a person: A psychotherapist's view of psychotherapy.* New York: Houghton Mifflin.

Rogers, C. R., Stevens, B., Gendlin, E. T., Shlien, J. M., & Van Dusen, W. (1967). *Person to person: The problem of being human: A new trend in psychology.* Lafayette, CA: Real People Press.

Child-Centered Play Therapy

Axline, V. (1969). *Play therapy* (rev. ed.). New York: Ballantine Books.

Landreth, G. L. (2012). *Play therapy: The art of the relationship* (3rd ed.). New York: Brunner-Routledge.

Ray, D. C. (2011). *Advanced play therapy: Essential conditions, knowledge, and skills for child practice.* New York: Routledge.

VanFleet, R., Sywaluk, A., & Sniscak, C. (2010). *Child-centered play therapy.* New York: Guilford Press.

COGNITIVE-BEHAVIORAL THEORY/ COGNITIVE-BEHAVIORAL PLAY THERAPY

Cognitive-Behavioral Theory

Beck, A. (1976). *Cognitive therapy and the emotional disorders.* New York: Meridian.

Burns, D. (1999). *Feeling good: The new mood therapy.* New York: New American Library.

Ellis, A. (2000). Rational emotive behavior therapy. In R. J. Corsini & D. Wedding (Eds.), *Current psychotherapies* (6th ed., pp. 168–204). Itasca, IL: F. E. Peacock.

Meichenbaum, D. (1986). Cognitive behavior modification. In F. H. Kanfer & A. P. Goldstein (Eds.), *Helping people change: A textbook of methods* (pp. 346–380). New York: Pergamon Press.

Cognitive-Behavioral Play Therapy

Cavett, A. M. (2015). Cognitive-behavioral play therapy. In D. A. Crenshaw & A. L. Stewart (Eds.), *Play therapy: A comprehensive guide to theory and practice* (pp. 83–98). New York: Guilford Press.

Knell, S. M. (1993). *Cognitive-behavioral play therapy.* Northvale, NJ: Jason Aronson.

Knell, S. M. (1994). Cognitive-behavioral play therapy. In K. O'Connor & C. Schaefer (Eds.), *Handbook of play therapy: Vol. 2. Advances and innovations* (pp. 111–142). New York: Wiley.

Knell, S. M. (2009). Cognitive-behavioral play therapy. In K. J. O'Connor & L. D. Braverman (Eds.), *Play therapy theory and practice: Comparing theories and techniques* (2nd ed., pp. 203–236). Hoboken, NJ: Wiley.

ECOSYSTEMIC PLAY THERAPY

Ecosystemic theory was created specifically for play therapy clients and therapists. There is not an overarching Ecosystemic theory.

O'Connor, K. (1993). Child, protector, confidant: Structured group exosystemic play therapy. In T. Kottman & S. Schaefer (Eds.), *Play therapy in action: A casebook for practitioners* (pp. 245–280). Northvale, NJ: Jason Aronson.

O'Connor, K. (2009). Ecosystemic play therapy. In K. J. O'Connor & L. D. Braverman (Eds.), *Play therapy theory and practice: Comparing theories and techniques,* (2nd ed., pp. 367–450). Hoboken, NJ: Wiley.

O'Connor, K. (2011). Ecosystemic play therapy. In C. E. Schaefer (Ed.), *Foundations of play therapy* (2nd ed., pp. 253–272). Hoboken, NJ: Wiley.

O'Connor, K. (2016). Ecosystemic play therapy. In K. O'Connor, C. Schaefer, & L. Braverman (Eds.), *Handbook of play therapy* (2nd ed., pp. 194–225). Hoboken, NJ: Wiley.

O'Connor, K., & Ammen, S. (2013). *Play therapy treatment planning and interventions: The Ecosystemic model and workbook.* Waltham, ME: Academic Press.

GESTALT THERAPY/GESTALT PLAY THERAPY

Gestalt Theory

Perls, F. (1970). Four lectures. In J. Fagan & I. L. Shepherd (Eds.), *Gestalt therapy now* (pp. 14–38). New York: Harper.

Perls, F., Hefferline, R. F., & Goodman, P. (1951). *Gestalt therapy: Excitement and growth in the human personality.* New York: Crown.

Gestalt Play Therapy

Carroll, F. (2009). Gestalt play therapy. In K. J. O'Connor & L. D. Braverman (Eds.), *Play therapy theory and practice: Comparing theories and techniques* (2nd ed., 283–314). Hoboken, NJ: Wiley.

Carroll, F., & Oaklander, V. (1997). Gestalt play therapy. In K. O'Connor & L. Braverman (Eds.), *Play therapy theory and practice: A comparative presentation* (pp. 184–203). New York: Wiley.

Oaklander, V. (1992). *Windows to our children: A Gestalt approach to children and adolescents.* New York: Gestalt Journal Press. (Original work published 1978)

Oaklander, V. (1994). Gestalt play therapy. In K. O'Connor & C. Schaefer (Eds.), *Handbook of play therapy* (pp. 142–156). New York: Wiley.

Oaklander, V. (2003). Gestalt play therapy. In C. Schaefer (Ed.), *Foundations of play therapy* (pp. 143–155). Hoboken, NJ: Wiley.

Oaklander, V. (2011). Gestalt play therapy. *International Journal of Play Therapy, 10,* 45–55.

Oaklander, V. (2015). Short-term Gestalt play therapy for grieving children. In H. Kaduson & C. Schaefer (Eds.), *Short-term play therapy for children* (3rd ed., pp. 28–52). New York: Guilford Press.

JUNGIAN THEORY/JUNGIAN PLAY THERAPY

Jungian Theory

Douglas, C. (2008). Analytical psychotherapy. In R. J. Corsini & D. Wedding (Eds.), *Current psychotherapies* (8th ed., pp. 107–140). Belmont, CA: Brooks/Cole.

Jung, C. G. (1969). Synchronicity: A causal connecting principle. In G. Adler, M. Fordham, W. McGuire, & H. Read (Eds.), & R. F. C. Hull (Trans.), *The collected works of C. F. Jung* (Vol. 8, pp. 419–519). Princeton, NJ: Princeton University Press.

Jungian Play Therapy

Allan, J. (1988). *Inscapes of the child's world: Jungian counseling in schools and clinics.* Dallas, TX: Springer.

Allan, J. (1997). Jungian play psychotherapy. In K. J. O'Connor & L. M. Braverman (Eds.), *Play therapy: A comparative presentation,* (2nd ed., pp. 100–130). New York: Wiley.

Allan, J., & Levin, S. (1993). "Born on my bum": Jungian play therapy. In T. Kottman & C. Schaefer (Eds.), *Play therapy in action: A casebook for practitioners* (pp. 209–244). Northvale, NJ: Jason Aronson.

Green, E. (2009). Jungian analytical play therapy. In K. O'Connor & L. Braverman (Eds.), *Play therapy theory and practice: Comparing theories and techniques* (2nd ed., pp. 100–139). Hoboken, NJ: Wiley.

Lilly, J. P. (2015). Jungian analytic play therapy. In D. Crenshaw & A. Stewart (Eds.), *Play therapy: A comprehensive guide to theory and practice* (pp. 48–65). New York: Guilford Press.

Peery, J. C. (2003). Jungian analytical play therapy. In C. E. Schaefer (Ed.), *Foundations of play therapy* (pp. 14–54). Hoboken, NJ: Wiley.

Punnett, A. (2016). Psychoanalytic and Jungian play therapy. In K. O'Connor, C. Schaefer, & L. Braverman (Eds.), *Handbook of play therapy* (2nd ed., pp. 61–92). Hoboken, NJ: Wiley.

NARRATIVE THEORY/NARRATIVE PLAY THERAPY

Narrative Theory

White, M. (2007). *Maps of narrative practice.* New York: Norton

White, M., & Epston, D. (1990). *Narrative means to therapeutic ends.* New York: Norton.

Zimmerman, J., & Dickerson, V. (1996). *If problems talked: Narrative therapy in action.* New York: Guilford Press.

Narrative Play Therapy

Cattanach, A. (2006). Narrative play therapy. In C. Schaefer & H. Kaduson (Eds.), *Contemporary play therapy: Theory, research, and practice* (pp. 82–99). New York: Guilford Press.

Cattanach, A. (2008). *Narrative approaches tin play therapy with children.* Philadelphia: Jessica Kingsley.

Mills, J. (2015). StoryPlay: A narrative play therapy approach. In D. Crenshaw & A. Stewart (Eds.), *Play therapy: A comprehensive guide to theory and practice* (pp. 171–185). New York: Guilford Press.

Mills, J., & Crowley, R. (2014). *Therapeutic metaphors for children and the child within* (2nd ed.). New York: Routledge.

Taylor de Faoite, A. (2011). *Narrative play therapy: Theory and practice.* Philadelphia: Jessica Kingsley.

PSYCHODYNAMIC THEORY/PSYCHODYNAMIC PLAY THERAPY

Psychodynamic Theory

Freud, S. (1949). *An outline of psycho-analysis* (J. Strachey, Trans.). New York: Norton.

Safran, J. D., & Kriss, A. (2014). Psychoanalytic psychotherapies. In D. Wedding & R. J. Corsini (Eds.), *Current psychotherapies* (10th ed., pp. 19–54). Belmont, CA: Brooks/Cole.

Psychodynamic Play Therapy

Cangelosi, D. (1993). Internal and external wars: Psychodynamic play therapy. In T. Kottman & C. Schaefer (Eds.), *Play therapy in action: A casebook for practitioners* (pp. 347–370). Northvale, NJ: Jason Aronson.

Mordock, J. B. (2015). Psychodynamic play therapy. In D. Crenshaw & A. Stewart (Eds.), *Play therapy: A comprehensive guide to theory and practice* (pp. 66–82). New York: Guilford Press.

Punnett, A. (2016). Psychoanalytic and Jungian play therapy. In K. O'Connor, C. Schaefer, & L. Braverman (Eds.), *Handbook of play therapy* (2nd ed., pp. 61–92). Hoboken, NJ: Wiley.

THERAPLAY

Theraplay is an approach to play therapy based on theories of attachment. It is not an independent theory.

Theraplay

Booth, P., & Jernberg, A. (2010). *Theraplay: Helping parents and children build better relationships through attachment-based play* (3rd ed.). San Francisco: Jossey-Bass.

Booth, P., & Winstead, M. (2015). Theraplay: Repairing relationships, helping families heal. In D. Crenshaw & A. Stewart (Eds.), *Play therapy: A comprehensive guide to theory and practice* (pp. 141–155). New York: Guilford Press.

Booth, P., & Winstead, M. (2016). Theraplay: Creating secure and joyful attachment relationships. In K. O'Connor, C. Schaefer, & L. Braverman (Eds.), *Handbook of play therapy* (2nd ed., pp. 164–194). Hoboken, NJ: Wiley.

Bundy-Myrow, S., & Booth, P. B. (2009). Theraplay: Supporting attachment relationships. In K. J. O'Connor & L. D. Braverman (Eds.), *Play therapy theory and practice: Comparing theories and techniques* (2nd ed., pp. 315–366). Hoboken, NJ: Wiley.

Jernberg, A., & Jernberg, E. (1993). Family Theraplay for the family tyrants. In T. Kottman & C. Schaefer (Eds.), *Play therapy in action: A casebook for practitioners* (pp. 45–96). Northvale, NJ: Jason Aronson.

Koller, T., & Booth, P. (1997). Fostering attachment through family Theraplay. In K. O'Connor & L. M. Braverman (Eds.), *Play therapy theory and application: A comparative presentation*. New York: Wiley.

Munns, E. (2011). Theraplay: Attachment-enhancing play therapy. In C. Schaefer (Ed.), *Foundations of play therapy* (2nd ed., pp. 275–296). Hoboken, NJ: Wiley.

INTEGRATIVE/PRESCRIPTIVE THERAPY

Corey, G. (2017). *Theory and practice of counseling and psychotherapy* (10th ed.). Boston: Cengage.

Jones-Smith, E. (2016). *Theories of counseling and psychotherapy: An integrative approach* (2nd ed.). Los Angeles: SAGE.

Norcross, J. C. (2005). A primer on psychotherapy integration. In J. C. Norcross & M. R. Goldfried (Eds.), *Handbook of psychotherapy integration* (2nd ed., pp. 3–23). New York: Oxford University Press.

Norcross, J. C., & Wampold, B. (2011). What works for whom?: Tailoring psychotherapy to the person. *Journal of Clinical Psychology in Session, 67*(2), 127–132.

INTEGRATIVE/PRESCRIPTIVE PLAY THERAPY

Drewes, A., Bratton, S., & Schaefer, C. (Eds.). (2011). *Integrative play therapy*. Hoboken, NY: Wiley.

Gil, E., Konrath, E., Shaw, J., Goldin, M., & Bryan, H. (2015). Integrative approach to play therapy. In D. Crenshaw & A. Stewart (Eds.), *Play therapy: A comprehensive guide to theory and practice* (pp. 99–113). New York: Guilford Press.

Gil, E., & Shaw, J. (2009). Prescriptive play therapy. In K. J. O'Connor & L. D. Braverman (Eds.), *Play therapy theory and practice: Comparing theories and techniques* (2nd ed., pp. 451–487). Hoboken, NJ: Wiley.

Schaefer, C., & Drewes, A. (2016). Prescriptive play therapy. In K. O'Connor, C. Schaefer, & L. Braverman (Eds.), Handbook of play therapy (2nd ed., pp. 227–240). Hoboken, NJ: Wiley.

APPENDIX B

Children's Books

MALADAPTIVELY PERFECTIONISTIC CHILDREN

Adderholdt, M., & Goldberg, J. (1999). *Perfectionism: What's bad about being too good?* Minneapolis, MN: Free Spirit.

Flanagan Burns, E. (2008). *Nobody's perfect: A story for children about perfectionism.* Washington, DC: Magination Press.

Greenspon, T. S. (2007). *What to do when good enough isn't good enough.* Minneapolis, MN: Free Spirit.

Manes, S. (1996). *Be a perfect person in just three days!* New York: Yearling.

McDonnell, P. (2014). *A perfectly messed-up story.* New York: Little, Brown.

Parr, T. (2014). *It's okay to make mistakes.* New York: Little, Brown.

Pett, M., & Rubinstein, G. (2011). *The girl who never made mistakes.* Naperville, IL: Sourcebooks.

Saltzberg, B. (2010). *Beautiful oops.* New York: Workman.

Shannon, D. (1998). *A bad case of stripes.* New York: Scholastic.

CHILDREN WHOSE PARENTS ARE DIVORCING

Abercrombie, B. (1995). *Charlie Anderson.* New York: Children's Publishing Division.

Brown, M. (1988). *Dinosaurs divorce: A guide for changing families.* New York: Little, Brown.

Coffelt, N. (2011). *Fred stays with me!* New York: Little, Brown.

Franz Ransom, J. (2000). *I don't want to talk about it.* Washington, DC: Magination Press.

Lansky, V. (1997). *It's not your fault, Koko bear: A read-together book for parents and young children during divorce.* Minnetonka, MN: Book Peddlers.

Spelman, C. M. (1998). *Mama and daddy bear's divorce.* Morton Grove, IL: Albert Whitman.

Stern, Z. (2008). *Divorce is not the end of the world: Zoe's and Evan's coping guide for kids*. Berkeley, CA: Tricycle Press.

Thomas, P. (1999). *My family's changing*. Hauppauge, NY: Barron Educational Series.

ANXIOUS CHILDREN AND CHILDREN WITH SPECIFIC FEARS

Cave, K. (2003). *You've got dragons*. Atlanta, GA: Peachtree.

Chung, A. (2014). *Ninja!* New York: Holt.

Cocca-Leffler, M. (2002). *Bravery soup*. Morton Grove, IL: Albert Withman.

Cook, J. (2012). *Wilma Jean and the worry machine*. Chattanooga, TN: National Center for Youth Issues.

Dewdney, A. (2005). *Llama llama red pajamas*. New York: Penguin Group.

Diesen, D. (2015). *Pout-pout fish and the big big dark*. New York: Macmillan Children's Publishing Group.

Duncan Edwards, P. (2003). *The worrywarts*. New York: HarperCollins

Emberley, E. (1992). *Go away, big green monster*. New York: Little, Brown.

Hadfield, C. (2016). *The darkest dark*. New York: Macmillan Children's Publishing Group.

Henkes, K. (1996). *Sheila Rae, the brave*. New York: HarperCollins.

Henkes, K. (2010). *Wemberly worried*. New York: HarperCollins.

Maier, I. (2006). *When Fuzzy was afraid of big and loud things*. Washington, DC: Magination Press.

Mayer, M. (1987). *There's an alligator under my bed*. New York: Penguin Groups.

Waber, B. (2002). *Courage*. New York: Houghton Mifflin.

Watt, M. (2008). *Scaredy squirrel*. Tonawanda, NY: Kids Can Press.

CHILDREN WHO STRUGGLE WITH PROBLEM SOLVING

Houghton, C. (2015). *Shh!: We have a plan*. Summerville, MA: Candlewick Press.

Jeffers, O. (2011). *Stuck*. New York: HarperCollins.

Klassen, J. (2016). *We found a hat*. Summerville, MA: Candlewick Press.

Parsley, E. (2015). *If you ever want to bring an alligator to school, don't!* New York: Little, Brown.

Reynolds, P. H. (2004). *Ish* (Creatrilogy). Summerville, MA: Candlewick Press.

Rubin, A. (2011). *Those darn squirrels!* New York: Houghton Mifflin.

Yamada, K. (2016). *What do you do with a problem?* London: Compendium.

CHILDREN WITH LOW SELF-IMAGE/SELF-CONFIDENCE OR NEED HELP WITH SELF-DOUBTS/BELIEVING IN THEMSELVES

Bakur Weiner, M. (2009). *I want your moo: A story about self-esteem*. Washington, DC: Magination Press.

Carlson, N. (1990). *I like me*. New York: Penguin Groups.

Diesen, D. (2014). *Pout-pout fish goes to school.* New York: Macmillan Children's Publishing Group.

Dyer, W. (2005). *Incredible you!* New York: Hay House.

Frasier, D. (2006). *On the day you were born.* New York: Houghton Mifflin.

Karst, P. (2000). *Invisible string.* Camarillo, CA: DeVorss.

Kranz, L. (2006). *Only one you.* Flagstaff, AZ: Northland.

Litwin, E. (2013). *Pete the cat and the magic sunglasses.* New York: HarperCollins.

Lucado, M. (1997) *You are special.* Wheaton, IL: Crossway.

MacDonald Denton, K. (1995). *Would they love a lion?* New York: Kingfisher.

Otoshi, K. (2010). *Zero.* Mill Valley, CA: KO Kids Books.

Palmer, P. (2011). *Liking myself.* Weaverville, CA: Boulden.

Petty, D. (2015). *I don't want to be a frog.* New York: Penguin Groups.

Piper, W. (2001). *The little engine that could.* New York: Platt & Munk.

Reynolds, P. (2012). *Sky color.* Summerville, MA: Candlewick Press.

Richmond, M. (2011). *I believe in you.* Naperville, IL: Sourcebooks

Schlein, M. (1993). *The way mothers are.* Morton Grove, IL: Albert Withman.

Spires, A. (2014). *Most magnificent thing.* Naperville, IL: Sourcebooks.

Stevins, E. (2013). *Mister D: A children's picture book about overcoming doubts and fears.* Charleston, SC: Create Space.

Wells, R. (2001). *Shy Charles.* New York: Penguin Groups.

CHILDREN WHO HAVE EXPERIENCED TRAUMA

Goodyear-Brown, P. (2003). *Gabby the gecko.* Self published: Paris Goodyear-Brown.

Haines, S. (2015). *Trauma is really strange.* Philadelphia: Singing Dragon.

Holmes, M. (2000). *A terrible thing happened.* Washington, DC: Magination Press.

Honda, L. (2014). *The cat who chose to dream.* Dixon, CA: Martin Pearl.

Schwiebert, P., & Deklyen, C. (2005). *Tear soup: A recipe for healing after loss.* Portland, OR: Grief Watch.

Sheppard, C. (1998). *Brave Bart: A story for traumatized and grieving children.* Albion, MI: National Institute for Trauma and Loss in Children.

Steele, W. (2016). *You are not alone.* Albion, MI: National Institute for Trauma and Loss in Children.

FOSTER AND ADOPTED CHILDREN

Gilman, J. (2008). *Murphy's three homes: A story for children in foster care.* Washington, DC: Magination Press.

Hampton, D. (2012). *My look-like-me mommy.* Mustang, OK: Tate.

Kasza, K. (1996). *A mother for Choco.* New York: Penguin Groups.

Oelschlager, V. (2010). *Porcupette finds a family.* Akron, OH: Vanita Books.

Paterson, K. (2004). *The great Gilly Hopkins.* New York: HarperCollins.

Pearson, J. (2016). *Elliot.* Ontario, Canada: Pajama Press.

CHILDREN BEING RAISED BY GRANDPARENTS

Byrne, G. (2009). *Sometimes it's grandmas and grandpas: Not mommies and daddies.* New York: Abbeville Kids.

Lovell, P. (2001). *Stand tall, Molly Lou Melon.* New York: G. P. Putnum's Sons.

Werle, S. (2016). *Our grandfamily.* Alberta, Canada: Children's Link Society.

CHILDREN WHO STEAL AND/OR LIE

Binkow, H. (2010). *Howard B. Wigglebottom and the monkey on his back.* San Diego, CA: Thunderbolt.

Cook, J. (2012). *Ricky sticky fingers.* Chattanooga, TN: National Center for Youth Issues.

Cook, J. (2015). *Lying up a storm.* Chattanooga, TN: National Center for Youth Issues.

Levins, S. (2012). *Bumblebee bike.* Washington, DC: Magination Press.

Lucado, M. (2006). *Flo the lyin' fly.* Nashville, TN: Thomas Nelson.

Segey, E. (2014). *Professor Ponzey and the truth potion.* Pines, FL: Mentalizer Education.

CHILDREN WITH ADHD/IMPULSIVE BEHAVIOR

Cook, J. (2006). *My mouth is a volcano!* Chattanooga, TN: National Center for Youth Issues.

Cook, J. (2007). *Personal space camp.* Chattanooga, TN: National Center for Youth Issues.

Cook, J. (2013). *I just want to do it my way!: My story about staying on task and asking for help.* Chattanooga, TN: National Center for Youth Issues.

Harris, R. H. (2010). *The day Leo said I hate you!* New York: Little, Brown.

Howard, A. (2003). *Cosmo zooms.* Orlando, FL: Harcourt Books.

Le, M. (2016). *Let me finish!* New York: Disney-Hyperion.

Lester, H. (1996). *Three cheers for Tacky.* New York: Houghton Mifflin.

Lester, H. (1997). *Listen, Buddy.* New York: Houghton Mifflin.

Underwood, D. (2013). *The quiet book.* New York: Houghton Mifflin.

Wells, R. (1999). *Noisy Nora.* New York: Penguin Groups.

CHILDREN WHO ARE UNCOMFORTABLE ABOUT BEING DIFFERENT/STRUGGLE WITH BELONGING

Andreae, G. (2012). *Giraffes can't dance.* New York: Cartwheel Books.

Dismondy, M. (2008). *Spaghetti in a hot dog bun: Having the courage to be who you are.* Chicago: Cardinal Rule Press.

Egan, T. (2007). *The pink refrigerator.* New York: Houghton Mifflin.

Esbaum, J. (2014). *I am cow, hear me moo!* New York: Penguin Groups.

Hall, M. (2015). *Red: A crayon's story.* New York: Greenwillow Books.

Henkes, K. (2008). *Chrysanthemum.* New York: Greenwillow Books.

John, J. (2016). *Quit calling me a monster!* New York: Random House.

Killer, K., & Lowe, J. (2016). *Hello, my name is Octicorn.* New York: HarperCollins Children's Books.

Ledwig, T. (2016). *The invisible boy.* New York: HarperCollins.

Lester, H. (2002). *Hooway for Wodney Wat.* New York: Houghton Mifflin.

Lester, H. (2015). *Score one for the sloths.* New York: Houghton Mifflin.

Lionni, L. (1997). *A color of his own.* New York: Dragonfly Books.

Offill, J. (2014). *Sparky!* New York: Random House.

Rousaki, M. (2003). *Unique Monique.* La Jolla, CA: Kane/Miller Book.

Simmons, S. J. (1997). *Alice and Greta: A tale of two witches.* Watertown, MA: Charlesbridge.

Venable, C. (2016). *Mervin the sloth is about to do the best thing in the world.* New York: Greenwillow Books.

CHILDREN WITH SOCIAL SKILLS AND FRIENDSHIP ISSUES

Bottner, B. (1997). *Bootsie Barker bites.* New York: Putnam and Grosset Group.

Campbell, S. (2014). *Hug machine.* New York: Atheneum Books.

Carlson, N. (1997). *How to lose all your friends.* New York: Penguin Books.

Cook, J. (2014). *Hygiene . . . you stink.* Boys Town, NE: Boys Town Press.

Coursen, V. (1997). *Mordant's wish.* New York: Holt.

Crimi, C. (2001). *Don't need friends.* New York: Random House.

Ferry, B. (2015). *Stick and stone.* New York: Houghton Mifflin.

Henkes, K. (1995). *A weekend with Wendell.* New York: Greenwillow Books.

Henkes, K. (1997). *Chester's way.* New York: Greenwillow Books.

Henkes, K. (2006). *Lilly's purple plastic purse.* New York: Williams Morrow.

Hutchins, H. J. (1991). *Katie's babbling bother.* Toronto, Ontario, Canada: Annick Press.

Janisch, H. (2012). *I have a little problem said the bear.* New York: NorthSouth Books.

Karst, P. (2000). *Invisible string.* Camarillo, CA: DeVorses.

Lester, H. (1995). *Me first.* New York: Houghton Mifflin.

Lester, H. (2016). *All for me and none for all.* New York: Houghton Mifflin.

O'Neill, A. (2002). *Recess queen.* New York: Scholastic.

Otoshi, K. (2010). *Zero.* Mill Valley, CA: KO Kids Books.

Otoshi, K. (2014). *Two.* Mill Valley, CA: KO Kids Books.

Pilkey, D. (1995). *Dragon's fat cat.* New York: Orchard Books.

Scheuer, K. (2014). *A bug and a wish.* Houston, TX: Strategic Book.

Watkins, R. (2015). *Rude cakes.* San Francisco: Chronicle Books.

Watt, M. (2011). *Scaredy squirrel makes a friend.* Tonowanda, NY: Kids Car Press.

CHILDREN WHO NEED HELP WITH RECOGNIZING AND EXPRESSING FEELINGS

Boynton, S. (2011). *Happy hippo, angry duck: A book of moods.* New York: Little Simon.

Cain, J. (2000). *The way I feel.* Seattle, WA: Parenting Press.

Curtis, J. L. (2007). *Today I feel silly and other moods that make my day.* New York: HarperCollins.

Diesen, D. (2013). *The pout-pout fish.* New York: Farrar, Straus and Giroux.

Goldblatt, R. (2004). *The boy who didn't want to be sad.* Washington, DC: Magination Press.

Hubbard, W. (1995). *C is for curious.* San Francisco: Chronicle Books.

Seuss, D. (2001). *My many colored days.* New York: Random House.

Vail, R. (2005). *Sometimes it's a bombaloo.* New York: Scholastic.

Witek, J. (2014). *In my heart: A book of feelings.* New York: Growing Hearts.

ANGRY AND AGGRESSIVE CHILDREN

Bang, M. (2004). *When Sophie gets angry . . . really, really angry.* New York: Blue Sky Press.

Blumenthal, D. (1999). *The chocolate-covered-cookie tantrum.* New York: Houghton Mifflin.

Lite, L. (2011). *Angry octopus: A relaxation story.* Marietta, GA: Stress Free Kids.

Mayer, M. (2000). *I was so mad.* New York: A Golden Book.

Shapiro, L. (1994). *The very angry day that Amy didn't have.* Plainview, NY: Childswork/Childsplay.

Silver, G. (2009). *Anh's anger.* Berkley, CA: Plumb Blossom.

Spelman, C. (200). *When I feel angry.* Parkridge, IL: Whitman, Albert & Co.

CHILDREN WITH BEHAVIOR PROBLEMS

Bogan, P. (2016). *Bossy Flossy.* New York: Holt.

Bottner, B. (1992). *The bootisie barker bites.* New York: Putnam & Grosset Group.

Byrne, R. (2016). *This book is out of control!* New York: Holt.

Carl, E. (2009). *The greedy python.* New York: Simon & Schuster.

Dewdney, A. (2012). *Llama llama time to share.* New York: Penguin Groups.

DiPucchio, K. (2016). *Dragon was terrible.* New York: Farrar, Straus and Giroux.

Gassman, J. (2013). *You get what you get.* Mankato, MN: Picture Window Books.

Geras, A. (2002). *Blossom's revenge: The cats of cuckoo square.* New York: Yearling.

Isern, S. (2016). *Raccoon wants to be first.* Madrid, Spain: NubeOcho.

Ludwig, T. (2011). *Better than you.* New York: Random House.

Manning, J. (2012). *Millie Fierce.* New York: Philomel Books.

O'Neill, A. (2002). *Recess queen.* New York: Scholastic.

Sendak, M. (2012). *Where the wild things are.* New York: HarperCollins.

Simmons, S. (1999). *Greta's revenge.* New York: Knopf Books.

Simon, F. (2001). *Horrid Henry's revenge.* London: Orion House.

Wagenbach, D. (2009). *The grouchies.* Washington, DC: Magination Press.

APPENDIX C

Professional Information

As of April 2017, according to the APT, a professional must meet the following standards in order to be credentialed as an RPT (Retrieved from *http://c.ymcdn. com/sites/www.a4pt.org/resource/resmgr/Credentials/RPTS_Guide_April_2017.pdf*):

1. Hold a current and active state license to independently provide mental health services.
2. Hold a master's or higher degree in a mental health field such as counseling, social work, psychology, and marriage and family counseling. Course work in specific areas must also be completed. The courses are outlined on APT's website (*www.a4pt.org*).
3. Have a minimum of 2 years and 2,000 hours of supervised clinical experience.
4. Take 150 hours of play therapy specific instruction from an approved provider or accredited university.
5. Provide 500 direct contact hours of play therapy alongside receiving 50 hours of play therapy specific supervision.

The requirements for becoming an SBRPT (Retrieved from *http://c.ymcdn. com/sites/www.a4pt.org/resource/resmgr/rpt_and_rpt-s_credentials/SB-RPT_Guide_ Nov_2016.pdf*) include:

1. Hold a current and active individual state license or certificate from the State Department of Education to independently practice as a school counselor or school psychologist.
2. Have earned a master's or higher mental health degree, with demonstrated coursework in child development, theories of personality, principles of psychotherapy, child and adolescent psychopathology, and ethics.

3. Have general clinical experience required by the State Department of Education, school counselor or school psychologist license/certification, and 2 years of continuous work in school setting post-licensure/certification.
4. Have taken 150 hours of play therapy specific instruction from institutions of higher education or APT-approved providers.
5. Have been supervised by an RPT-S for a period of no less than one school year during which the applicant documents a minimum of 600 direct client contact hours utilizing play therapy plus 50 hours of concurrent supervision.

The standards also describe the requirements to become an RPT-S, which are the same as those for the RPT, with the addition of the following (Retrieved from *http://c.ymcdn.com/sites/www.a4pt.org/resource/resmgr/Credentials/RPTS_ Guide_April_2017.pdf*):

1. Have an additional three (3) years and 3,000 direct client contact hours of clinical experience after initial full licensure.
2. Required supervisor training, which can be either completing six (6) hours of play therapy specific supervisor training *and* (a) demonstrating completion of either state board requirements for supervisor training *or* (b) completing APT's supervisor requirements (24 hours of supervisor training).

From APT's Position Paper on Touch:

Play therapists recognize that touch comes in many forms and occurs in many contexts within the play session. Oftentimes, the use of touch is foreseeable, such as when a child asks for a 'high five' or wants to sit on the therapist's lap while reading a story, or in physically based approaches (i.e., therapist and child thumb wrestling). Other times, the child may spontaneously touch the therapist when giving an unsolicited hug, wishing to be escorted to the bathroom, or climbing onto the therapist's lap without warning. Unpredictable circumstances may arise in which the therapist may need to touch the child to provide supportive guidance in physical activities, provide nurturing touch in emotional situations, or to otherwise tend to the emotional and physical safety of the child (i.e. when a child bolts from the playroom, climbs up shelves or locks themselves [*sic*] into various spaces). In any or all of these circumstances, the play therapist carefully monitors his/her touch response, utilizes touch with a clear rationale and appropriate intensity and acts in the most judicious manner in order to maintain safe conditions for the child and/or comfortable/acceptable boundaries for him/herself. All incidents of any of these examples of touch are to be documented and discussed with the child's guardian. (Association for Play Therapy, 2015, p. 2)

From APT's Best Practices document in connection with deciding who the client is in play therapy:

Play therapists working with minor clients understand the unique nature of working with a client whose legal consent is given by another party having power in the client's life. The therapist understands that the minor is their [*sic*] client and represents the minor client, not the legal guardian, in clinical decision making. The play therapist provides a professional disclosure statement that includes information regarding the responsibilities and expectations of the guardian, client and play therapist. (Association for Play Therapy, 2016, p. 2)

From the Best Practices document related to client confidentiality in play therapy:

Clients have the right to expect confidentiality and to be provided with an explanation of its limitations, including disclosure to appropriate legal guardian(s), disclosure as legally required and for safety when an immediate safety risk is revealed, suspicion of child abuse or other safety issue, supervision and/or treatment teams case reviews, and requests made by the payer, and/or governmental authority and/or by court order to obtain information about any documents or documentations in their case records. Play therapists seek legal guardian signature on all consents, including for treatment whenever applicable and when not constricted by state or federal laws. (APT, 2016, p. 4)

References

Adler, A. (1954). *Understanding human nature* (W. B. Wolf, Trans.). New York: Fawcett Premier. (Original work published 1927)

Adler, A. (1958). *What life should mean to you.* New York: Capricorn. (Original work published 1931)

Allan, J. (1988). *Inscapes of the child's world: Jungian counseling in schools and clinics.* Dallas, TX: Springer.

Allan, J. (1997). Jungian play psychotherapy. In K. J. O'Connor & L. M. Braverman (Eds.), *Play therapy: A comparative presentation* (2nd ed., pp. 100–130). New York: Wiley.

Allan, J., & Levin, S. (1993). "Born on my bum": Jungian play therapy. In T. Kottman & C. Schaefer (Eds.), *Play therapy in action: A casebook for practitioners* (pp. 209–244). Northvale, NJ: Jason Aronson.

Ansbacher, H., & Ansbacher, R. (Eds.). (1956). *The individual psychology of Alfred Adler: A systemic presentation in selections from his writings.* San Francisco: Harper & Row.

Arrien, A. (1993). *The four-fold way: Walking the paths of the warrior, teacher, healer, and visionary.* New York: HarperCollins.

Ashby, J., Kottman, T., & DeGraaf, D. (2008). *Active intervention for kids and teens.* Alexandria, VA: American Counseling Association.

Association for Play Therapy. (2015). Paper on touch: Clinical, professional, and ethical issues. Retrieved from *http://c.ymcdn.com/sites/www.a4pt.org/resource/resmgr/Publications/Paper_On_Touch_2015.pdf.*

Association for Play Therapy. (2016). Play therapy best practices: Clinical, professional and ethical issues. Retrieved from *http://c.ymcdn.com/sites/www.a4pt.org/resource/resmgr/publications/Best_Practices_Sept_2016.pdf.*

Association for Play Therapy. (2017). Play therapy defined. Retrieved from *www.a4pt.org/?page=WhyPlayTherapy.*

Axline, V. (1969). *Play therapy.* New York: Ballantine Books.

Beaudion, M., & Walden, S. (1998). *Working with groups to enhance relationships.* Duluth, MN: Whole Person Associates.

Beck, A. (1976). *Cognitive therapy and the emotional disorders.* New York: Meridian.

Behnke, S., & Warner, E. (2002). Confidentiality in the treatment of adolescents. *Monitor on Psychology, 33*(3), 4.

Bixler, R. (1949). Limits are therapy. *Journal of Consulting Psychology, 13,* 1–11.

Blanco, P., & Ray, D. (2011). Play therapy in the schools: A best practice for improving academic achievement. *Journal of Counseling and Development, 89,* 235–242.

Boik, B., & Goodwin, E. (2000). *Sandplay therapy: A step-by-step manual for psychotherapists of diverse orientations.* New York: Norton.

Booth, P., & Jernberg, A. (2010). *Theraplay: Helping parents and children build better relationships through attachment-based play* (3rd ed.). San Francisco: Jossey-Bass.

Booth, P., & Winstead, M. (2015). Theraplay: Repairing relationships, helping families heal. In D. Crenshaw & A. Stewart (Eds.), *Play therapy: A comprehensive guide to theory and practice* (pp. 141–155). New York: Guilford Press.

Booth, P., & Winstead, M. (2016). Theraplay: Creating secure and joyful attachment relationships. In K. O'Connor, C. Schaefer, & L. Braverman (Eds.), *Handbook of play therapy* (2nd ed., pp. 164–194). Hoboken, NJ: Wiley.

Bratton, S., Ray, D., Rhine, T., & Jones, L. (2005). The efficacy of play therapy with children: A meta-analytic review of treatment outcomes. *Journal of Professional Psychology Research and Practice, 36*(4), 376–390.

British Association for Play Therapy. (2014a). Play therapist personal qualities. Retrieved from *www.bapt.info/play-therapy/play-therapy-core-competences.*

British Association for Play Therapy. (2014b). Play therapy defined. Retrieved from *www.bapt.info/play-therapy/history-play-therapy.*

Brody, V. (1978). Developmental play: A relationship-focused program for children. *Journal of Child Welfare, 57,* 591–599.

Brody, V. (1993). *The dialogue of touch: Developmental play therapy.* Treasure Island, FL: Developmental Play Training Associates.

Brooke, S. (2004). *Tools of the trade: A therapist's guide to art therapy assessments* (2nd ed.). Springfield, IL: Charles C Thomas.

Brooks, R. (1981). Creative characters: A technique in child therapy. *Psychotherapy, 18,* 131–139.

Brown, S., & Vaughn, C. (2009). *Play: How it shapes the brain, opens the imagination, and invigorates the soul.* New York: Penguin.

Buchalter, S. (2009). *Art therapy techniques and applications.* Philadelphia: Jessica Kingsley.

Bundy-Myrow, S., & Booth, P. B. (2009). Theraplay: Supporting attachment relationships. In K. J. O'Connor & L. D. Braverman (Eds.), *Play therapy theory and practice: Comparing theories and techniques* (2nd ed., pp. 315–366). Hoboken, NJ: Wiley.

Burns, D. (1999). *Feeing good: The new mood therapy* (rev. ed.). New York: New American Library.

Cangelosi, D. (1993). Internal and external wars: Psychodynamic play therapy. In T. Kottman & C. Schaefer (Eds.), *Play therapy in action: A casebook for practitioners* (pp. 347–370). Northvale, NJ: Jason Aronson.

Carey, L. (2008). *Sandplay: Therapy with children and families.* Lanham, MD: Rowman & Littlefield.

Carlson, J., & Englar-Carson, M. (2017). *Adlerian psychotherapy*. Washington, DC: American Psychological Association.

Carmichael, K. (2006). *Play therapy: An introduction.* Upper Saddle River, NJ: Pearson.

Carnes Holt, K., & Bratton, S. (2015). The efficacy of child parent relationship therapy for adopted children with attachment disruptions. *Journal of Counseling and Development, 92,* 328–337.

Carroll, F. (2009). Gestalt play therapy. In K. J. O'Connor & L. D. Braverman (Eds.), *Play therapy theory and practice: Comparing theories and technique* (2nd ed., pp. 283–314). Hoboken, NJ: Wiley.

Carroll, F., & Oaklander, V. (1997). Gestalt play therapy. In K. O'Connor & L. Braverman (Eds.), *Play therapy theory and practice: A comparative presentation* (pp. 184–203). New York: Wiley.

Cattanach, A. (2006). Narrative play therapy. In C. Schaefer & H. Kaduson (Eds.), *Contemporary play therapy: Theory, research, and practice* (pp. 82–99). New York: Guilford Press.

Cattanach, A. (2008). *Narrative approaches tin play therapy with children.* Philadelphia: Jessica Kingsley.

Cavett, A. M. (2015). Cognitive-behavioral play therapy. In D. A. Crenshaw & A. L. Stewart (Eds.), *Play therapy: A comprehensive guide to theory and practice* (pp. 83–98). New York: Guilford Press.

Chapman, G. (1992). *The five love languages: Secrets to love that lasts.* Chicago: Northfield.

Chapman, G. (2000). *The five love languages of teenagers.* Chicago: Northfield.

Chapman, G., & Campbell, R. (1997). *The five love languages of children.* Chicago: Northfield.

Corey, G. (2017). *Theory and practice of counseling and psychotherapy* (10th ed.). Boston: Cengage.

Corey, G., Corey, M., & Callanan, P. (2011). *Issues and ethics in the helping professions* (8th ed.). Belmont, CA: Brooks/Cole.

Covey, S. R. (2013). *The 7 habits of highly effective people: Powerful lessons in personal change.* New York: Simon & Schuster.

Crenshaw, D., Brooks, R., & Goldstein, S. (Eds.). (2015). *Play therapy interventions to enhance resiliency.* New York: Guilford Press.

Czyszczon, G., Riviere, S., Lowman, D., & Stewart, A. (2015). In D. Crenshaw & A. Stewart (Eds.), *Play therapy: A comprehensive guide to theory and practice* (pp. 186–200). New York: Guilford Press.

DeDomenico, G. (1995). *Sand tray world play: A comprehensive guide to the use of the sand tray in psychotherapeutic and transformational settings.* Oakland, CA: Vision Quest.

Des Lauriers, A. (1962). *The experience of reality in childhood schizophrenia.* New York: International Universities Press.

Developmental Therapy Institute. (1992). *Developmental teaching objectives rating form-revised* (4th ed.). Athens, GA: Developmental Therapy Institute.

Devereaux, C. (2014). Moving with the space between us: The dance of attachment security. In C. Malchiodi & D. Crenshaw (Eds.), *Creative arts and play therapy for attachment problems* (pp. 84–99). New York: Guilford Press.

Dewey, E. (1978). *Basic applications of Adlerian psychology for self-understanding and human relationships.* Coral Springs, FL: CMI Press.

Dillman Taylor, D., & Meany-Walen, K. K. (2015). Investigating the effectiveness of Adlerian play therapy with children with disruptive behaviors: A single-case research design. *Journal of Child and Adolescent Counseling, 1*(2), 81–99.

Douglas, C. (2008). Analytical psychotherapy. In R. J. Corsini & D. Wedding (Eds.), *Current psychotherapies* (8th ed., pp. 107–140). Belmont, CA: Brooks/Cole.

Dreikurs, R., & Soltz, V. (1964). *Children: The challenge.* New York: Hawthorn/Dutton.

Eckstein, D., & Kern, R. (2009). *Psychological fingerprints* (6th ed.). Dubuque, IA: Kendall/Hunt.

Ellis, A. (2000). Rational emotive behavior therapy. In R. J. Corsini & D. Wedding (Eds.), *Current psychotherapies* (6th ed., pp. 168–204). Itasca, IL: F. E. Peacock.

Evers-Fahey, K. (2016). *Towards a Jungian theory of the ego.* New York: Routledge.

Fall, K., Holden, J. M., & Marquis, A. (2010). *Theoretical models of counseling and psychotherapy* (2nd ed.). New York: Routledge.

Freud, S. (1949). *An outline of psycho-analysis* (J. Strachey, Trans.). New York: Norton.

Frey, D. (2015). Play therapy interventions with adults. In D. Crenshaw & A. Stewart (Eds.), *Play therapy: A comprehensive guide to theory and practice* (pp. 452–464). New York: Guilford Press.

Gallo-Lopez, L., & Schaefer, C. (2005). *Play therapy with adolescents.* Lanham, MD: Jason Aronson.

Gardner, B. (2015). Play therapy with adolescents. In D. Crenshaw & A. Stewart (Eds.), *Play therapy: A comprehensive guide to theory and practice* (pp. 439–451). New York: Guilford Press.

Gardner, R. A. (Ed.). (1993). *Storytelling in psychotherapy with children.* Northvale, NJ: Jason Aronson.

Gaskill, R. L. (2010, December). Neurobiology of play therapy. *Play Therapy.* Retrieved from *www.mlppubsonline.com/article/Neurobiology_Of_Play_Therapy/558446/53463/article.html.*

Gil, E. (2014). The creative use of metaphor in play and art therapy with attachment problems. In C. Malchiodi & D. Crenshaw (Eds.), *Creative arts and play therapy for attachment problems* (pp. 159–177). New York: Guilford Press.

Gil, E., Konrath, E., Shaw, J., Goldin, M., & Bryan, H. (2015). Integrative approach to play therapy. In D. Crenshaw & A. Stewart (Eds.), *Play therapy: A comprehensive guide to theory and practice* (pp. 99–113). New York: Guilford Press.

Glover, G., & Landreth, G. (2016). Child-centered play therapy. In K. O'Connor, C. Schaefer, & L. Braverman (Eds.), *Handbook of play therapy* (2nd ed., pp. 93–118). Hoboken, NJ: Wiley.

Gonsher, A, (2016). Limit-setting in play therapy. In K. O'Connor, C. Schaefer, & L. Braverman (Eds.), *Handbook of play therapy* (2nd ed., pp. 53–428). Hoboken, NJ: Wiley.

Goodyear-Brown, P. (2010). *Play therapy with traumatized children: A prescriptive approach.* Hoboken, NJ: Wiley.

Grant, R. J. (2017). *Play-based interventions for autism spectrum disorder and other developmental disabilities.* New York: Routledge.

Green, E. (2009). Jungian analytical play therapy. In K. O'Connor & L. Braverman

(Eds.), *Play therapy theory and practice: Comparing theories and techniques* (2nd ed., pp. 100–139). Hoboken, NJ: Wiley.

Green, E., Baggerly, J., & Myrick, A. (Eds.). (2015). *Counseling families: A play-based treatment*. New York: Rowman & Littlefield.

Green, E., Drewes, A., & Kominski, J. (2013). Use of mandalas in Jungian play therapy with adolescents diagnosed with ADHD. *International Journal of Play Therapy, 22*(3), 159–172.

Griffith, J., & Powers, R. L. (2007). *The lexicon of Adlerian Psychology: 106 terms associated with the Individual Psychology of Alfred Adler* (2nd ed.). Port Townsend, WA: Adlerian Psychology Associates.

Guerney, B. (1964). Filial therapy: Description and rationale. *Journal of Consulting Psychology, 28,* 304–310.

Guerney, L. (2013). *Group filial therapy: The complete guide to teaching parents to play therapeutically with their children*. Philadelphia: Jessica Kingsley.

Homeyer, L., & Sweeney, D. (2017). *Sandtray: A practical manual* (3rd ed.). New York: Routledge.

James, O. (1997). *Play therapy: A comprehensive guide*. Northvale, NJ: Jason Aronson.

Jernberg, A. (1979). *Theraplay: A structured new approach for problem children and their families*. San Francisco: Jossey-Bass.

Jernberg, A., & Jernberg, E. (1993). Family Theraplay for the family tyrant. In T. Kottman & C. Schaefer (Eds.), *Play therapy in action: A casebook for practitioners* (pp. 45–96). Northvale, NJ: Jason Aronson.

Jung, C. G. (1969). Synchronicity: An acausal connecting principle. In G. Adler, M. Fordham, W. McGuire, & H. Read (Eds.), & R. F. C. Hull (Trans.), *The collected works of C. F. Jung* (Vol. 8, pp. 419–519). Princeton, NJ: Princeton University Press.

Karges-Bone, L. (2015). *Bibliotherapy*. Dayton, OH: Lorenz Educational Press.

Karpman, S. (1968). Fairy tales and script drama analysis. *Transactional Analysis Bulletin, 26*(7), 39–43.

Kenney-Noziska, S., Schaefer, C., & Homeyer, L. (2012). Beyond directive and nondirective: Moving the conversation forward. *International Journal of Play Therapy, 21*(4), 244–252.

Kfir, N. (1989). *Personality and priorities: A typology*. Bloomington, IN: Author House.

Kfir, N. (2011). *Personality and priorities: A typology*. Bloomington, IN: Author House.

Kissel, S. (1990). *Play therapy: A strategic approach*. Springfield, IL: Charles C Thomas.

Knell, S. M. (1993). To show and not tell: Cognitive-behavioral play therapy. In T. Kottman & S. Schaefer (Eds.), *Play therapy in action: A casebook for practitioners* (pp. 169–208). Northvale, NJ: Jason Aronson.

Knell, S. M. (1994). Cognitive-behavioral play therapy. In K. O'Connor & C. Schaefer (Eds.), *Handbook of play therapy: Vol. 2. Advances and innovations* (pp. 111–142). New York: Wiley.

Knell, S. M. (2009). Cognitive-behavioral play therapy. In K. J. O'Connor & L. D. Braverman (Eds.), *Play therapy theory and practice: Comparing theories and techniques* (2nd ed., pp. 203–236). Hoboken, NJ: Wiley.

Knell, S. (2016). Cognitive-behavioral play therapy. In K. O'Connor, C. Schaefer, & L. Braverman (Eds.), *Handbook of play therapy* (2nd ed., pp. 118–133). Hoboken, NJ: Wiley.

Knoff, H., & Prout, H. (1985). *Kinetic drawing system for family and school: A handbook.* Los Angeles: Western Psychological Services.

Koller, T., & Booth, P. (1997). Fostering attachment through family Theraplay. In K. O'Connor & L. M. Braverman (Eds.), *Play therapy theory and application: A comparative presentation* (pp. 204–233). New York: Wiley.

Kottman, T. (2011). *Play therapy: Basics and beyond* (2nd ed.). Alexandria, VA: American Counseling Association.

Kottman, T., & Ashby, J. (2015). Adlerian play therapy. In D. Crenshaw & A. Stewart (Eds.), *Play therapy: A comprehensive guide to theory and practice* (pp. 32–47). New York: Guilford Press.

Kottman, T., Ashby, J., & DeGraaf, D. (2001). *Adventures in guidance: How to integrate fun into your guidance program.* Alexandria, VA: American Counseling Association.

Kottman, T., & Heston, M. (2012). The child's inner life and a sense of community. In J. Carlson & M. Maniacci (Eds.), *Alfred Adler revisited* (pp. 115–128). New York: Routledge.

Kottman, T., & Meany-Walen, K. K. (2015). Adlerian family play therapy. In E. Green, J. Baggerly, & A. Myrick (Eds.), *Counseling families: A play-based treatment* (pp. 71–87). New York: Rowman & Littlefield.

Kottman, T., & Meany-Walen, K. (2016). *Partners in play: An Adlerian approach to play therapy* (3rd ed.). Alexandria, VA: American Counseling Association.

Lakoff, G., & Johnson, M. (2003). *Metaphors we live by* (rev. ed.). Chicago: University of Chicago.

Landgarten, H. (1981). *Clinical art therapy: A comprehensive guide.* New York: Brunner/Mazel.

Landreth, G. L. (2012) *Play therapy: The art of the relationship* (3rd ed.). New York: Brunner-Routledge.

Landreth, G. L., & Bratton, S. C. (2006). *Child–parent relationship therapy: A 10-session filial therapy model.* New York: Taylor & Francis.

Lankton, C., & Lankton, S. (1989). *Tales of enchantment: Goal-oriented metaphors for adults and children in therapy.* New York: Brunner/Mazel.

LeBlanc, M., & Ritchie, M. (2001). A meta-analysis of play therapy outcomes. *Counseling Psychology Quarterly, 14,* 149–163.

Lee, A. C. (2009). Psychoanalytic play therapy. In K. J. O'Connor & L. D. Braverman, *Play therapy theory and practice: Comparing theories and techniques* (2nd ed., pp. 25–82). Hoboken, NJ: Wiley.

LeFeber, M. (2014). Working with children using dance/movement. In E. Green & A. Drewes (Eds.), *Integrating expressive arts and play therapy with children and adolescents* (pp. 124–148). New York: Wiley.

Lerner, M., Mikami, A., & Levine, K. (2011). Socio-dramatic affective-relational intervention for adolescents with Asperger syndrome and high functioning autism: Pilot study. *Autism, 15*(1), 21–42.

Lew, A., & Bettner, B. L. (1998). *Responsibility in the classroom: A teacher's guide to understanding and motivating students.* Newton Centre, MA: Connexions Press.

Lew, A., & Bettner, B. L. (2000). *A parent's guide to understanding and motivating children.* Newton Centre, MA: Connexions Press.

Lewin, K. (1951). *Field theory in social science.* New York: Harper & Brothers.

Lilly, J. P. (2015). Jungian analytic play therapy. In D. Crenshaw & A. Stewart (Eds.), *Play therapy: A comprehensive guide to theory and practice* (pp. 48–65). New York: Guilford Press.

Lin, Y., & Bratton, S. (2015). A meta-analytic review of child-centered play therapy approaches. *Journal of Counseling and Development, 93*(1), 45–58.

Malchiodi, C. (2007). *Art therapy sourcebook.* New York: McGraw-Hill.

Malchiodi, C. (Ed.). (2015). *Creative interventions with traumatized children* (2nd ed.). New York: Guilford Press.

Malchiodi, C., & Ginns-Gruenberg, D. (2008). Trauma, loss, and bibliotherapy: The healing power of stories. In C. Malchiodi (Ed.), *Creative interventions with traumatized children* (pp. 167–188). New York: Guilford Press.

Maniacci, M. P., Sackett-Maniacci, L., & Mosak, H. H. (2014). Adlerian psychotherapy. In D. Wedding & R. Corsini (Eds.), *Current psychotherapies* (10th ed., pp. 55–94). Belmont, CA: Brooks/Cole.

Manly, L. (1986). Goals of misbehavior inventory. *Elementary School Guidance and Counseling, 21,* 160–161.

Marschak, M. (1960). A method for evaluating child–parent interaction under controlled conditions. *Journal of Genetic Psychology, 97,* 3–22.

McCalla, C. L. (1994). A comparison of three play therapy theories: Psychoanalytical, Jungian, and client-centered. *International Journal of Play Therapy, 3,* 1–10.

Meany-Walen, K., Bratton, S., & Kottman, T. (2014). Effects of Adlerian play therapy on reducing students' disruptive behavior. *Journal of Counseling and Development, 92,* 47–56.

Meany-Walen, K. K., Kottman, T., Bullis, Q., & Dillman Taylor, D. (2015). Adlerian play therapy with children with externalizing behaviors: Single case design. *Journal of Counseling and Development, 93*(2), 418–428.

Meichenbaum, D. (1986). Cognitive behavior modification. In F. H. Kanfer & A. P. Goldstein (Eds.), *Helping people change: A textbook of methods* (pp. 346–380). New York: Pergamon Press.

Merriam-Webster Dictionary. (n.d.). Play therapy. Retrieved August 18, 2017, from *www.merriam-webster.com/dictionary/play therapy.*

Metcalf, L. (2006). *The miracle question: Answer it and change your life.* Bethel, CT: Crown House.

Mills, J. (2015). StoryPlay: A narrative play therapy approach. In D. Crenshaw & A. Stewart (Eds.), *Play therapy: A comprehensive guide to theory and practice* (pp. 171–185). New York: Guilford Press.

Mills, J., & Crowley, R. (2014). *Therapeutic metaphors for children and the child within* (2nd ed.). New York: Routledge.

Mordock, J. B. (2015). Psychodynamic play therapy. In D. Crenshaw & A. Stewart (Eds.), *Play therapy: A comprehensive guide to theory and practice* (pp. 66–82). New York: Guilford Press.

Mosak. H., & Maniacci, M. (1999). *A primer of Adlerian psychology.* Philadelphia: Brunner/Mazel.

Moustakas, C. (1997). *Relationship play therapy.* New York: Rowman & Littlefield.

Munns, E. (2011). Theraplay: Attachment-enhancing play therapy. In C. Schaefer (Ed.), *Foundations of play therapy* (2nd ed., pp. 275–296). Hoboken, NJ: Wiley.

Munns, E., & Munns, C. (2015). Including families in Theraplay with children. In E. Green, J. Baggerly, & A. Myrick (Eds.), *Counseling families: A play-based treatment* (pp. 21–34). New York: Rowman & Littlefield.

Naranjo, C. (1970). Present centeredness: Technique, prescription and ideal. In J. Fagan & I. L. Shepherd (Eds.), *Gestalt therapy now* (pp. 47–69). New York: Harper.

Nash, J. B., & Schaefer, C. (2011). Play therapy: Basic concepts and practices. In C. Schaefer (Ed.), *Foundations of play therapy* (2nd ed., pp. 3–13). Hoboken, NJ: Wiley.

Nelsen, J., Nelsen Tamborski, M., & Ainge, B. (2016). *Positive discipline: Parenting tools.* New York: Harmony Books.

Nemiroff, M., & Annunziata, J. (1990). *A child's first book about play therapy.* Washington, DC: American Psychological Association.

Netto, R. (2011). *Easy guide to Jungian psychology.* York Beach, ME: Nicolas-Hays.

Norcross, J. C. (2005). A primer on psychotherapy integration. In J. C. Norcross & M. R. Goldfried (Eds.), *Handbook of psychotherapy integration* (2nd ed., pp. 3–23). New York: Oxford University Press.

Nurse, A. R., & Sperry, L. (2012). Standardized assessment. In L. Sperry (Ed.), *Family assessment: Contemporary and cutting-edge strategies* (2nd ed., pp. 53–82). New York: Routledge.

Oaklander, V. (1992). *Windows to our children: A Gestalt approach to children and adolescents.* New York: Gestalt Journal Press. (Original work published 1978)

Oaklander, V. (1993). From meek to bold: A case study of Gestalt play therapy. In T. Kottman & C. Schaefer (Eds.), *Play therapy in action: A casebook for practitioners* (pp. 281–300). Northvale, NJ: Jason Aronson.

Oaklander, V. (1994). Gestalt play therapy. In K. O'Connor & C. Schaefer (Eds.), *Handbook of play therapy* (pp. 142–156). New York: Wiley.

Oaklander, V. (2003). Gestalt play therapy. In C. Schaefer (Ed.), *Foundations of play therapy* (pp. 143–155). Hoboken, NJ: Wiley.

Oaklander, V. (2011). Gestalt play therapy. *International Journal of Play Therapy, 10,* 45–55.

Oaklander, V. (2015). Short-term Gestalt play therapy for grieving children. In H. Kaduson & C. Schaefer (Eds.), *Short-term play therapy for children* (3rd ed., pp. 28–52). New York: Guilford Press.

O'Connor, K. (1993). Child, protector, confidant: Structured group exosystemic play therapy. In T. Kottman & S. Schaefer (Eds.), *Play therapy in action: A casebook for practitioners* (pp. 245–280). Northvale, NJ: Jason Aronson.

O'Connor, K. (2000). *The play therapy primer* (2nd ed.). New York: Wiley.

O'Connor, K. (2002). The value and use of interpretation in play therapy. *Professional Psychology: Research and practice, 33*(6), 523–528.

O'Connor, K. (2009). Ecosystemic play therapy. In K. J. O'Connor & L. D. Braverman (Eds.), *Play therapy theory and practice: Comparing theories and techniques* (2nd ed., pp. 367–450). Hoboken, NJ: Wiley.

O'Connor, K. (2011). Ecosystemic play therapy. In C. E. Schaefer (Ed.), *Foundations of play therapy* (2nd ed., pp. 253–272). Hoboken, NJ: Wiley.

O'Connor, K. (2016). Ecosystemic play therapy. In K. O'Connor, C. Schaefer, & L.

Braverman (Eds.), *Handbook of play therapy* (2nd ed., pp. 194–225). Hoboken, NJ: Wiley.

O'Connor, K., & Ammen, S. (1997). *Play therapy treatment planning and interventions: The ecosystemic model.* San Diego, CA: Academic Press.

Ojiambo, D., & Bratton, S. C. (2014). Effects of group activity play therapy on problem behaviors of preadolescent Ugandan orphans. *Journal of Counseling and Development, 92*(3), 355–365.

Paré, M. A. (2015). Psyche and system: Integrating Jungian play therapy into family counseling. In E. Green, A. Myrick, & J. Baggerly (Eds.), *Counseling families: Play-based treatment* (pp. 53–69). Lanham, MD: Rowman & Littlefield.

Peery, J. C. (2003). Jungian analytical play therapy. In C. E. Schaefer (Ed.), *Foundations of play therapy* (pp. 14–54). Hoboken, NJ: Wiley.

Perls, F. (1970). Four lectures. In J. Fagan & I. L. Shepherd (Eds.), *Gestalt therapy now* (pp. 14–38). New York: Harper.

Perls, F., Hefferline, R. F., & Goodman, P. (1951). *Gestalt therapy: Excitement and growth in the human personality.* New York: Crown.

Punnett, A. (2016). Psychoanalytic and Jungian play therapy. In K. O'Connor, C. Schaefer, & L. Braverman (Eds.), *Handbook of play therapy* (2nd ed., pp. 61–92). Hoboken, NJ: Wiley.

Raskin, N., Rogers, C., & Witty, M. (2014). Client-centered therapy. In D. Wedding & R. Corsini (Eds.), *Current psychotherapies* (10th ed., pp. 95–145). Belmont, CA: Brooks/Cole.

Ray, D. C. (2011). *Advanced play therapy: Essential conditions, knowledge, and skills for child practice.* New York: Routledge.

Ray, D. C., Armstrong, S. A., Balkin, R. S., & Jayne, K. M. (2015). Child-centered play therapy in the schools: Review and meta-analysis. *Psychology in the Schools, 52l,* 107–123.

Ray, D. C., & Landreth, G. (2015). Child-centered play therapy. In D. Crenshaw & A. Stewart (Eds.), *Play therapy: A comprehensive guide to theory and practice* (pp. 3–16). New York: Guilford Press.

Robins, C., & Rosenthal, M. Z. (2011). Dialectical behavior therapy. In J. Herbert & E. Forman (Eds.), *Acceptance and mindfulness in cognitive behavioral therapy* (pp. 164–192). Hoboken, NJ: Wiley.

Rogers, C. (1951). *Client-centered therapy: Its current practice, implications and theory.* London: Constable.

Rogers, C. R. (1961). *On becoming a person: A psychotherapists view of psychotherapy.* Boston: Houghton Mifflin.

Rohnke, K. (1991). *Bottomless baggie.* Dubuque, IA: Kendall/Hunt.

Rohnke, K. (2004). *Funn 'n games.* Dubuque, IA: Kendall/Hunt.

Safran, J. D., & Kriss, A. (2014). Psychoanalytic psychotherapies. In D. Wedding & R. J. Corsini (Eds.), *Current psychotherapies* (10th ed., pp. 19–54). Belmont, CA: Brooks/Cole.

Schaefer, A. (2011). *Ain't misbehavin': Tactics for tantrums, meltdowns, bedtime blues, and other perfectly normal kid behaviors.* Ottawa, Ontario, Canada: Wiley.

Schaefer, C. (Ed.). (2003). *Play therapy with adults.* New York: Wiley.

Schaefer, C. E., & Drewes, A. A. (Eds.). (2014). *The therapeutic powers of play: 20 core agents of change* (2nd ed.). Hoboken, NJ: Wiley.

Schaefer, C., & Drewes, A. (2016). Prescriptive play therapy. In K. O'Connor, C.

Schaefer, & L. Braverman (Eds.), *Handbook of play therapy* (2nd ed., pp. 227–240). Hoboken, NJ: Wiley.

Schoel, J., & Maizell, R. (2002). *Exploring islands of healing: New perspectives on adventure based counseling.* Beverly, MA: Project Adventure.

Schottelkorb, A., & Ray, D. (2009). ADHD symptom reduction in elementary students: A single-case effectiveness design. *Professional School Counseling, 13,* 11–22.

Shelby, J. (2015). Family-based cognitive behavioral therapy. In E. Green, A. Myrick, & J. Baggerly (Eds.), *Counseling families: Play-based treatment* (pp. 3–20). Lanham, MD: Rowman & Littlefield.

Snow, M., Winburn, A., Crumrine, L., Jackson, E., & Killian, T. (2012). The iPad playroom: A therapeutic technique. *Play Therapy, 7*(3), 16–19.

Swan, K., & Ray, D. (2014). Effects of child-centered play therapy on irritability and hyperactivity behaviors of children with intellectual disabilities. *Journal of Humanistic Counseling, 53,* 120–133.

Sweeny, D., & Landreth, G. (2009). Child-centered play therapy. In K. J. O'Connor & L. D. Braverman (Eds.), *Play therapy: Theory and practice* (2nd ed., pp. 123–162). Hoboken, NJ: Wiley.

Taylor de Faoite, A. (2011). *Narrative play therapy: Theory and practice.* Philadelphia: Jessica Kingsley.

Trippany-Simmons, R., Buckley, M., Meany-Walen, K., & Rush-Wilson, T. (2014). Individual psychology. In R. Parsons & N. Zhang (Eds.), *Counseling theory: Guiding reflective practice* (pp. 109–139). Los Angeles: SAGE.

Turner, B. (2005). *The handbook of sandplay therapy.* Cloverdale, CA: Temenos.

VanFleet, R. (2013). *Filial therapy: Strengthening parent–child relationships through play* (3rd ed.). Sarasota, FL: Professional Resource Press.

VanFleet, R., Sywaluk, A., & Sniscak, C. (2010). *Child-centered play therapy.* New York: Guilford Press.

VanFleet, R., & Topham, G. L., (2016). Filial therapy. In L. McMahon (Ed.), *Handbook of play therapy and therapeutic play* (2nd ed., pp. 135–165). New York: Routledge.

Vygotsky, L. (1978). *Mind in society: The development of higher psychological processes.* Cambridge, MA: Harvard University Press.

Watts, R. (2013). Adlerian counseling. In B. Irby, G. Brown, & S. Jackson (Eds.), *The handbook of educational theories for theoretical frameworks* (pp. 459–472). Charlotte, NC: Information Age.

White, M. (2007). *Maps of narrative practice.* New York: Norton

White, M., & Epston, D. (1990). *Narrative means to therapeutic ends.* New York: Norton.

Wilson, K., & Ryan, V. (2005). *Play therapy: A non-directive approach for children and adolescents* (2nd ed.). Burlington, MA: Elsevier.

Wood, D., Bruner, J. S., & Ross, G. (1976). The role of tutoring in problem-solving. *Journal of Child Psychology and Psychiatry, 17,* 89–100.

Yasenik, L., & Gardner, K. (2012). *Play therapy dimensions model: A decision-making guide for integrative play therapists.* Philadelphia: Jessica Kingsley.

Zimmerman, J., & Dickerson, V. (1996). *If problems talked: Narrative therapy in action.* New York: Guilford Press.

Index